The HEALING GIFT

"David Freud makes a compelling case as he demonstrates that his wife Linda's ability to channel incredibly accurate medical information often results in extraordinary healing. This may be the long awaited breakthrough in consciousness so urgently needed in a world gone mad. What emerges is a unique integration of science, holistic medicine, and ancient spiritual knowledge involving angels and Kabbalah into a new unified approach for healing chronic disease and optimizing wellness. As her dramatic case histories presented here show, Linda Freud is far beyond the level of any medical intuitive that I am aware of. I highly recommend *The Healing Gift* as a paradigm breakthrough in holistic healing."

—Gabriel Cousens, M.D., M.D.(H.), is diplomat of American Board of Integrative Holistic Health, diplomat of Ayurveda, director of The Tree of Life Rejuvenation Center (www.treeoflife.nu), and author of *There Is a Cure for Diabetes, Conscious Eating,* and *Spiritual Nutrition.*

"Linda Freud, with whom I have worked for several years, adds an important therapeutic dimension to the emotional and spiritual healing of chronically ill patients. My clinical experience has shown that the severity of the disease state is often matched by the severity of negative emotions and spiritual imbalances. Linda has made a major contribution in treating negative emotions, removing earthbound spirits, and identifying past life issues that may exacerbate chronic illness. While the origin and nature of her channeling gift may be highly mystical, the healing that ensues is completely results oriented. She is a true original."

—Thomas Rau, M.D., is chief medical director of the Paracelsus Clinic in Lustmühle, Switzerland, and the Paracelsus al Ronc Clinic in Castaneda, Switzerland (www.paracelsus.ch), founder of the Biological Medical Network in Europe and America (www.drrausway.com), and author of *The Swiss Secret to Optimal Health: Dr. Rau's Diet for Whole Body Healing.*

"Linda has made a major contribution to the science of detoxifying mercury, a root cause of much chronic degenerative disease. I find her level of diagnostic accuracy and attention to detail in the healing process to be astonishing. Linda is blessed with a prodigious gift of healing."

—Dietrich Klinghardt, M.D., is lead clinician at the Comprehensive Medical Center in Bellevue, Washington, director of the Klinghardt Academy of Neurobiology (www.klinghardt.org), and recipient of the 2007 Physician of the Year Award from the Global Foundation of Integrative Medicine.

"Linda Freud is simply amazing at what she does. I've never seen someone who is so accurate and complete with her medical diagnosis and recommendations. In addition to being warm, compassionate, and caring, she is consistently as precise and on the mark with her diagnoses as if she had performed a battery of laboratory tests and diagnostic images. In fact, she derives information that goes far beyond the one-dimensional nature of what certain traditional lab tests are capable of doing."

—Thom Lobe, M.D., is director of Beneveda Medical Group, Beverly Hills, California (www.beneveda.com)

"After undergoing a battery of expensive physical and energetic tests performed by a leading German doctor several years ago, I saw Linda Freud who without any previous knowledge of my test results proceeded to not only duplicate the results of my medical tests, but took the entire process even further to provide me with valuable medical information. I have done my due diligence and am astonished at the accuracy of her healing gift."

—Burton Goldberg (www.burtongoldberg.com) is author/editor of many books, including *Alternative Medicine: The Definitive Guide*, and creator of DVDs on the latest advances in stem cells and in curing depression, addiction, and cancer.

"In the nearly ten years I have known Linda and David Freud, I have watched with awe and amazement as Linda is able, through her intuitive gifts, to reveal the most precise detail of information regarding health conditions—matching or surpassing any health practitioner whom I am aware of. I am confident that *The Healing Gift* will catapult Linda into becoming an internationally acclaimed personality."

—Hyla Cass, M.D., is a practitioner of integrative medicine and psychiatry in Pacific Palisades, California (www.cassmd.com), a former assistant clinical professor of psychiatry at UCLA School of Medicine, author of *Supplement Your Prescription: What Your Doctor Doesn't Know About Nutrition* and *8 Weeks to Vibrant Health,* and a frequently quoted authority, television commentator, and speaker on integrative medicine.

"Linda's expertise in healing chronic degenerative conditions stems from her extraordinary ability to identify and detoxify environmental toxins and pathogens that are difficult to detect through traditional lab testing. In *The Healing Gift,* David Freud provides stunning testimonials of healing that defy conventional logic and reveal his wife to be a gifted and knowledgeable healer."

—Elson M. Haas, M.D., is medical director of the Preventive Medical Center of Marin in San Rafael, California, and author of *Staying Healthy with Nutrition* (www.elsonhaas.com).

"Linda's ability to detect and treat environmental toxicity that is the root cause of so many "undiagnosable" chronic conditions is unique. Her amazing gift, coupled with a deep understanding of natural healing modalities, allows her to achieve incredible results even in complicated cases."

—Uzzi Reiss, M.D., is director of the Beverly Hills Anti-Aging Center for Men and Women and author of *Natural Hormone Balance for Women* and *The Natural Superwoman* (www.uzzireissmd.com).

"Linda Freud stands apart from other medical intuitives in terms of the results, the thoroughness, the completeness of what she can accomplish."

—Vernon Erwin, D.D.S., is a founding member of the International Academy of Biological Dentistry and Medicine (www.drerwin.com).

"I am convinced that Linda Freud's claim of channeling angels and spirits is authentic. In addition to her providing valuable and accurate information on my health, I have witnessed her shake when she receives medical and spiritual information from the angelic realms. The shaking phenomenon is a trait consistent with what is described by rabbinic and kabbalistic authorities as a key attribute of the Hebrew prophets. Clearly, something extraordinary is going on here."

—Rabbi Matityahu Glazerson (www.glazerson.com) is a leading rabbinic scholar on the Torah Codes and prolific author of over 30 books, including the co-authored *Torah Codes: A Glimpse Into the Infinite, The Holocaust in Torah Codes,* and *The Mayan Culture and Judaism.*

The
HEALING GIFT

THE REMARKABLE WORLD
OF A MEDICAL INTUITIVE

DAVID FREUD with LINDA FREUD
Foreword by Hyla Cass, M.D.

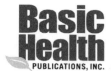

**Basic
Health**
PUBLICATIONS, INC.

The information contained in this book is based upon the research and personal and professional experiences of the authors. It is not intended as a substitute for consulting with your physician or other healthcare provider. Any attempt to diagnose and treat an illness should be done under the direction of a healthcare professional.

The publisher does not advocate the use of any particular healthcare protocol but believes the information in this book should be available to the public. The publisher and authors are not responsible for any adverse effects or consequences resulting from the use of the suggestions, preparations, or procedures discussed in this book. Should the reader have any questions concerning the appropriateness of any procedures or preparation mentioned, the authors and the publisher strongly suggest consulting a professional healthcare advisor.

Basic Health Publications, Inc.
28812 Top of the World Drive
Laguna Beach, CA 92651
949-715-7327 • www.basichealthpub.com

Library of Congress Cataloging-in-Publication Data
Freud, David
    The healing gift : the remarkable world of a medical intuitive / David Freud with Linda Freud.
        p. cm.
    Includes bibliographical references and index.
    ISBN 978-1-59120-201-1 (alk. paper)
    1. Freud, Linda 2. Women healers—Biography. 3. Intuition.
I. Freud, Linda II. Title.
    RZ408.F735   2010
    615.8'528—dc22

                                                        2010013636

Editor: Susan E. Davis
Copyeditor: Cheryl Hirsch
Typesetting/Book design: Gary A. Rosenberg
Cover design: Mike Stromberg

Printed in the United States of America

10   9   8   7   6   5   4   3   2   1

Contents

Foreword

When David Freud approached me about writing the Foreword for this book, I was delighted and honored. I feel blessed to be a small part of what I consider to be a reality-busting, history-making phenomenon of a book. In the nearly ten years I have known Linda and David Freud, I have watched with awe and amazement as Linda is able, through her intuitive gifts, to reveal the most precise detail of information regarding health conditions—matching or surpassing any health practitioner that I am aware of. Along with other physicians in the Los Angeles area and throughout the country, I, in my practice as an integrative medical doctor and psychiatrist, have referred very challenging cases to her for feedback, and have yet to be disappointed in the results. Since I also create new formulas for the supplement market, I have consulted her many times for her opinions of them, and again, her accuracy is proven by their clinical effectiveness.

Linda attributes her success as a healer to channeling angels and spirits through the use of a pendulum. They direct her to diagnostic information derived from a series of databases that contain extremely thorough information on physical, emotional and spiritual issues. The resulting treatment recommendations are a blend of Western and Eastern natural healing modalities. These include protocols for detoxifying different pathogens and environmental toxins and enhancing the body's natural functions and energies through orthomolecular nutrition, anti-aging protocols, and customized healing diets.

Linda works exclusively with natural remedies—vitamins, minerals, amino acids, essential fatty acids, probiotics, glandulars, natural hormone precursors, as well as herbal remedies, homeopathy, and diet. If Linda channels that a pharmaceutical approach is needed, she refers the client to one of the other integrative (or holistic) or mainstream medical doctors she works with in the Los Angeles area. In addition to me, these include Dr. Thom Lobe, under whose license she operates, and who specializes in nutritional and energy medicine; Dr. Uzzi Reiss, a specialist in endocrinology and gynecology; Dr. Karl Epstein, who practices orthopedics and sports medicine; Dr. Gary Bellack, an ear, nose, and throat specialist; Dr. Cynthia Watson, whose family practice utilizes integrative medicine; and Dr. Vernon Erwin, who specializes in biological dentistry.

While skeptics may question Linda's explanation for her gift, no one has yet been able to disprove her gift or come up with a different explanation of how she is able to accomplish what she does. As a result, her healing gift forces us to stretch our preconceived notions of what is possible. What I have observed leads me to conclude that Linda has a uniquely advanced level of connection to higher truths and realities. This makes her gift revolutionary in its implications for both healing and human consciousness.

In writing this book, David faced the enormous problem of how to present Linda and her amazing gift to the world. In order to be taken seriously, the burden of proof was on him to first establish scientific credibility for her channeled medical information. To convince a skeptical scientific community and public of her accuracy, he systematically leads the reader down what he calls "the path of verification." Toward this end, I feel that he has accomplished his goal brilliantly.

As a result of this process, what logically emerged was an integration of two separate books, addressing the two types of information that Linda channels—objective and subjective. Once her channeling of highly accurate medical information can be accepted as scientifically objective, then the subjective information she channels (reincarnation, conversing with angels and spirits, and future predictions) must also be taken seriously, for, as David so aptly describes it, "these all come from the same spigot."

Since the book contains such a voluminous amount of amazing information on a wide range of topics, some readers may prefer to focus on the healing section of the book (Chapters 1–13, 15–16), while others may want to focus on Linda's most remarkable metaphysical pursuits (Chapters 14, 17–21). Both sections, however, are fascinating, and together they create a cohesive whole story that you won't want to miss. I highly recommend reading the Preface and A Guide to Reading This Book for information that will provide assistance in this endeavor.

A psychiatrist by training, I studied Freudian psychoanalysis, as well as the works of Carl Jung. Their channeled presence in Chapter 17, Sigmund Freud Speaks, can only be described as thoroughly original and revolutionary in scope. Without giving away the revelations, which will surely generate enormous controversy, it gives us a much richer impression of who they were as individuals and how they are still working on their relationship on the other side (how human!). It's good to know, too, that their present "thinking" appears to be a natural evolution of their original philosophies. As for psychoanalysis, just as psychiatry hasn't remained wedded to the "Freudian school," neither has Freud!

In summary, it's my pleasure to introduce you to both this remarkable book and to my dear friends, Linda and David Freud. Their efforts here will undoubtedly create quite a stir not only with the public, but also in many scientific, academic, and religious quarters. Even more importantly, it would appear that Linda's gift validates the long sought-after link between science and spirituality. David and Linda have told me they welcome the massive scientific scrutiny that will undoubtedly result from this book. This new paradigm of medical insight will have a profound effect on how medicine is practiced and will catapult Linda into becoming an internationally acclaimed personality in a manner she so richly deserves.

Hyla Cass, M.D.
Pacific Palisades, California

Preface

In 2004, medical researcher Burton Goldberg wrote a very positive article on Linda for the July–August edition of *Alternative Medicine* magazine entitled "Channeling Help from Afar" after experiencing the miracle of her gift first-hand. His article, which can be found on Linda's website, www.thehealing-gift.com, generated enormous interest in her work. He is truly responsible for putting Linda on the map.

I had known Burton years earlier when he worked in Beverly Hills, California, overseeing the production of what would become his landmark book *Alternative Medicine: The Definitive Guide*. After that, he moved away and we fell out of touch. In 2004, when I bumped into him at the Natural Products Expo West in Anaheim, he told me he had just undergone a very rigorous and complete physical by Dr. Bruno Kessler, an integrative medical doctor from Germany who also used many esoteric energetic testing protocols found in German Biological Medicine (see Chapter 1). Burton declared, in his inimitable manner, that Kessler was "the greatest medical diagnostician I have ever seen." I asked if he had heard about Linda, and he responded that he had heard great things about her through his grapevine of medical associates, but he was unaware of what her capabilities really were. I invited him to have a health reading with Linda. After spending approximately two hours with Linda, he announced that he was "utterly overwhelmed" by what he had experienced, exclaiming that *"Linda not only got the same results that Dr. Kessler had obtained, she had gone even further!"* He decided then and there that he had to write an article for his magazine even if it meant being held up to ridicule. Little did he know that the article would lead a significant number of desperately sick people to Linda whose medical conditions she was able to cure.

A year later I met cardiologist Dr. Stephen Sinatra, author of *The Sinatra Solution* and *Reverse Heart Disease Now*, at an American Academy of Anti-

Aging Medicine conference in Chicago. We immediately connected, and when I showed him the article, he expressed interest in seeing Linda to learn more about her gift. After flying to Los Angeles to see Linda, he proclaimed that he was "astonished by what I have just witnessed." He and his business associate Stanley Jankowitz subsequently approached Norman Goldfind, publisher of Basic Health Publications, and announced that he simply *had* to publish a book on this most remarkable gift. Thus this book was conceived.

How I Wrote This Book

The challenges of trying to figure out how to present Linda and her astonishing gift to the world were enormous. As Dr. Hyla Cass correctly points out in the Foreword, my primary purpose is to substantiate the audacious claims we make in such a way that Linda's gift is taken seriously by medical doctors, research scientists, and alternative health care practitioners, as well as the public at large. For her gift truly represents a verifiable breakthrough in human consciousness. We are prepared to be held up to rigorous scientific scrutiny by serious and sincere researchers who, without preconceived notions, seek the truth, wherever it may lead. We have no fear of this, as we are well aware of who is buttering our bread. However, to reach the point where we are taken seriously, the burden of proof is on me to establish a path of verification that is acceptable to a skeptical scientific community.

Among the claims we, and a growing chorus of doctors and theologians, are making is:

• While Linda has limited formal medical training, she may very well be the most advanced medical diagnostician and practitioner in the world. Her many years of rigorous medical study in conjunction with channeling have given her extensive experience in medical matters.

• Linda has achieved consistent communication with angels and the spirits of the departed that reveal not only medical and other types of scientific information, but what can only be described as enlightened or even otherworldly levels of information on a wide range of emotional, spiritual, and metaphysical issues.

My initial challenge in climbing this literary Mt. Everest is that these seemingly disparate claims involve two diametrically opposite types of information: objective and subjective. After much careful deliberation and several false starts, I realized that the only logical way to accomplish my goal was, in essence, to merge together two books: one containing objective medical information, the other containing subjective emotional, metaphysical, and spiritual information. Integrating the two was necessary to show the full flower of what Linda is truly capable of doing. Therefore, in order to be taken seriously, I had to present *a case for establishing scientific credibility that the medical information that Linda channels is objective.* Only then could I dare discuss the extraordinary spiritual and metaphysical revelations contained in the second part of the book. Once a consensus of mainstream and integrative doctors, alternative health care providers, and medical researchers accepts the medical information as objective, then the subjective channeled information cannot be rejected out of hand as fanciful or delusional notions. *It must, in fact, be taken seriously for it all comes from the same spigot.*

Ostensibly, metaphysics, reincarnation, and the like seem unrelated to physical health, and generally they are—but not always. How, you may ask, could metaphysical information impact a chronic degenerative condition? Here is a typical example: Linda may channel that a cofactor in her client's arthritic back pain is due to mercury toxicity that has a negative bearing on the methylation process affecting the phase II detoxification pathways of the liver. Later in the same session, it may be revealed that another cofactor of the same condition—the root cause of the problem–is an unresolved pain or emotional issue from a past life when that individual, as part of Napoleon's infantry, suffered a gunshot wound in the back. Though one cofactor may be considered objective and the other subjective, both types of information are derived from the same angelic source.

The task of presenting the medical information as "objective" was daunting. Some of the science that we utilize is either unknown or not necessarily accepted as valid in traditional medical circles. Yet Linda (working under the guidance of Dr. Thom E. Lobe, M.D., who is discussed below) is able to dramatically improve and often heal many forms of chronic degenerative disease that frequently elude both allopathic and alternative practitioners. In Chapter 10, for example, Linda shows the complexity of the unconventional healing variables she integrates to successfully treat cases of ulcerative colitis, herpes, arthritis, chronic arrhythmia, and male infertility. In fact, most of the testimonials in this book are from clients who came to Linda only after conventional allopathic or alternative approaches had failed them. Since Linda accomplishes such cures with methods that most practitioners are unfamiliar with, one of my goals was to bridge the gap by presenting alternative methods of diagnosing and treating chronic degenerative conditions in a way that naturally skeptical medical professionals and laypeople would take her work seriously.

The question quickly became "objective by whose standards?" Certainly, the way a clinically trained allopathic physician views a patient's health problems is usually quite different from the way an integrative medical physician, acupuncturist, chiropractor, or homeopath views the same patient's condition. The difficulties in explaining Linda's process to the allopathic medical community were magnified by the fact that Linda does not work with pharmaceutical drugs, but *only* with natural remedies. My job would have been very much easier if Linda channeled, "Take one erythromycin and call me in the morning." Therefore, the onus was on me to show that combining various types of natural remedies along with the appropriate diet are capable of controlling or curing a significant number of chronic degenerative diseases. As a result, I had to bridge the gap between the ways that allopathic and alternative medicine address certain health issues. Whenever possible, I cited scientific studies from well-known journals, books, and laboratories to back up a particular thesis. In other cases, I cited studies from highly regarded sources in the alternative health care community.

Medical knowledge is a bit like theater of the absurd—what one person considers objective, another considers subjective. Acupuncture is based on several thousand years of anecdotal experience. The track record of homeopathy or chiropractic is far shorter but nonetheless similarly impressive. The yardstick of what constitutes success for these modalities is simple: Does the patient's health improve from these therapies or remedies? Yet, what is effective for one group of people is ridiculed as unscientific by narrow-minded people unwilling to integrate new or old ideas, wherever they come from. In this book, we are asking the reader to be open to an entirely new possibility of scientific reality—one that includes a spiritual reality. Is there a historical precedent for such a request?

Though we are hardly putting ourselves, even remotely, in the same category, history is replete with examples of scientific geniuses such as Albert Einstein, who sought to reconcile their natural scientific curiosity with their equally natural spiritual leanings. The greatest example of that is Sir Isaac Newton, undoubtedly one of the most brilliant scientists in history, who fathered a thought process that embraced the logic of a mechanized clockwork universe—the foundation of Newtonian physics. It's deeply ironic, therefore, that he was also simultaneously ensconced in the occult, alchemy, and mysticism—ideas held up to ridicule by the scientific establishment. As Michael

White observes in *Isaac Newton: The Last Sorcerer*, Newton's vast library of secret writings revealed that he spent a great deal of time studying the Bible, examining prophecy, investigating natural magic, and attempting to unravel the secrets of alchemy. According to White, Newton's early biographers were so shocked and embarrassed by what they discovered that they suppressed his secret writings as "the obvious production of a fool and a nave."

Linda had an important role in the writing of this book. Besides reviewing each chapter, Linda called upon her angelic and spirit guides to channel each paragraph of the metaphysically oriented chapters to make sure the flow and direction of the writing passed upper-world muster. Her attention to detail proved invaluable. However, her channeling tour de force was Chapter 17, Sigmund Freud Speaks, where she channeled Sigmund, our principal spirit guide, hour after hour, day after day, to get the information needed for me to assemble the historically important evidence for what is revealed in that chapter.

Before reading this book, I urge you to study A Guide to Reading This Book, as well as our website, www.thehealinggift.com, to find out how best to approach the vast array of different subject matter. Not all readers will be interested in the same topics. Many readers may choose to start at the beginning and focus on how Linda channels angels and spirits to achieve medical miracles as well as explore the alternative science that is utilized to accomplish this. The goal here is to lead the reader down the path of verification to establish both her approach and the science as objective. Others may prefer to jump right to the miraculous metaphysical information (Chapters 14, 17–21) that Linda is able to channel through her discourse with angels and spirits.

Linda's Medical Partner: Dr. Thom E. Lobe, M.D., and the Beneveda Medical Group

When she was not assisting me with the book, Linda is an employee of the Beneveda Medical Group in Beverly Hills, California (www.beneveda.com), where she works directly with and under the medical license of founder and director Dr. Thom E. Lobe, M.D., F.A.C.S., F.A.A.P., and his medical staff. Linda became affiliated with Dr. Lobe after she discovered that his vision of healing was in sync with her own. In addition, his wide array of equipment centering on energy medicine provides beneficial results for her clients that complement her work.

Dr. Lobe earned his medical degree at the University of Maryland School of Medicine where he graduated cum laude with special honors in pediatrics in 1975. After training with former Surgeon General Dr. C. Everett Koop, M.D., as well as with other leading physicians at Harvard, Johns Hopkins, and Ohio State University, he acquired an international reputation as an innovator in groundbreaking surgical techniques that has led him to be one of the most sought-after pediatric surgeons in the world. For example, as chief of pediatric surgery at the University of Texas Medical Branch in Galveston, he made national news by being one of the first doctors to successfully separate a particularly difficult variety of Siamese twins. A prolific author of more than 200 books, book chapters, and peer-reviewed articles, Dr. Lobe is also the founder and editor of the first medical journal devoted to advanced surgical techniques in children.

But those accomplishments were not enough. After searching for alternative and complementary approaches to solving complex medical problems, Dr. Lobe earned a naturopathic degree and passed his boards in medical hypnosis and medical acupuncture. This led him to become an advisor to the Institute for the Study of Traditional Chinese Medicine at the Chinese University of Hong Kong. All these experiences led him to form the Beneveda Medical Group, where he has established a new paradigm involving the best of complementary and alternative medicine to treat the whole person—body, mind, and spirit. In so doing, he has established a new template for the enlightened practice of medicine in the 21st century. This new paradigm is broadly referred to as energy medicine (see Chapter 2). In addition to using Linda's prodigious healing gift as described throughout this book, the Beneveda Medical Group utilizes several cutting-edge diagnostic and treatment therapies that involve the transmission of subtle or vibrational energies that can have a quantum effect on the physical, emotional, and even spiritual aspects of healing. Linda is proud to work with Dr. Lobe in this endeavor.

In Linda Freud, Dr. Lobe immediately noted the same degree of medical miracle and brilliance that other leading doctors, medical researchers, and healing centers around the world with whom she has occasionally worked have come to recognize. In addition to Dr. Stephen Sinatra, M.D., and Burton Goldberg, these include Dr. Dietrich Klinghardt, M.D., of the Klinghardt Academy of Neurobiology; Dr. Thomas Rau, M.D., of the Paracelsus Clinic in Lustmühle, Switzerland; psychiatrist and author Dr. Hyla Cass, M.D.; healer and author Dr. Gabriel Cousens, M.D., of the Tree of Life Rejuvenation Center in Patagonia, Arizona; gynecologist and author Dr. Uzzi Reiss, M.D.; Dr. Hans Gruenn, M.D., of the Longevity Clinic of Los Angeles; ear, nose, and throat specialist Dr. Gary Bellack, M.D.; Dr. Elson Haas, M.D., of the Preventive Medical Center of Marin in San Rafael, California; biological dentists Dr. Hal

Huggins, D.D.S., and Dr. Vernon Erwin, D.D.S.; orthopedics and sports medicine specialist Dr. Karl Epstein, M.D.; Dr. Steven Small, N.M.D.; and biochemist Stephen Levine, Ph.D., former president of Allergy Research Group, a prominent supplement manufacturer in Alameda, California. Working in conjunction with Dr. Lobe, Linda sees clients at the Malibu Beach Recovery Center, a facility recognized for its unique holistic approach to drug and alcohol rehabilitation.

But Linda's support team goes beyond some of the brightest medical doctors in the integrative medical community. Linda's gift for channeling angels has been recognized and accepted by important rabbis from Jerusalem, including Rabbi Matteyahu Glazerson, Rabbi Moshe Schatz, and Rabbi Nachum Chaimowitz. In addition, Linda works within the parameters of Orthodox Jewish religious beliefs and under the guidance and auspices of Rabbi Aaron Parry of *Ohr Marpeh* (The Healing Light), a nonprofit religious corporation in Los Angeles.

Linda's word-of-mouth reputation was built mainly on her abilities as a medical intuitive. However, she also sees clients for a range of channeled emotional, spiritual, and metaphysical services described on her website and in the sections on the Emotional Database (see Chapters 15–16) and the Metaphysical Database (see Chapter 18). The most common topics her clients wish to have channeled involve such real-world issues as relationships, finances, and careers as well as esoteric issues including past-life research. Although many of Linda's clients continue to see her long after they are healed of a physical ailment, her first job is, as she readily admits, "to put out the physical fire first and ask metaphysical questions later."

A Matter of Clarification

I must clear up a source of confusion that may exist regarding my name before we begin this most extraordinary journey of healing. I was born Steven David Freud and never had a problem or issue with my first name. In fact, I have a rather pleasant association with it, as it is the first name of interesting people like Spielberg, Sondheim, Jobs, and McQueen.

In 2006, I was starting a channeling session with Linda when suddenly her pendulum started moving back and forth in a static manner indicative of a pattern where she was temporarily not receiving any answers to my health inquiries. Something was clearly wrong as this had never happened before. Linda briefly went into trance and announced that her angelic guides "were no longer interested in talking to Steven." I began to panic and asked what I had done wrong. After she channeled again, Linda announced, "You have not done anything wrong. They are just not interested in speaking with Steven any longer. They are interested in talking to David, your middle name."

After breathing a quizzical sigh of relief, I inquired why. "They no longer wish to refer to you as Steven; they wish to call you by your middle name. In fact, they want you to go to the synagogue and have your Hebrew name Schmuel changed [through a ceremony] to David. It is indicative of a metaphysical transformation in you that will occur as you write this book." It is understood in Kabbalah (an ancient Jewish mystical tradition) that names have certain energy attached to them. Furthermore, it is taught that by changing your name, you can change your destiny. Since beginning the process of writing this book, I have made a gradual transition among those who know me to David. And so it is.

Acknowledgments

In the early 1990s, my life lay in ruins due to a series of misdiagnosed illnesses that had completely incapacitated me. During this time I endured the most physically brutal, lonely, and financially exhausting experiences of my life. It was a time when I lost everything a man could lose—career, personal life, and finances—and still be standing. Yet, within my misfortune and through the grace of God, I arose from those written off in life and slowly began crawling and then walking on my journey back to health. I was to learn that the proverb "That which does not kill me strengthens me" is true. Yet, in spite of the suffering, I would not change what happened to me for anything in the world. For you could not put a price tag on the body of spiritual and medical knowledge that I acquired in those years. That knowledge was to become the foundation of my newly reinvented life that lay ahead. All the glory truly is to God.

Just when I reached my lowest ebb in 1992, my prayers began to be answered when I met Linda, whom I was quick to recognize as my soul mate. Though also coping with illness, she began to experience transcendent miracles as her healing gift emerged. To her I owe everything including my very life. After marrying in 1995, we were blessed in 1999 with the birth of our miracle boy, Aryeh, to whom Linda gave birth at age 44 against all odds. In addition, our beloved 13-year-old singing miniature schnauzer Schnitzel patiently lay by my feet, keeping me company as I metaphorically stumbled up this literary Mt. Everest. My family has been exceedingly patient during the extended period of time it took me to write this admittedly unusual book. I am most grateful for their support.

It is with enormous gratitude that Linda and I thank my precious mother Millie, who against all odds provided emotional and financial support when I was deathly ill in the early 1990s and during a lengthy recovery and rebuilding process. It took many, many years for me to fully regain my health and reestablish a new life from ground zero. Linda and I are incredibly grateful for the confidence that she exhibited in our ability to rise from the ashes, build a new life together, and serve God in a most unique way. We love you, Mom. I also wish to honor my father, Dr. William I. Freud, of blessed memory, who always wanted me to be a doctor. In addition, we wish to thank Linda's parents, Martin and Lois Riemer, for their encouragement.

In addition to the healers discussed in Chapter 1, in particular Dr. Daniel Reeves, Dr. Edward Smith, and Dr. Vaughn Harada, we must mention such individuals as Bella Karish, of blessed memory, Tom and Janet Sexton, Warren Barigian, and Klaus Puhlmann, who were very important to us in the early years. There is also a group of friends in America, Europe, and Israel who are members of what we refer to as "a loose confederation of metaphysical researchers," some of whom we have known and worked with since the early 1990s. These include Rabbi Moshe Schatz, Rabbi Matityahu Glazerson, Rabbi Aaron Parry, Richard Burnstein, Sari Katz, and Arjang and Nicole Zendehdel. They have provided lasting support and friendship, never wavering in their convictions that they have witnessed authentic miracles through Linda's channeling. For this we are most grateful.

There are friends in Switzerland with whom we share both gratitude and special memories. These include Dr. Thomas and Elizabeth Rau at the Paracelsus Clinic, Mario Binetti at the Kientalerhof Center for Wellbeing, Arnold Smayers in Zurich, and Thomas Baechler and Helga Sieber in Lindau, Germany.

There were other people whose friendship was very much appreciated during the writing of this book. These include Dr. Thom E. Lobe, Dr. Hyla Cass, Dr. Vernon Erwin, Dr. Kirk Slagel, Dr. Naweed Syed from the University of Calgary, Dr. Dietrich Klinghardt, Robert Eanes of VeraDyne Corp., Richard Lord of Metametrix Laboratories, Dr. Stephen Small, Joseph Gong, James Haig, Robert Johnstreet, Rowena Gates of Eng 3 Corp., Rowan Farber, Ken Dao, Stephen Levine, Karl Epstein, Ann Jerome, Paul Robison, Scott Moyer, Compton Rom Bada, Chrystyne Jackson, Ernestine Stowell, Pam Wall of Fitch Creative, Diego Valobra of www.pirolabs.it, Carolyn L. Winsor of the Occidental Institute Research Foundation, and Shelagh Bellack, Christina Scherer, Rabbi Zelig Pliskin, Donald Friedmann, Lloyd and Ruth Straits, and our talented copyeditor Cheryl Hirsch. We are also are grateful to the Freud Museum in London and the C. G. Jung Library in Los Angeles.

Linda and I wish to profoundly thank Burton Goldberg, a medical research pioneer who put Linda on the map with his wonderful article in *Alternative Medicine* magazine. We are most grateful to Dr. Stephen Sinatra and

Stanley Jankowitz who introduced us to Norman Goldfind, publisher of Basic Health Publications. Norman gave us a wonderful opportunity to tell a most extraordinary story. We must thank him for the patience and support he showed us during the time it took to write this book.

At our first production meeting, Linda asked Norman to bring a list of editors who worked for him. When he showed Linda the list, she channeled that Susan E. Davis would be the best possible editor for this project. It proved to be a wonderful decision as Susan provided invaluable assistance in helping me craft this book. Being an old soul herself, she not only realized early on the uniqueness of Linda, but exhibited a sensitivity toward the difficult hurdles that needed to be overcome as I presented Linda to the world. She patiently gave me enough leeway to creatively explore how to accomplish this, while keeping me focused on the big picture. The book would not have been the same without her expertise, guidance, and attention to detail.

A Guide to Reading This Book

Before embarking on this unique journey of healing, I urge you to read the Foreword by Dr. Hyla Cass, M.D., the Preface, and our www.thehealing gift.com website as they contain valuable information about the purpose and thought process behind this book. So much information is contained on such a wide range of topics that it is necessary to provide a guide to the book. As explained in both the Foreword and Preface, this book is actually an integration of two separate books. Some readers will naturally gravitate toward Chapters 1–13, 15, and 16 which begin the journey down the scientific path of verification and are, in large part, devoted to proving that the medical information Linda channels is accurate and objective. This validates not only the healing miracles Linda is able to accomplish, but also the theories and methods behind the forms of alternative medicine that she uses. Other readers will gravitate toward the extraordinary emotional, metaphysical, and spiritual revelations in Chapters 14 and 17–21 that are certain to spark enormous controversy. However, to gain a complete picture of what Linda is capable of accomplishing requires that the whole book be read.

Introducing Linda's Gift and Her Alternative Healing Process (Chapters 1–3)

The book opens with a description of the extraordinarily difficult and complex health problems I faced in the early 1990s (Chapter 1, Discovery of Linda's Gift). My healing journey led up several blind alleys until I stumbled onto several obscure diagnostic and treatment modalities in America, Germany, and Switzerland. In 1992, during the course of those discoveries, I met Linda, my soulmate, who was also seriously ill. After the incredible process by which her healing gift emerged, we were startled to discover the striking similarities between her approach of channeling angels and the methods of the Hebrew prophets. Her gift, along with the healing knowledge I had amassed, eventually helped save both of our lives.

What emerged was a healing philosophy (Chapter 2, Our Healing Philosophy) borne from our sometimes tumultuous personal experiences with allopathic medicine. That led us to discover the multiple modalities of alternative medicine, which treat the whole person through an integration of body/mind/spirit. This involved a particular emphasis on detoxification of environmental toxins and common pathogens, enhancement of brain and organ function with an increase in energy through many forms of natural supplements, and adherence to a healing diet. To this Linda later added various meditation processes and metaphysical research to help achieve a higher spiritual alignment.

This, in turn, led to the development of Metaphysical Systems Engineering^{SM}, Linda's unique diagnostic approach (Chapter 3, An Introduction to Metaphysical Systems Engineering). Linda utilizes three comprehensive databases of information—physical, emotional, and metaphysical—from which she channels angels and spirits by means of a pendulum to receive incredibly accurate diagnostic information and treatment protocols. This has brought about life-changing results for many of Linda's clients who had serious, complicated medical conditions. Although there is some overlap, the rest of the book, in broad strokes, covers the Physical Databases (Chapters 4–13); the Emotional Database (Chapters 14–16); the Metaphysical Database (Chapters 17–18), which is focused on reincarnation and other spiritual issues; a discourse on angels, the source of Linda's gift (Chapters 19–20); and one of Linda's important past life incarnations that is, in part, the basis for her gift (Chapter 21).

Part One: Physical Healing (Chapters 4–13)

These chapters deal with issues related to physical healing and include numerous examples of how Linda uses the Physical Databases to diagnose and treat the most common variables she sees in her practice—heavy metals and other environmental toxins, acidosis, fungi, parasites, bacteria, and miasms—with a range of natural modalities. *These are often significant cofactors in many chronic degenerative conditions and are often overlooked by doctors whose only or principal means of treatment is with pharmaceutical drugs. As a result, this information should prove invaluable for someone who has had only limited or no success with the traditional allopathic approach.*

• Chapter 4, The Physical Databases, provides a detailed description of how Linda uses them. A case history illustrates how she works with the cardio-vascular database in her process.

• Chapter 5, Fungal Disease: The Modern Consequence of Environmental Toxicity, and Chapter 6, Pleomorphism: The Lost Chapter of Biology, are devoted to the scourge of fungal disease and acidosis, two of the root causes of much chronic degenerative disease. This is primarily brought on by environmental toxicity, poor lifestyle choices, and diet, which are often ignored or misunderstood by allopathic doctors. Linda has enjoyed enormous success in treating candida and other common fungal forms using an obscure, nontoxic homeopathic approach called pleomorphism.

• Chapter 7, Parasites: Stealth Marauders of Disease, shows how Linda diagnoses and treats parasite disease, a very common and difficult-to-diagnose cofactor in many forms of chronic degenerative disease. Parasite infestation is often misunderstood or ignored by many allopathic physicians, who mistakenly believe that it primarily exists only in third world countries. A remarkable testimonial from a client shows how parasitic infection was a hidden cause of unwanted weight gain.

• Chapter 8, Miasms: The Invisible Enemy in Chronic Disease, discusses the fascinating and little understood homeopathic concept of genetically inherited miasms—vibrational resonances derived from various infectious diseases (typically tuberculosis, syphilis, gonorrhea, and staphylococcal and streptococcal infections) that can span multiple generations. These inherited resonances do not mean that the individual suffers from a particular infectious condition. Rather, it is often the underlying causal factor for a medical condition that runs in a family. The origin of certain difficult-to-diagnose medical conditions can often be traced back to miasms. More importantly, they are one of the key barriers to detoxification because they bind in different types of heavy metal toxins and prevent them from being excreted from the body.

• So serious and misunderstood is the relationship between mercury toxicity and chronic degenerative disease, and so central is it to Linda's work, that it was necessary to devote four chapters (9–12) to it. Chapter 9, Mercury: The

Thousand-Headed Monster of Chronic Degenerative Diseases, provides a detailed overview of mercury toxicity, describing the scope of the problem as well as widespread ignorance that still exists despite overwhelming scientific evidence. While mercury comes from many different environmental sources, the chronic leakage of mercury from silver amalgam mercury fillings is clearly the most dangerous and misunderstood source of the problem. The difficulty in diagnosing low-level leakage of mercury from silver fillings is due to the fact that it burrows in body or brain tissue and does not generally show up in conventional blood, urine, or saliva tests. Readers may be shocked by the chart, which identifies a huge number of illnesses where mercury toxicity may be a cofactor.

• Chapter 10, How the Monster Rears Its Head, describes the many ways that mercury causes major devastation by disrupting core biochemical processes in the body on a cellular level. This chapter also provides remarkable testimonials describing how Linda successfully treats such conditions as arthritis, herpes, and ulcerative colitis when the core causal factor involves mercury toxicity. There is a particularly heartwarming story about a couple, desperate to have a baby, who were unable to conceive due to the husband's deformed sperm that rendered him infertile. After the in vitro fertilization process failed, they came to see Linda as a last resort. Linda channeled a detoxification program that eliminated mercury from his testicles and elsewhere in his body. Several months later the couple conceived beautiful twins.

• Chapter 11, Neurotoxicity and Mercury: The Brain Polluter of Chronic Wasting Diseases, documents the overwhelming link between mercury and a spate of serious neurological conditions such as multiple sclerosis, Alzheimer's disease, autism, and Parkinson's disease. These include many emotional conditions that conventional mental health professionals are still woefully ill-prepared to treat effectively due to a lack of understanding about the dangers of neurotoxins.

• Chapter 12, Chelating Mercury Out of the Darkness: Linda's Rules for Mercury Detoxification, describes the body/mind/spirit processes that Linda uses to detoxify mercury out of the body. It also serves as a basic primer on the overall process for both health practitioners and patients.

• Chapter 13, A World of Natural Supplements, is a very brief overview of the main categories of supplements that Linda utilizes in her work. We review the many and varied reasons why people with chronic degenerative disease should take natural supplements. A future book is planned with an in-depth investigation of all that we have learned about natural supplements, the true relationship between diet and healing, and the many components that constitute a physically and emotionally healthy lifestyle.

Part Two: Emotional Healing (Chapters 14–16)

The Emotional Database is a blend of objective and subjective information. Chapter 14, Our Work with Sigmund Freud: A Preamble to the Emotional Database, is an introduction to our ongoing and close personal relationship with Sigmund Freud, our primary spirit guide, who provided invaluable assistance in both the assemblage and usage of the Emotional and Metaphysical Databases that Linda channels from. His goal in working with Linda is to help reshape the field of psychology in the 21st century with discoveries he has made in the spirit world. In what is the first of several shocking revelations to come forth from Sigmund, it is revealed that two of Linda's clients are actually the reincarnations of two of Sigmund's close friends and associates whom he guided to Linda!

Sigmund Freud was instrumental in guiding Linda to treat the neurological and physiological components behind certain emotional problems. In addition to a discussion on his approach to neurotoxins, Chapter 15, The Emotional Database, contrasts the pharmaceutical approach in treating depression with various natural methods, including cutting-edge nutraceuticals. These neurological "construction materials" are precursors to important neurotransmitters that control depression—serotonin and dopamine. Chapter 16, The Connection Between Emotions and Women's Hormones, delves into the role and relationship of hormones to a woman's emotional and physical well-being. Disruptions of the endocrine system due to a maze of environmental toxins wreak emotional and physical havoc for many women who suffer from premenstrual syndrome and during menopause.

Part Three: Spirit, Metaphysics, and Reincarnation (Chapters 17–18)

The Metaphysical Database contains information that currently must be regarded as subjective, but over time will hopefully be regarded as objective. It covers reincarnation, paranormal phenomenon, and spiritual issues that are revolutionary in their implications.

• In what will surely be considered the crown jewel of the book, Chapter 17, Sigmund Freud Speaks: A Preamble to the Metaphysical Database, contains an astonishing discourse in which Sigmund reveals the importance of reincarnation in resolving deep-seated issues in personal relationships. Drawing on his failed relationship with Carl Jung, he shows, in great detail, how the origins of his problems with Jung were a karmic replay of another equally famous and historic past life the two of them shared. The preponderance of evidence for the existence of these particular past lives and its bearing on the Freud/Jung breakup is so overwhelming that it literally flips the fields of religion, psychology, and literature upside down.

• Chapter 18, The Metaphysical Database, explores the purpose of reincarnation for the soul and the framework through which Linda conducts past-life research. In addition there is a discussion of paranormal phenomenon involving earthbound spirits, which in Hebrew are called *dybbuks*. Parasitic in nature, dybbuks require a host body so they can continue their negative behaviors at the expense of an unwitting victim. Three case histories describe how these disembodied spirits attached themselves to the auric fields of unsuspecting individuals, causing them to experience severe emotional problems or even "phantom" health problems that were undiagnosable. Although not a common phenomenon, dybbuk possession is quite real, but far more subtle than portrayed in movies like *The Exorcist*. Linda has found that it can appear as a cofactor in chronic alcoholism, drug addiction, and stress. Like religious figures from different faiths and bygone eras, she performs a ritual ceremony that removes the dybbuk and sends it back to the light.

In what can only be described as a complete shock, Linda received, just prior to the book's completion, a totally unexpected visitation from the spirit of pop singer Michael Jackson following his tragic and untimely death. His overdose on Propofol did not merely kill him, but continues to negatively affect his soul as it remains on the earth plane, unable to ascend to the light. Michael came to Linda to request that she help him in that endeavor.

Part Four: The Source of Linda's Gift— Communicating with Angels (Chapters 19–21)

While some readers may consider the ability to communicate with angels an utter impossibility and completely subjective, others will find the discourse based on ancient and long-established rabbinic commentary—ranging from the Talmud to the Zohar (the principal book of Kabbalah)—a wellspring of spiritual knowledge. Communication with angels was the exclusive province of the Hebrew prophets and the source of their visions. These visions have stood the test of time and are regarded as crucial to both the Jewish and Christian faiths.

• Starting with a recent study showing a significant majority of people believe in angels (collective unconscious archetypes) and followed by a discussion of the spiritual implications of the anthropic principle, the case is made for the existence of angels in Chapter 19, Belief in Angels: A Common Bond of the World's Religions. Various rabbinic texts are cited regarding the significance of one's personal guardian angels, an important component in Linda's spiritual work. An analysis of the Hebrew prophet Ezekiel's Vision of the Chariot (*Merkabah*) then identifies the various angelic hierarchies that collectively function as an angelic communications network. The numerous functions that angels perform as well as their appearance and various personality attributes are discussed in detail. In a fascinating testimonial, Linda channeled information for a client regarding the unfortunate manner in which angelic justice was meted out to his dying uncle after a verdict was reached by the archangelic court. Our subsequent research showed this to be consistent with the manner described in various Kabbalistic texts.

• Chapter 20, Meet the Archangels: A Guide to Those Angels That Speak to Linda, is a discussion of the five most important archangels who speak with Linda. Our understanding of these archangels is through Kabbalah, which reveals their veiled existence in the Old Testament (Torah) and in the writings of the Hebrew prophets. Linda also received a dramatic angelic visitation in the Swiss Alps where the divine hand behind earth changes was revealed.

• Chapter 21, Metaphysical Patterns in Time: Soul Connections Revealed, explores two of Linda's many past lives. The context for this occurs after Linda helped one of her favorite clients deal with a debilitating condition and a frightening poltergeistian experience that spanned two continents. While investigating her client's past lives, it became evident why it was "karmically" correct for Linda to heal her: She had been Linda's aunt in one life and her benefactress in another. Linda's life as a major ancient queen is then revealed which helps to explain why she has her extraordinary gift.

CHAPTER 1

Discovery of Linda's Gift

Do not go where the path may lead,
go instead where there is no path and leave a trail.
—RALPH WALDO EMERSON

IMAGINE THE FOLLOWING SCENARIO and see if you relate: You have been suffering for years with a mysterious ailment that has radically affected the quality of your life. You have bounced around from doctor to doctor only to receive little or no relief. In fact, your overall condition continued to deteriorate under their care. You paid for a battery of expensive diagnostic tests that one doctor had recommended and your treatment was based on those results. After several months, you still had no energy to do anything but drag yourself through the day. Your assorted aches, pains, migraines, insomnia, low sex drive, and other unpleasant and debilitating health problems persisted despite many doctors' best efforts. In fact, one of the drugs prescribed to control your problem was now disagreeing with you. On your last ten-minute visit, all you were told was to lower your dosage for that drug and take another drug to counteract the effects of the first one. The first twinge of doubt had set in. You were beginning to lose faith that doctors could help you.

Though well-intentioned, your current doctor was also becoming frustrated with your lack of progress and suggested that perhaps your problems were psychosomatic in nature. Now you began to question your own sanity. You were depressed and riddled with anxiety. The confidence you once had was fading fast, your career aspirations were not working out, you were now broke, and your relationship had ended. Your significant other did not know how to cope with your health/emotional issues, so he or she threw in the towel. In desperation you did some research on the Internet and decided to give alternative medicine a whirl. After all, what the doctors did had made you sicker. You had nothing to lose, even if the doctors ridiculed your new ideas. A friend told you about an acupuncturist or chiropractor who had helped him or her so you figured you'd give that practitioner a try. Twenty-five sessions and thousands of dollars later you did feel a little better but certainly nowhere near the way the practitioner had promised you'd feel by this time. It seemed like your new healer was getting a piece of the puzzle right, but not the whole puzzle. Perhaps the doctors who said you were crazy were right. The old doubts begin to creep in. Oh, well, at least your doctor will renew your prescription for Prozac.

Congratulations! If you identify with any part of this scenario, you are a candidate to see Linda Freud. This description is a composite of literally hundreds of clients who have come to see her over the years. They had already burned through a considerable number of allopathic and alternative doctors and were truly desperate. Linda was their last hope.

LINDA'S GIFT AS A MEDICAL INTUITIVE

In 1993 Linda discovered that she could use a pendulum coupled with sophisticated medical databases of information to intuitively diagnose and recommend treatment for medical conditions. In a broad sense she follows in a tradition pioneered by mystic visionary Edgar Cayce and most recently embodied by Carolyn Myss, who coined the phrase "medical intuitive." Myss is the author of such best-selling books as *Anatomy of the Spirit* and *Sacred Contracts*. Over the course of this book, we will show that *Linda makes contact with the angelic realms and spirit guides who direct her work as a medical intuitive to effectuate real healing by working with all aspects of the mind/body/spirit connection in a uniquely accurate way.*

Here's a very brief overview of how Linda works. Linda uses her process called Metaphysical Systems Engineering℠, a comprehensive psychic channeling system derived from physical, emotional, and metaphysical information. Introduced in Chapter 3, that process provides a clear picture of the client's health. Treatment involves identifying the optimal natural supplements and therapies for each individual in each stage of the healing process. Linda's expansive repertoire of healing modalities includes orthomolecular nutrients, herbal medicine, homeopathy, flower and gem essences, and diet, all of which are discussed in subsequent chapters. These are used to detoxify toxins, eliminate pathogens, and correct energetic, biochemical, and nutritional imbalances. As healing begins to unfold and symptoms begin to abate, Linda's clients are awed by the creative solutions to their physical problems channeled from the spirit world.

Sometimes her results can be verified through traditional laboratory analysis. However, when they are not verifiable through these methods, it is not due to any deficiencies in Linda's process. It is due to one of two reasons:

1. A disconnect exists among disparate healing modalities because they view the same health condition through different sets of lenses. Completely valid and time-honored concepts of energetic medicine are simply not acknowledged in the allopathic world. For example, no lab test exists that can quantify how the gall bladder acupuncture meridian is functioning. The healing action of homeopathic remedies cannot be quantified through lab analysis, and yet they have a profound effect on healing. In such cases, anecdotal confirmation from the client that he or she is feeling dramatically better confirms the accuracy of what Linda has channeled.

2. The one-dimensional nature of certain lab tests reflects their inability to detect a pathogen, toxin, or imbalance that may be the root cause of a condition. For example, it is very difficult to detect the presence of neurotoxins in the deep recesses of the brain.

The bottom line is this: While skeptics may discount the spiritual source of her work, *they cannot discount the astonishing healing success she achieves as a medical intuitive.* Yet the question remains: Why Linda? The simple answer is that some people are more sensitive to energy than others. Different people perceive nuances of subtle energy to varying degrees and in different ways. Metaphysics (meta + physics) teaches that there tends to be a relationship between the number of times a soul has reincarnated and the level of accumulated wisdom that soul has (hopefully) acquired along the way. The wisdom of an old soul often manifests as a heightened ability to sense subtle energies. This explains why most people would not perceive a miracle even if they were whacked over the head with it.

Woody Allen is the quintessential skeptic whose personal foibles mirror those of people who doubt the existence of God. A constant theme in his movies and essays is the preconditions he puts on God, requiring miraculous proof of his existence before he will commit to the rigors of belief. If only God would give him some clear sign, he suggests, like making a large deposit in his name at a Swiss bank, uttering a few words, or moving a lamp on the dresser.

In his 1986 movie *Hannah and Her Sisters*, when proof fails to materialize, he lapses into cynicism while watching a Marx Brothers' movie and concludes, "I should stop ruining my life searching for answers I'm never going to get and just enjoy myself."

Cynicism makes the nonbeliever insensitive to subtle energies, causing him or her to ridicule metaphysics, a highly evolved hybrid spiritual and scientific process, which adheres to the proposition that although there are simple truths, the ultimate truth is not simple. With proper spiritual discipline and training , certain very old souls can perceive the glory and grandeur of God's logic to varying degrees. Linda Freud is such a soul. Through Linda's gift, those who work with her have first-hand knowledge that a higher being exists. We do not believe He exists; we *know* He exists. *Linda has seen the lamp move on the dresser.*

PRELUDE TO THE GIFT

Most people assume that Linda was born with her gift, which she actively developed as a child and young adult. Nothing could be further from the truth. Linda showed no signs that she would one day possess what a growing number of well-respected doctors now believe is the most astonishing and prodigious medical diagnostic gift in the world. A friend of ours, who witnessed this unfold from the beginning, has jokingly remarked that "Linda could not channel rain in a monsoon storm before she met David."

This is why it is important to understand that my healing story and Linda's healing story are inexorably bound together, as well they should be for we are soul mates who have been married to or have known each other in multiple lifetimes. Truly ours is a metaphysical love story. Her gift only emerged after meeting me when I was very ill. Linda and other psychics have channeled that it was her karmic destiny to save my life. I truly believe that I would have died years ago if not for her prodigious gift. Therefore, the story of her healing gift is inseparable from my personal healing and vice versa. This is the real reason why I am the only person who could write this book. We are team partners in this endeavor as I provide ongoing research for the expansion of the databases that are critical to Linda's work. Linda likens what I do to running the IT (Information Technology) Department of Metaphysical Systems Engineering. Certain information about our health must now be revealed to show that our knowledge of healing was not gained in a vacuum. This was not a hobby or our trained profession; this was knowledge needed to save our very lives.

Illness Derails David's Life

Without a doubt, the years from 1989 to 1992 were the worst years of my life. How I survived the brutal beating my health took still astonishes me. Looking back in hindsight, however, I can clearly see that within my misfortune, I was somehow being guided to make medical and spiritual discoveries that would later become the driving forces behind Linda's work. At the time, there were metaphysical forces at work that I was utterly unaware of, though I would not realize this until one year later when Linda's gift burst through.

By the close of the 1980s, I had spent well over a decade honing my skills as a singer-songwriter. I had been actively playing the piano since age six, and music had been the grand obsession of my life ever since. I had received my bachelors of music degree from California Institute of the Arts in 1975. I possessed the ability to play and compose many genres of music, holding my own as a classical or jazz pianist and popular song stylist. Although I had briefly dabbled in film scoring and as a record producer, I spent many years focused on song writing as well as performing my songs in restaurants and bars in the Los Angeles area. I even traveled to Japan in 1982 to perform my solo act. My music was a mix of rock and roll and rhythm and blues. I was the "Piano Man" in a vein somewhat similar to that of Billy Joel or Elton John.

I had a master plan for success. Supporting myself with my day job—selling commercial and residential real estate—I took all my commissions and poured them into my music, recording a series of very expensive 24-track masters that I wrote, produced, and financed. I hired prominent LA studio musicians and backup singers to perform on my album in the hope of securing a record contract with a major label. My manager and attorney had arranged for auditions with major labels upon completion of my record.

Then in 1988, while in the middle of recording my album, I suddenly took ill, forcing me to stop work. My manager and attorney kept patiently waiting for me to recover and complete the album. This never happened as my health deteriorated at a rapid rate in spite of my frantic efforts to turn it around. I could not understand what had happened to me as I did not use drugs, smoke, or drink. I was emotionally crushed, believing that my entire life had been a preparation for a career as a performer. I had run through all my money and was completely broke. There was no backup plan.

Suddenly my priorities changed. Music, which had been my entire life, was no longer relevant. Now the question was: Would I live or would I die? In 1990, as I became even more incapacitated, the music simply died in me. It was a cruel and bitter pill to swallow. As my life force ebbed, I was reduced to a survival existence, completely consumed with beating this mysterious set of illnesses that had befallen me. (As I was to discover years later, Linda and other psychics all channeled that my music career was not allowed to happen because that was not meant to be my life's calling. Although it took a while to emotionally accept this reality, I finally made peace with it, holding no animosity or bitterness. I now understand a deeper purpose and karma—the medical and spiritual research I do in conjunction with Linda's gift is precisely what I am supposed to be doing during this phase of my life.)

Life throws us many curve balls that we do not understand at the time they're happening. However, when people have faith in God, they can weather any storm and know that everything that happens is for the best. I now realize that I am actually the most fortunate man in the world, as I get a ringside seat to witness Linda channeling angels and spirits that produced the healing miracles documented in this book.

The Nightmare of David's Multiple Health Conditions

Although I was not exactly a picture of glowing health growing up, nothing I had previously experienced prepared me for the physical onslaught I was about to endure. Other than having childhood allergies, an auto accident when I was thirteen, and my gallbladder removed as an adult, I had no particular history of disease other than the flus, colds, and infections that most people get from time to time.

What happened in 1989 was that I began to experience a severe numbness and pressure in my jaw and brain. My head felt like it was locked in a vise. Over the next year, my health worsened as the undiagnosed trauma in my head caused periodic blackouts, fainting spells, tremors, and convulsions that occurred with increasing regularity. I also experienced inexplicable tremors in my hands and arms that looked like the beginning stages of Parkinson's disease. I endured horrible insomnia that made me wake up feeling exhausted, and I suffered from massive tachycardia (rapid heart beat) for no apparent reason. If I was stressed, it came on more easily, but it happened even if I wasn't stressed. Soon I was in the throes of extreme exhaustion, experiencing a constant chronic and throbbing ache in my kidneys and adrenal glands. My compromised immunity brought on a series of seemingly endless bacterial, fungal, and viral infections. I also endured chronic dental infections and tooth pain as many of my teeth were beginning to rot and die.

I was diagnosed as having the catchall condition called chronic fatigue syndrome, otherwise known as "the flu that never ends." After suffering from bacterial pneumonia treated by antibiotics, my life force waned and I could no longer function. But it was the constant numbness in my brain, fainting spells, and blackouts that worried me most. For years thereafter I fainted daily, passing out unconscious for hours at a time in the mid- to late-afternoon.

I saw a neurologist in Beverly Hills about the intense numbness in my brain, my inability to think clearly, and the blackouts and fainting spells. He ordered a SPECT (single photon-emission computed tomography) study, an EEG (electroencephalogram), and a MRI (magnetic resonance imaging) scan. I will never forget the quizzical look on his face when he tried to describe what the test results showed. "Mr. Freud, the tests show that you are suffering from MS-like symptoms." "Does that mean I have MS?" I asked frantically. "Mr. Freud, the tests show brain patterns that are fairly consistent to what we see in MS patients, although I am not yet prepared to say you have MS." There I was, poised for my moment of medical truth, and instead was hearing some double-speak gobbledygook that still left me holding the bag. While acknowledging that something was clearly wrong with my brain, the neurologist cleverly danced his way around a precise diagnosis. What was not illusionary, however, was the constant assault my brain and body were under. I went back to see him soon after that as my problems were intensifying. He was a sympathetic man who had done his best by admitting that diagnosing multiple sclerosis was anything but easy. He explained that it was actually a process of eliminating all other possibilities and that reaching a definitive conclusion could take months or even years.

At the close of the 1980s, I had gone to several prominent doctors in Los Angeles and was getting progressively weaker and dysfunctional. My doctors, though sympathetic to my suffering, were completely clueless as to why I was in such a run-down condition. After batteries of expensive tests, no clear diagnosis had been made. Every round of antibiotics and anti-inflammatory steroids ultimately backfired as new health problems surfaced. My health was spiraling out of control, my career lay in ruins, and my finances were decimated. Fighting for my life, I prayed for a miracle to save me.

Beginning to Find Answers

My prayers were finally answered by an utterly obscure technology called Electroacupuncture According to Voll (EAV). EAV is the diagnostic centerpiece of a holistic healing system called German Biological Medicine. (See "The Importance of EAV or Voll Testing.") My introduction to EAV came about quite accidentally in 1989 when my voice teacher recommended I see a chiropractor, whom I will call Dr. Jonah Clark, who used a completely different diagnostic approach from the conventional methods that had failed me. As the son of an internal medicine doctor, I was naturally quite skeptical. But I was now desperate and had nothing left to lose.

I will never forget our first meeting. After testing me on his computerized Voll device, Dr. Clark declared that the core of my problems was a mouthful of silver amalgam fillings and infected root canals. I was completely caught off guard. This was the first time I had ever heard of such a diagnosis. After pondering my fate for a moment, I blurted out, "Dr. Clark, you are either some sort of medical genius, who is far more advanced than any of the doctors I've seen, or you are a complete charlatan who should be run out of town. I don't know which."

I left his office feeling dazed and confused but also overwhelmed and excited. What he had told me was completely different from anything my other doctors had told me. How could my doctors view my health problems so differently? Yet an inner voice told me that I had just witnessed a diagnostic miracle. Dr. Clark's whole perspective and approach were so fresh and original. Perhaps this would work. Time would tell; either he was right or he was wrong. As I continued seeing Dr. Clark for several months, I began to see slow but steady improvement for the first time. Certainly the severity of my immediate health crisis was beginning to dissipate. I was fascinated by EAV as I realized that it was far more accurate than anything else I had found. The homeopathic remedies Dr. Clark prescribed were finally providing a small measure of relief for my kidneys and my immune system. I decided to stop seeing the doctors with whom I had spent a considerable sum of money with nothing to show for it.

My problem was this: How could I verify the accuracy of a diagnostic modality that was essentially unknown in America? I certainly was not prepared to start my healing process by spending a small fortune, which I did not have, to remove a mouthful of silver amalgam fillings.

The Importance of EAV or Voll Testing

There are two reasons why it is necessary to discuss this amazing technology in detail. For those readers who do not require a technical explanation, feel free to skip this inset.

1. Electroacupuncture According to Voll (EAV) was essential in shaping the process of

how Linda does her diagnostic detective work. The holistic protocols of German Biological Medicine, involving the integration of homeopathy, acupuncture, herbal medicine, orthomolecular nutrients, and diet, became the framework for using the various databases I assembled over the years.

2. For people who are unable to work with Linda, the next best diagnostic approach is to have a full workup with a practitioner proficient in EAV. This is not meant to replace traditional lab testing but to complement it by providing valuable information about toxicity and other imbalances that are otherwise undiagnosable. In addition, it promotes the unique healing perspective of energetic medicines such as acupuncture and homeopathy. My story exposes the deficiencies of conventional diagnostic protocols and the narrow-minded belief system that can sometimes result from it. My hope is that people who have not found relief through conventional medicine investigate the miracle of Voll testing.

Electroacupuncture According to Voll was the brainchild of the German medical doctor Dr. Reinhold Voll (1909–1989), who had a most unusual background. Trained as an electrical engineer, he later switched to medicine, eventually becoming a professor of anatomy. Combining an amazingly eclectic blend of left- and right-brain abilities, Dr. Voll also worked as an acupuncturist and was proficient with the pendulum (see Figure 1-1). His research in the 1940s and 1950s led him to develop a stunning, noninvasive diagnostic instrument that, along with treatment protocols, married acupuncture meridians and homeopathy with modern electrical engineering. This is called Voll testing, electrodermal screening, or a similar approach called Vega test. Documented and proven effective in over a decade of hospital studies in Germany, EAV is widely used today throughout Europe by over 25,000 medical practitioners.[1] Although known principally in alternative medical circles, it has not gained widespread acceptance in

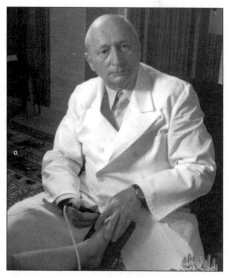

FIGURE 1-1. Dr. Reinhold Voll.

the United States for several reasons, despite its brilliance as a diagnostic instrument.

Dr. Voll researched the effects of electricity on the body using a technique called electrical conductivity metering. Though it was well known that skin is very resistant to electrical current, Dr. Voll discovered a new "biological circuit" originating from the acupuncture meridian channels located beneath the skin. (Meridians are invisible energetic pathways in the body that conduct the flow of energy called *Qi* to every organ, gland, and system in the body. They form the basis of acupuncture, the ancient Traditional Chinese Medicine system that is thousands of years old.) Dr. Voll proved that skin exhibited higher levels of electrical conductivity (lower electrical resistance) at the precise location of acupuncture points on meridians compared with other areas of the skin. His revolutionary discovery revealed the potential of using the acupuncture meridian system as both a diagnostic and a therapeutic interface.

Based on this discovery, Dr. Voll developed a sophisticated voltage-metering device that he called the Dermatron to measure the skin resistance of acupuncture points and corresponding diagnostic protocols (see Figure 1-2). Dr. Voll had the patient hold a small brass cylinder called a hand mass in one hand that was charged with a very low current and was connected by cable to the Dermatron. Dr. Voll held a brass-tipped probe, also attached by cable to the Dermatron, with which he touched acupoints located on the patient's hands, feet, and skull. That complete electrical circuit allowed Voll to measure changes in electrical conductivity, giving him an accurate picture of the functional status of all the acupuncture points and meridians. Dr. Voll was thus able to electronically "read" the functional level of Qi energy of every organ, gland, and system through the corresponding meridians.

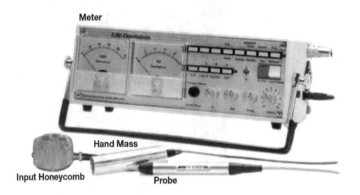

FIGURE 1-2.
An example
of an older EAV
device that is still
widely utilized
throughout
Europe.

Dr. Voll found 21 basic EAV meridians (Chinese doctors typically use 12), each corresponding to a specific organ, gland, or system in the body. He then identified acupuncture points along each meridian associated with a specific functional area of that organ, gland, or system. For example, there is a specific point along the endocrine meridian associated with adrenal gland function and another associated with thyroid function. Dr. Voll found that when a meridian tested out of balance, that indicated the organ, gland, or system was in a disease state. He understood that changes in resistance of electrical conductivity were caused by such inflammatory processes or disturbances as pathogens, toxins, allergies, or emotions, which affected the ability of the organ, gland, or system to conduct electricity.

Dr. Voll developed a conductivity scale from 1 to 100 to fit the needs of the medical parameters he was testing. He found that a reading of 50 reflected a functionally healthy and balanced meridian corresponding to a functionally healthy and balanced organ, gland, or system. A reading higher than 60 indicated an underlying inflammatory process in that organ, gland, or system. The higher the number above 60, the greater the inflammation.

Conversely, Dr. Voll found that a degenerative state caused cellular activity to stagnate, making it more difficult for a normal level of electrical conductivity to flow through the circuit. When this happened, a reading below 30 indicated a severely compromised meridian. When the measurement of a meridian climbed up but then fell steadily downward, Dr. Voll observed that the site was no longer capable of sustaining a consistent level of electrical conductivity, indicating a functional weakening of the meridian. Dr. Voll referred to this disease discovery process as an "indicator drop."

Using his device, Dr. Voll was able to take readings of each of the 21 meridians within a few minutes. Readings ranged from normal (around 50) to high (inflammation at 60 or higher) to low (30 or below). This gave him an understanding of the functional status of all the major organs, glands, and systems in the patient's body. This was a major breakthrough in medical technology in the early 1950s.

But the usefulness of the Dermatron didn't stop there. Voll found that the meridian points were extremely sensitive to remedies. When he brought a remedy within close proximity of the patient's energetic field, he found it could alter acupoint readings. This knowledge gave Voll the ability to use the device to measure the effect of a remedy on a meridian. Let's say, for example, that the patient has an inflammation reading of 75 in the kidney meridian. Dr. Voll then placed a test ampoule of Solidago, a common herbal kidney drainage remedy, in an aluminum "honeycomb" that is electrically connected to the hand mass and retested the kidney meridian point. (Due to its electromagnetic properties, the honeycomb acts like an antenna, transmitting the energetic signature of the remedy to the patient.) Dr. Voll could now determine if Solidago was the proper remedy to correct the imbalance. If the reading dropped toward 50, then Solidago was the appropriate one. Dr. Voll consistently found that when a remedy substantially improved a reading, it also improved the health of the affected organ when taken by the patient. Dr. Voll discovered that such testing could be done with any type of remedy—herbal, homeopathic, nutritional supplements, and pharmaceuticals.

What's more, Dr. Voll found this method of remedy testing could assist in diagnosing the cause of illness by discovering how the body reacted to ampules of pathogens, toxins, and allergens. For example, if Dr. Voll wished to test for the presence of hepatitis in the liver, he had the patient hold a glass vial of a homeopathic hepatitis remedy, called a hepatitis nosode, while he took another reading on the liver meridian point. A significant improvement in the reading closer to the balance value of 50 indicated the presence of hepatitis in the liver as well as the benefit of treating with that particular nosode remedy.

As surreal as Voll testing sounds, the science behind it is quite logical. The notion of utilizing an electronic biofeedback device to analyze some aspect of biological functioning is a well-established concept. Cardiologists routinely utilize an electrocardiograph (ECG) to measure heart rhythms, neurologists rely on the electroencephalograph (EEG), and psychologists use neurofeedback equipment. To the layperson, Voll testing is analogous to a mechanic using a computerized diagnostic tuning system on an automobile. He hooks up a probe through the ignition system to digitally analyze the health of various parameters of the engine or other systems in the automobile. Why then is an EAV device not found in every medical office?

The downside to EAV is that it is not a completely objective measuring system because it is operator-dependent. An EAV tester must develop a tactile sensitivity with the probe to accurately measure meridian points. This is an acquired skill with a steep learning curve, requiring dedication and practice before a practitioner is able to get consistently accurate and repeatable readings. It is akin to a dentist successfully learning how to manipulate a high-speed drill or a pianist achieving precise tactile mastery over the keyboard that allows him or her to express a specific musical effect. In addition, EAV references a type of cellular communication through forms of energy found in acupuncture and homeopathy that conventional medicine does not recognize, let alone understand. From the economic perspective of the practitioner, the length of time required to perform a basic EAV test is lengthy (up to 45 minutes), and it is not covered by insurance.

As a result, EAV has not caught on with mainstream practitioners despite its extraordinary potential. However, in the hands of the small number of skilled practitioners using this unique diagnostic

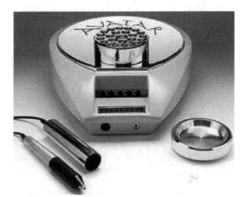

Figure 1-3. Avatar computerized EAV device.

method, an EAV device can produce consistent, reproducible results that stand up to scientific scrutiny when compared to standardized medical-testing procedures.

In recent years, EAV systems have been superseded by newer types of computerized information medical devices such as the Avatar Testing System by VeraDyne Corporation (see Figure 1-3). *The results with this equipment when compared to Voll's original device are medically akin to a brilliant violinist playing a Mozart concerto with a Stradivarius as opposed to a violin bought from a mass-market retailer.* Our hope is that this miraculous testing method will one day become standard medical procedure.

Shortly after receiving this diagnosis from Dr. Clark, I told my father about my possible diagnosis of mercury toxicity from mercury amalgam fillings as the core cause of my multiple medical conditions. He was highly dubious and suggested that I consult the head of nephrology whom he knew at Century City Hospital in Los Angeles. When I saw Dr. G, I told him about this mysterious computerized device called EAV and the chiropractor who had administered the test, although I did not mention his name. Needless to say, Dr. G had never heard of such a device and told me that I had been swindled and was gullible because I was desperate. He attempted to convince me that mercury toxicity from amalgam fillings could not be the cause of the constant pain in my kidney area.

"Mr. Freud, I am an expert on heavy metal toxicity, and I can assure you that the symptoms you describe could not possibly be from your fillings. But if you really need to have it proven to you, I will arrange to get a urine sample from you and have it sent to the lab at the hospital for testing. If you have mercury poisoning in your kidneys, it will show up in a urine test."

That certainly seemed like a plausible, rational explanation so I immediately agreed to it. He then said to me, "Who is this man who told you such rubbish and performed some voodoo test on you that I've never heard of? Why he's not even a medical doctor. He's only a chiropractor. To be honest, if he's filling your head with such tripe, he should have his medical license revoked. You'd probably be doing a whole lot of people a favor if you would just report him to the medical boards! Your father also tells me that you have been under a great deal of stress, and from what I can see he is right. It looks to me like you might be a hypochondriac. Have you thought about going to a psychiatrist?"

When the test results came back a few days later, they were negative. I spoke to Dr. G by telephone, and in a cocksure manner he said he was now convinced more than ever that I needed psychiatric help. Given all I had suffered, his condescending nature was painful to deal with. However, out of deference to my father, I did not respond. Still, in the back of my mind, I just knew that Dr. Clark had been correct in his diagnosis. But how to prove it?

Through another doctor, I was able to obtain a powerful oral chelator, a substance that can be either pharmaceutical or natural, that binds to heavy metals and other minerals as it pulls them out of tissues in the body and brain from which they are then excreted through the various processes of elimination. After ingesting it and waiting 45 minutes, I urinated into a specimen jar. I will never forget the horrific pain and discomfort I felt in my kidneys, but I toughed it out, determined to get to the bottom of my medical mystery. I sent the specimen jar to another laboratory and waited for the results. *When it came back, I was shocked. The lab results showed a 600 percent increase in the level of mercury in my urine over my previous test!* I went back to Dr. G and showed him the lab results. As his jaw dropped open from shock, he babbled something about how surprised he was. In a rare display of anger, I shouted at him, "Who is the charlatan now?" I stormed out of his office and never looked back. I had experienced a medical epiphany and witnessed a higher truth. I was now a wiser man. I had graduated.

This knowledge, however, came at a steep price. Although I had proved to Dr. G and my father that amalgam fillings were the only possible explanation for the extraordinarily high levels of mercury in my urine, I was to suffer from severe kidney disease due to my kidneys' inability to filter out this insidious poison. From this painful lesson, I learned never to begin chelation unless all mercury fillings have been removed and the kidneys are detoxed before dumping more poison into them.

I was now hooked on Voll diagnosis and treatment, so I began to research other alternative healing modalities, including herbal remedies and amino acid therapies. (See "Introduction to German Biological Medicine.") I was then introduced to another healer, whom I will call Dr. Edward Smith. A naturopath who worked with a similar EAV computerized system of diagnosis, Dr. Smith also incorporated several other types of supplements, including a broad range of orthomolecular nutrients and herbal remedies in addition to homeopathic remedies.

Introduction to German Biological Medicine

Although I was making progress with Dr. Smith, I had made little headway on my debilitating neurological problems. Emboldened by my recent successes with German Bio - logical Medicine, I eagerly read a wonderful publication called *Explore* magazine (www.explorepub.com) that contained articles translated from German describing the latest research findings in the field. In 1991 I decided to visit several doctors in Germany whose work was described in the magazine as they possessed more advanced diagnostic and treatment protocols than those available in America.

I saw Dr. Max Daunderer, M.D., in Munich (www.toxcenter.de), who was considered by many to be the foremost researcher on amalgam toxicity. A full-mouth panorex x-ray showed that on the upper-right side of my mouth where I had a root canal, the dentist had put a silver amalgam on the tip of the root instead of the usual gutta-percha. Dr. Daunderer said the mercury was leaching out of the root canal socket and going across the blood-brain barrier into many regions of my brain. My convulsions, tremors, fainting attacks, numbness, and depression were all directly traced to this! In addition, other amalgam fillings were releasing deadly mercury vapors, the core cause of my chronic fatigue syndrome, kidney disease, and tachycardia. Dr. Daunderer urged me upon my return to California to see a biological dentist as soon as possible and have the root canal entirely extracted and all amalgam fillings removed. He emphatically explained that only a biological dentist had the special training and protocols required to safely remove the fillings without spreading mercury vapors up my nose and into the brain or down my throat and into the body (see Chapter 12).

I then went to Baden-Baden to see Dr. Helmut Schimmel, M.D., inventor of the Vega test (www.vegatest.com), an offshoot of the Voll test. From him, I learned the relationship between genetically inherited miasms (energetic imbalances) and heavy metals (see Chapters 8–12). He agreed with Dr. Daunderer that I had to see a biological dentist trained in German Biological Medicine as soon as possible. He recommended Dr. Vaughn Harada, D.D.S., who practiced in Santa Monica, California. I gasped in amazement at the bizarre synchronicity of it all. I had come half way around the world only to learn that the dentist I needed to see worked only about a mile from where I lived!

I then traveled to the small town of Hohenlimburg to see Dr. Wilhelm Langreder, M.D., whose work I had read about in *Explore*. I intuitively felt that the methods of this brilliant German doctor might hold the key to my neurological issues. After studying with Dr. Voll, Dr. Langreder developed a form of medicine called Micro-Magnetic Medicine that used the Dermatron device in a unique way so that the patient did not take oral remedies. He used another German frequency device called the Mora to electronically imprint vibrational information of specific homeopathic remedies into small glass vials he called contactors that the patient simply held in his or her hand. Dr. Langreder used this form of electronic homeopathy to systematically move toxins out of cells and then out of the body in a totally brilliant and sequential manner. I am also convinced that Dr. Langreder had a more advanced understanding of the relationship between teeth and organs than any physician or dentist whom I am aware of.

He was a true genius, and I received more neurological relief from his therapies than from anyone else. I hope that someday practitioners will revive his work (www.m-m-m-online.de).

The first time I met Dr. Langreder, I was just recovering from one of my frequent fainting spells. Unfortunately, his command of English was minimal and his accent was thick. His instructions on how to use the contactors were convoluted, and I got flustered trying to follow them. He finally grew exasperated with our miscommunication and walked out of the room, exclaiming in broken English, "How can you not understand me! You are a relative of Sigmund Freud!"

Just then a tall, skinny man appeared out of nowhere to rescue me. Speaking in a soft, low voice in perfect English he said, "Don't worry. We in the office have a hard time understanding him too. I'll explain how it works over lunch." This man, whom I will call Dr. Hans Dorfmann, M.D., was a doctor in private practice from nearby Düsseldorf. However, he spent a lot of time studying with Dr. Langreder to learn his methods. He asked what was wrong, and I told him my tale of woe. He recommended the work of another brilliant doctor in Switzerland, Dr. Bruno Haefeli, N.D., who had developed proprietary blood staining techniques for analyzing fungi.[2,3] Dr. Dorfmann invited me to his office where he took a blood sample to send to Dr. Haefeli for analysis. When the results of the blood test came back, it confirmed Dr. Dorfmann's worst suspicions. I was absolutely loaded with various forms of fungi, which undoubtedly was a major component in my health condition. This was completely new to me, and after taking various homeopathic remedies for fungi that Dr. Haefeli himself made, I started to feel better.

Out of Dr. Dorfmann's initial act of unfettered kindness, we developed a strong bond of friendship. However, the most astonishing aspect of our relationship was the subsequent disclosure of a metaphysical past-life relationship he had with Sigmund Freud, who was to become Linda's principal spirit guide. The deeper nature of our relationship is explained in Chapter 14.

Upon my return from Germany, I went to see Dr. Vaughn Harada, the dentist who successfully removed the entire root canal as well as my amalgam fillings. This was a watershed event in my healing process. My real healing could not begin until this step was taken. But I was hardly finished with dentistry. Over the next decade I spent a veritable fortune on dental work as I continued to suffer from chronic dental infections. Many of my teeth were rotting out. Over time, I was to lose the entire upper-right side of my mouth through extractions and another root canal. In fact, with the exception of my front teeth, all of my remaining teeth were literally ground down to the nubs. Another unforeseen consequence of mercury poisoning.

Dr. Edward Smith turned out to be an important figure in Linda's and my life from a medical perspective as well as a personal perspective. Not only was he instrumental in improving my health, but he also became a close friend and confidant. In June 1992, after a tumultuous breakup with my girlfriend, he gave me the greatest gift of all. He introduced me to Linda, who was also his patient. Linda had been suffering for years with a complicated case of chronic fatigue syndrome and migraines. A few years earlier, she had gone to the Mayo Clinic for treatment of her migraines. Despite extensive treatment, the doctors were unable to help her. The chief neurologist told her that she belonged to that 10 percent category of migraine sufferers for whom they had no idea what causes the problem or how to treat it. Our early dates went like this: "How are you feeling?" "Not too good. How are you feeling?" "Not too good." "OK, let's stay in."

Within two months of meeting, we took a trip to Germany to continue the work I had started with most of the healers I had seen on my first trip. Dr. Schimmel found that Linda had a number of miasms through a blood test he performed. (The relationship between miasms and chronic degenerative diseases would later become an important aspect of her work.) Dr. Haefeli also analyzed her blood and found high levels of different forms of fungi. What we learned from Dr. Dorfmann and Dr. Haefeli was an incredible appreciation for the role that fungi play in so many forms of chronic degenerative disease. As a result Linda has made the removal of these fungi an integral part of her work.

As we became familiar with Dr. Smith's naturopathic approach to medicine, we were continually amazed at how he used his computerized Voll device to delve deeply into the complexities of our multiple health conditions. We cannot underestimate the impact this had on us. Although Voll testing is not of the spirit world, for us it was a bridge to that world. The understanding of subtle energy was a necessary prerequisite to Linda's gift being revealed. We appreciated that Dr. Smith gave us a blend of orthomolecular nutrients, herbs, and homeopathy in accordance with what energetically tested best for us. Most importantly, he shared his knowledge of EAV and the accompanying treatment protocols of German Biological Medicine. As her gift expanded, Linda integrated this knowledge into Metaphysical Systems Engineering.

When her gift burst through, there was mutual agreement between us that the time had come for Linda to take over our medical management from Dr. Smith. She was now traversing time-space dimensions and worlds to receive even greater, more detailed levels of medical, emotional, and spiritual information from the angelic realms. Linda had become the human embodiment of the EAV device and so much more! However, we will always remain grateful for all Dr. Smith did for us. What we learned from him about how to organize diagnostic processes in accordance with EAV principles proved indispensable.

THE ORIGINS OF LINDA'S GIFT

It all started innocently enough. In the summer of 1993, Linda and I went to an alternative health show in Pasadena, California. As we walked the aisles of exhibitors, we soaked in the array of natural remedies, crystals, organic foods, and the like. Ever on the lookout for remedies or other body/mind/spirit approaches to alleviate our still-serious health issues, we hoped against hope that we would discover some combination lock of supplements to end our constant suffering.

We stopped by a booth run by a kindly old German fräulein named Hanna Kroeger to see if any of her assorted herbal and homeopathic remedies might address our health issues. Suddenly, Linda spied a small silver pendulum on a narrow silver chain. She was fascinated by it and mentioned that pendulums had intrigued her for years. She had always wanted one, but for one reason or another had never gotten around to getting one. I immediately plunked down $18 to buy one for her. If this would bring her some happiness, no matter how crazy it might seem to me, why not do it? Isn't that what being in love is all about? Neither of us had any idea that this seemingly innocuous act would be the beginning of a journey that would revolutionize our very lives and provide unique levels of healing for so many people.

Over the next few weeks and months Linda picked up the pendulum and positioned it over various bottles of supplements that either she or I were taking. She would ask very straight-ahead questions such as "Is this remedy good for me or not?" and "If so, what is my proper daily dosage?" She did not wait long for a response. In answer to the first question, if the pendulum moved clockwise, that meant "yes." If it moved counterclockwise, it meant "no." If it moved straight back and forth, that meant either rephrase the question or that she was not asking the right question. If it moved in a small circle-eight configuration, that meant the question was not particularly relevant or, as the French say, *comme ci, comme ça.*

Linda eagerly demonstrated her latest discoveries to me. I indulged her because I was in love. Quite candidly, however, I was inwardly skeptical and gently admonished her not to take her newfound fascination with the pendulum too seriously. I attempted to reason with her that it was all right to regard dowsing with the pendulum as an armchair curiosity, but she should not take anything she got about diagnosis or supplementation too seriously because she did not have any credentials in the health care field. Still, thank God, her fascination with dowsing not only remained intact, it continued to grow exponentially as her proficiency with the pendulum grew.

Over the next couple of months, Linda periodically explained to me that she had developed her own "vocabulary" of responses that she could get from the pendulum. She said, "Such and such remedy is good for you, see?" I watched as the pendulum began to circle to the right. As she continued to practice her peculiar craft, her abilities grew. She held a bottle of supplements in her left hand with the pendulum suspended above it in her right hand and asked, "Is this remedy effective for you and is this remedy tolerated by you?" She explained that "guides" told her that a remedy could be effective but not tolerated, it could be tolerated but not effective, or it could not be effective or tolerated. All these outcomes were unacceptable. Any remedy must pass both tests. (See "A Major Influence on Linda.")

A Major Influence on Linda

Dr. Daniel S. Reeves, D.C., is another healer we saw in the early 1990s who was critical to our health. Both the man and his healing methods had an indelible impact on our lives (see Figure 1-4). Although trained as a chiropractor, he transcended that label; he was a true energy medicine healer. He utilized a purely energetic form of chiropractic technique called total body modification, or TBM (www.tbmseminars.com/ faq.asp). As of 2010, Dr. Reeves is 94 years old and still going strong, though he has retired from his healing practice.

Originally developed by Dr. Victor Frank, D.C., TBM is an advanced form of applied kinesiology, also called muscle testing, which is used for both diagnosis and treatment. Dr. Reeves characterizes it as tapping into the energy systems of various organs much the same way as one uses a computer. However, he took it a step further than other practitioners by combining it with a channeling process he had perfected that allowed him to get superior and extraordinary results. It is absolutely no exaggeration to say that he was routinely able to knock out bacterial and viral conditions and much more with his bare hands in one healing

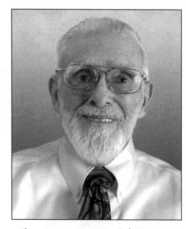

Figure 1-4. Dr. Daniel Reeves.

session! Through him we saw a level of healing that was possible if one could harness and cultivate one's spiritual energies. He was unquestionably the greatest muscle tester and mover of healing energy whom Linda and I have ever seen. The healing miracles we experienced and witnessed in those years are indelibly etched in our minds and will never be forgotten.

One of Dr. Reeves' great attributes was his ability to reduce his ego and become a pure vessel to receive "instructions" from the higher realms he was channeling. We attribute his unique ability to the fact that he is an incredibly old soul who has reincarnated many times as a physical and spiritual healer, along with having a pristine personal character in this lifetime. Never did we hear a disparaging word regarding other lesser healers. Although a most humble and gracious man, he was a giant among the healers who knew him and could accomplish feats of healing that, with the exception of what later happened with Linda, we had never seen before. His greatness stemmed from his humility, and he always gave credit to God and the spiritual world, maintaining that he was just the vessel through which the diagnostic information and healing energies flowed. He viewed his healing gift as the best way for him to serve God and do his work. He was to serve as a role model for Linda.

During this time, I pioneered a technique where Dr. Smith initially provided a Voll assessment of what was wrong with either Linda or me. We then handed Dr. Reeves this "laundry list" of information so he could then devote the entire hour to healing us with channeled TBM technology instead of first having to diagnose using applied kinesiology. After Linda's gift burst through, she took over this function and prepared an equivalent list from which Dr. Reeves worked. The astonishing thing is that Dr. Reeves and Linda were consistently in 99 percent psychic agreement about the diagnostic results that she got. It therefore came as no surprise when Linda channeled some time later that among the many past-life connections we had with Dr. Reeves, in one past life he had been her father. Our deep metaphysical connection through several lifetimes had continued.

Here is a dramatic example of Dr. Reeves' prodigious gift that had a profound impact on Linda and me. One day, as we were getting ready to see Dr. Reeves, Linda announced that she thought she might be pregnant. I asked her to confirm that with the pendulum. But the pendulum went back and forth in an unusual manner, indicating that we were either asking the wrong question or that the question needed to be rephrased. No matter how we asked the question, the response from the pendulum was the same. When we saw Dr. Reeves, Linda told him about what had happened. Dr. Reeves briefly went into trance, silently asking his spirit guides what the issue was. After a moment, he nodded his head as if he understood the problem and proceeded to do a complicated energetic TBM movement on Linda. When he muscle-tested her, he beamed a bright smile and said, "Now channel to see if you are pregnant." When she did, the pendulum swung wildly to the right. We both jumped up and down, tears of joy streaming down our faces. After trying to get pregnant for years with no success, suddenly at age 43, she was pregnant—and without fertility drugs! Our prayers had finally been answered.

After regaining our composure, we asked Dr. Reeves what he had done to change the reading. He said, " You were right to sense that you were technically pregnant. However, the reason that you had a cryptic response from the pendulum was that the fertilized egg was stuck in your left fallopian tube and had not moved down to the uterus. The energy work that I did caused the fertilized egg to move down on its own accord into your uterus." Still a bit shaken by the miracle we had witnessed, we stopped off at a local pharmacy to pick up a home pregnancy test. The results were positive! Nine months later, at age 44, Linda gave birth to our precious son Aryeh.

LINDA'S SHAKING: THE STARTLING CONFIRMATION OF HER ANGELIC CONNECTION

And then I saw it. One day in the spring of 1994 I was sitting with Linda while she used the pendulum to go over some remedies for my health based on the new database I was putting together. Suddenly, without warning, she started shaking violently in an involuntary manner from side to side. The shaking lasted only a few seconds, but it was profoundly noticeable before it subsided. My most immediate concern was that Linda had just experienced an epileptic attack. I asked her, rather frantically, if she was feeling all right. After she regained her composure, she told me that she was OK but that she had felt an electrical jolt of energy go through her central nervous system from her head down through her spinal cord. At this point, I asked her to check the Physical Databases to see if what she had experienced was an epileptic seizure. She reported that it was not. However, we were both a bit frightened. With all that she had going on with her health, this was the last thing she needed.

Since Linda seemed to have completely recovered from momentary but somewhat violent convulsions, we decided to see if it recurred before going to Dr. Smith, Dr. Reeves, or a neurologist to check it out. Over the following weeks she continued to periodically experience this violent aberration. Each episode lasted only a few seconds, although it was definitely perceptible to anyone present that something was certainly amiss. However, since she promptly made a complete recovery each time and there appeared not to be any lingering side effects, we decided not to consult a doctor.

One aspect of the shaking was most puzzling. *Linda only had these "attacks" when she was channeling with the pendulum in her hand.* My research revealed that epileptic seizures occur in a completely random manner, and doctors are still unclear as to what exactly triggers them. While it might have been logical to assume that stress or negative emotions could exacerbate such an attack, Linda assured me that simply was not so. What was unfathomable was how could holding a small pendulum in her hand trigger such reactions? We remained concerned but decided to take a wait-and-see attitude.

At about this time, we were already deeply absorbed in studying Kabbalah and were regularly attending Shabbat services at the Kabbalah Center in Los Angeles. The extent and complexity of our illnesses helped to galvanize our spiritual awareness as never before. Both of us are products of a more modern form of the Jewish faith called the conservative movement. For those who do not know, this form of Judaism is midway between the more secularized reform movement and the more observant traditional orthodox movement.

A startling episode of synchronicity occurred one day shortly after the seizures started that I will never forget. I was reading *Meditation and the Bible,* which was to finally provide the needed breakthrough that explained the bizarre nature of Linda's shaking. The book was written by Rabbi Aryeh Kaplan, a highly regarded contemporary rabbinic scholar and author of forty-seven books.

Among the many subjects covered in the book are not only the importance of meditation in the Jewish faith, but commentary on what the prophetic experience entailed for Hebrew prophets. Rabbi Kaplan utilized serious rabbinic commentary from such highly esteemed traditional sources as Rabbi Moses Maimonides (1137–1204) and Rabbi Chaim Luzzatto (1707–1746) in his analysis. This proved to be important because too often, as we repeatedly discovered, we had obtained information on various aspects of Kabbalah from new age sources that later proved to be erroneous or to contain half-truths. In our quest for higher spiritual truths of Kabbalah, it had become quite clear who the real authorities were and who, though well meaning, spread misinformation that seems to abound on the subject.

When I read the following excerpt from *Meditation and the Bible,* which quoted Rabbi Luzzatto, a great Italian rabbi and scholar of Kabbalah, I was stunned: "When God reveals Himself and bestows His influence, the prophet is greatly overwhelmed. His body and his limbs immediately begin to tremble, and he feels as though he is being turned inside out. This, however, is due to the nature of the physical. It [the body] cannot tolerate the revelations of the spiritual, and this is particularly true when it comes to the revelations of God's own Glory. The prophet's senses cease to operate, and his mental faculties can no longer function independently. They have all become dependent on God and the influx that is being bestowed."[4]

In the same chapter, Rabbi Maimonides repeated this claim in similar language: "Prophecy is also a very traumatic experience. The prophet's limbs tremble, his body becomes faint, and he loses control of his stream of consciousness. All that remains in his conscious mind is a clear understanding of what he is experiencing at the time."[5]

Without revealing what I had just read, I turned to Linda and asked her to describe what the shaking felt like. She thought about it for a few seconds and replied, "I feel like I am being turned inside out." When I pressed her, she said, "I temporarily lose total control over my body and am powerless to stop it." I then showed her the two quotes. Immediately after reading them, she started shaking uncontrollably, with an intensity that, up to now, I had not witnessed. We then knew, with absolute certainty, that this was angelic verification of what was really happening.

As we continued to read Rabbi Luzzatto's discourse, we came to understand more of what Linda was experiencing. Rabbi Luzzatto writes: "The prophetic experience must come about through intermediaries. A human being cannot directly attach himself to God's Glory, perceiving it as one sees a man standing in front of him. The perception of God involved in true prophecy must therefore come through God's servants, whose task it is to provide such a vision.

"These individuals then act as lenses through which the individual sees the Glory. What the prophet actually perceives, however, is the Glory itself, and not something else. The way one sees it, however, depends on the particular intermediary involved, just as what one would see through a lens would depend on the particular type of lens.

"There are therefore many degrees of perception, depending on the [spiritual] lens [*ispaklaria* in Hebrew] involved. It may cause the subject to appear far away or very close. There can furthermore be different degrees of transparency or opaqueness in the lens itself."[6]

Rabbi Maimonides also quoted two examples from scripture that he says are representative of the trembling phenomenon:

1. "[Abraham fell into a trance,] and a great dark dread fell upon him." (Genesis 15:12)

2. Daniel described his vision: "[I saw this great vision and I became powerless.] My appearance was destroyed, and my strength deserted me. [I heard the sound of His words, and I fell on the ground in a trance]." (Daniel 10:8)[7]

As best as we can determine, the words of Rabbis Maimonides and Luzzatto have never been challenged in the religious literature. One key aspect of the Hebrew prophets that delineates them from other types of individuals who channel the higher realms was the ability to tremble or shake at the time of receiving actual prophecy. We are not aware of any commentary, rabbinic or otherwise, that contradicts this assertion. In addition, several very well-respected rabbis from Israel and America who have seen Linda as clients and have witnessed the shaking are convinced that what was described in *Meditation and the Bible* is akin to what Linda is experiencing. They assert that the incredible accuracy of her medical information is proof that what she is doing is real.

THE MEANING OF LINDA'S GIFT

The next big scientific discovery isn't a new type of computer chip or even a new type of subatomic particle, but a new, profoundly deeper understanding of our very relationship with God. Today we live in a world dominated by scientific discovery and thought processes. Religion and even the very existence of God are now openly questioned in certain scientific circles. Science has been elevated to the status of God, instead of being viewed as a tool of God, created by God. This has caused a paradoxical conflict on two levels for humanity in this information age. Though science has brought enormous benefit to humanity in countless ways, man-made toxicity has also polluted our environment and poisoned our inner ecology. An additional and unintended emotional consequence of technology has occurred in the process. It has inflated our egos and fostered arrogance to the point where we have lost sight of our humanity and our God-given spiritual essence.

In such a hostile and skeptical world, any new form of prophecy that emerges today must be able to withstand scientific scrutiny and be verifiable in accordance with prevailing scientific norms before it is universally accepted. (See "The Capacity of the Soul to Perceive Higher Scientific Truths.") Our path of verification of Linda's gift stems from two perspectives: direct scientific evidence and confirmations from historical texts on the Hebrew prophets.

Our specific claim is that Linda's gift represents the first real connection in the modern age with a form of prophecy that existed thousands of years ago in Israel. The primary method by which she receives diagnostic and treatment information is through communication with angels and spirits. She is not channeling her "higher self" as new age mediums do. This is why we have devoted Chapters 19 and 20 to an understanding of angels within the Hebrew tradition.

It is not the purpose of this book is to claim that Linda Freud is a Hebrew prophet. Readers can draw their own conclusions for themselves. What can be said with conviction is that:

• Many people, ranging from prominent doctors to her clients from all walks of life, believe that Linda has a most prodigious gift of healing—a unique level of diagnostic accuracy combined with consistently superior healing results with the natural remedies available to her.

• She claims that the information is channeled from angels and spirits.

• She exhibits the specific characteristic of shaking during the most poignant moments of the channeling process. This is absolutely consistent with what has historically been written about the Hebrew prophets by the highest and most reliable religious sources of the Jewish faith.

Hers is a new type of prophecy for our era, intended for those who demand scientific exactitude. In this way Linda's work differs from the traditional approach of the Hebrew prophets who often relied on the language of allegory and metaphor. However, in the current scientific climate, language that is open to interpretation is not an option if one wishes to be taken seriously. It is important to remember that the very foundation of Christianity is based on Christians' interpretations of the Hebrew prophets.

The Capacity of the Soul to Perceive Higher Scientific Truths

A younger soul who has not reincarnated very often is more likely to connect with science from a limited Newtonian, materialistic perspective as opposed to an older soul who has a higher capacity to grasp the Einsteinian quantum view of reality. While a certain degree of skepticism is healthy, one who is excessively skeptical becomes cynical, causing a spiritual blockage in the soul that impairs the development of intuition necessary to align with higher spiritual realities. Unwilling to remove their blinders and break free of the shackles of the materialistic view of reality, atheists are conditioned to seek simplistic Newtonian answers by their stubborn insistence on "seeing is believing" instead of "believing is seeing."

For most people of faith, "believing" conditions the soul to a state where believing becomes the "seeing." This subtle process occurs in an incremental manner over time. It can be cultivated through a spiritual practice and purification of one's inner space through prayer, meditation, or a physical discipline such as yoga.

A nonbeliever fails to grasp the limitations of scientific methods such as a hypothetical experiment that relies only on the five senses. It amazes us that the spiritual implications of bellwether theories of quantum physics such as Werner Heisenberg's Uncertainty Principle are conveniently ignored: If a tree falls down in a forest and nobody hears it, does it make a noise? There must be an observer to hear it; otherwise nothing is heard. The very act of divine or human observation—or "consciousness"—affects that which one is observing.

Recent advances in quantum physics such as superstring theory present a dilemma for the scientist because they cannot be accessed or proven through a hypothetical experiment. Like our search for God, they exist outside the physical world of time and space. Both remain an abstraction because we cannot see, touch, smell, or otherwise physically interact with them. Yet, this is hardly a limitation of the spirit world or superstring theory. It is a limitation of our five senses, which cannot connect to either of them. Atheists ignore this inconvenient truth as they advocate the teaching of unprovable theories at leading universities while denying the existence of God. They criticize those who seek a divinely inspired moral order and seek to replace it with "deadness," a vacuum devoid of spiritual meaning, as the underlying logic for our ultimate origin and destiny.[8] There is no heaven, no hell, certainly no karmic retribution for bad behavior—just science.

Great scientific discoveries share a common thread. What start out as far-fetched notions eventually become the norm after a protracted scientific or religious struggle. Science has always thrived when researchers have been willing to explore far-fetched notions and integrate them as they become proven. As the testimonials in this book demonstrate, we are merely "early adopters" of a *spiritual technology based on ancient knowledge.* Linda has crossed the threshold into a higher consciousness that integrates meta + physics. The irony is that we are great believers in the scientific method and support the teaching of superstring theory because we recognize this theory lends great credence to the existence of God. As quantum physicists knock on heaven's door, their scientific discoveries raise new questions that demand spiritual answers! Based on our work on biological systems, we are prepared to show skeptics of any persuasion what we have found.

The testimonials in this book attest to Linda's unique diagnostic gifts. They are medically or anecdotally verifiable, making them impossible to deny.

The vast majority of people who adhere to the often-rigorous healing protocols channeled by Linda experience a significant improvement in their health. A considerable number are healed. When there is full compliance, I do not know of any doctor or healer who has a higher percentage track record of success than Linda.

The central idea the reader should come away with is that it is not Linda's unique gift of accurate medical diagnosis that is most important. What is of far greater significance are the reasons why she is able to do what she does. Linda's claim, which is the central thesis of this book, is that all of this uniquely accurate information is channeled directly from her angelic and spirit guides. That is why many people now believe that her gift represents a unique opportunity for humanity to peer beyond the veil of hidden knowledge to grasp how angels function in our world.

As her gift becomes properly understood and verified by the medical community, people of all faiths will have the ability to challenge nonbelievers with conviction. We will confront an increasingly atheistic society *with science.* We have thrown down the gauntlet. This is our steadfast position.

God's angels are extending an olive branch of hope to skeptical, embittered, downtrodden, very sick people too cynical or tired to believe in God and his healing miracles. By using Linda as the vessel for receiving information leading to miraculous healings that are both scientifically and/or anecdotally verifiable, God has truly given us a gift and reason to hope. All this at a time when our entire planet has been plunged into a crisis of confidence on every level—moral, spiritual, economic, military, political, medical, and environmental. For He has apparently determined that for humans consumed by the incredible looming darkness of world events, it is now time for the angels to make their presence known to people who live their lives with spiritual conviction as well as to the skeptical masses who are clueless regarding the presence of God. It is truly a time for people of faith to refute an increasingly atheistic society that worships at the alter of science. The significance of Linda's gift of accessing a unique and higher level of medical truth is that it proves that God is the driving force behind science. His angelic messengers seek to share this aspect of His divinity with us.

CHAPTER 2

Our Healing Philosophy

Sickness is the vengeance of nature for the violation of her laws.
—CHARLES SIMMONS

LOOKING BACK ON OUR LIVES, it now seems obvious that our outlook on health and healing has been heavily influenced by both the initial failures and ultimate successes we experienced in overcoming our own severe health problems. When Linda and I first met, the last thing on our minds was that she would establish a career as a healer while I would become a medical researcher. Our decision to become proactively involved in researching our own health conditions resulted from the utter failure of the pharmaceutical approach to improve our health. Urgent necessity became the mother of invention as our deteriorating health conditions forced us to look outside mainstream medicine. However, this journey to alternative medicine began with great reluctance, as it was utterly foreign and uncharted territory. For me, in particular, this was challenging and difficult because I had been raised in the world of mainstream medicine.

As the son of an internal medicine doctor, there were always pharmaceutical drugs around the house. I grew up thinking that the way to achieve optimal health was to take more pharmaceuticals. I have a memory as a boy of going to my father's office and watching the drug company account executive extol the virtues of the latest and greatest pharmaceutical drugs as he dumped a pile of samples on Dad's desk. My father generally accepted his explanation as gospel and waxed rhapsodically about the latest advances in drug therapy and high-tech surgical wizardry with wonder in his eyes. I listened and believed. When I got very ill in 1990, my father recommended that I see certain high-priced doctors in Los Angeles. I assumed he knew. Why wouldn't I? I adored and trusted him. It wasn't until I got deathly ill that I realized that the drugs prescribed for me were contributing to my rapid decline. Quite by accident I stumbled into the world of natural healing supplements. I immediately felt their power and never looked back.

In the ensuing years, Linda and I became voracious researchers of new supplements and alternative healing methods. While Linda's diagnostic gift is probably unique in the world, it is actually only half of the healing equation. The other half of the equation for any healer, regardless of diagnostic approach, is this: What do you actually do for the patient? *How do you treat?*

EXPOSING THE LIMITATIONS OF CONVENTIONAL MEDICINE

The most basic tenet of medical management was espoused thousand of years ago by the Greek healer Hippocrates: "Above all else, do no harm." Although it sounds old-fashioned and out of step with the times, it is still the gold standard of medical advice. We paid a price for this medical epiphany with our own health, having driven down several blind alleys, passively witnessing our doctors make mistake after mistake. Only then did we realize just how much of what passes for real healing is more like the emperor's new clothes.

Far too many consumers become confused and disappointed by their doctors' lack of success in treating chronic degenerative diseases. (This excludes the miracles of emergency room medicine and other critical care situations where surgery is the only answer.) After all, doctors are bright, well-meaning people. Anyone who endured the rigors of medical school and passed a state medical license must have amassed an impressive body of knowledge. Why then does a doctor not have the same stellar track record as, say, the muffler repair man? The reason the muffler repair shop can give you a lifetime warranty is because the automobile is a Newtonian device, made up of easily diagnosed, interconnected parts. Obviously, the body is radically different than an automobile. Yet the prevalent belief in allopathic medicine is that the body conforms to the Newtonian model so that it can be broken down into isolated subspecialties. Such thinking, however, can be short-sided and naive. For example, while a heart condition may be due to a breakdown of heart physiology, it may also be exacerbated by difficult-to-diagnose heavy metal toxicity causing infection, an endocrine imbalance such as low testosterone, or a hypothyroid condition. A specialist, depending on his or her training/ bias, may not even know to look for these possibilities. The body as a whole interconnected system is not being fully examined. This is just one of several reasons why he or she can offer very few guarantees on anything.

Economic and political considerations also determine a doctor's scientific outlook. For example, the official position of the American Dental Association as of 2010 is that mercury from dental amalgam generally poses no health danger. Therefore, a doctor or dentist who buys into that party line would scoff at a patient's concerns about removing amalgam fillings. Consumer awareness of that type of bias has led to a growing disillusion with conventional medicine, causing many people to look to alternative medicine for answers.

Reliance on One-Dimensional Lab Tests

Obviously, the more information available, the better the likelihood of a meaningful diagnosis. Conventional laboratory tests are essential in establishing the patient's health profile. However, while they often provide valuable information showing the effects of a cause, they do not necessarily reveal the actual cause. In far too many cases these tests provide only partial information that does not sufficiently connect the dots to reveal the true origin of the patient's illness. The reason is that certain traditional tests are only one-dimensional in nature, meaning information derived from them is not enough to determine *why a person has a condition—just that the person has a condition.* Failure to get to why a person has a condition results in a lack of critical knowledge that prevents the doctor from addressing the problem from a holistic perspective. This partial knowledge often relegates doctors to only being able to mask or treat symptoms.

An example of an incomplete diagnosis is a patient treated for a reoccurring infection with antibiotics. A simple lab test shows the presence of a reoccurring infectious bacterium but does not reveal the cofactors that indicate why the infection has reoccurred, after it was treated with antibiotics, just that it has reoccurred. From our perspective, doctors who rely solely on conventional diagnostic tests to formulate treatment protocols are at a distinct disadvantage compared to those who integrate them with energetic testing protocols such as EAV. Doctors who combine allopathic and energetic testing methods are able to develop a more comprehensive healing game plan for curing their patients.

When new clients come to Linda with a battery of tests from their previous healer, they are often amazed when an undiagnosed environmental toxin is revealed as the origin of the condition. Despite all the tests, the doctor still did not find the core issue. Current lab testing techniques have shortcomings in identifying certain types of environmental toxicity in body and brain tissues, which is often the core causal factor behind much chronic degenerative disease that commonly goes undetected. A consequence of this missing data is that many doctors are not necessarily able to discover the underlying origin behind an illness and are not aware of the detoxification protocols needed to treat it.

Another key differentiation in testing between the allopathic and holistic medical models is the lack of agreement on the definition of a toxin or pathogen. For example, in the allopathic model, a toxin or a pathogen must be physical and identifiable through traditional lab tests. In homeopathy, a toxin or a pathogen can be either physical or energetic. Treatment protocols can be deduced by consulting the *Materia Medica*, a lexicon of homeopathic remedies, or using such energetic testing techniques as Voll, Vega, pendulum, muscle testing or, in certain cases such as miasms, a blood test (see Chapter 8). Since the pharmaceutical model does not acknowledge the possibility of an energetic toxin or pathogen, traditional doctors can't go there. If doctors were only aware of diagnostic alternatives that complement conventional laboratory testing methods, they could develop a more comprehensive game plan for curing their patients.

Reliance on Pharmaceutical Drugs

Although the typical doctor may perform the latest high-tech diagnostic tests, the primary treatment modality in his or her healing repertoire is pharmaceutical drugs. At the end of the day, no matter what else doctors might know or how well-intentioned they may be, they are still primarily in the business of treating or masking the patient's symptoms. As a consequence, a real disconnect exists between the results achieved by a diagnostic test and the modality ultimately used to treat problems revealed by the test. The reason is that doctors are often unaware that other nontoxic, natural approaches exist to treat the same condition. Their medical, and far too often economic, allegiances are to what they learned in medical school—pharmaceutical drugs and surgery. However, if one becomes a real student of natural healing, it is possible to eliminate the need for pharmaceuticals a majority of the time.

Let us be clear: We do not preach that there is not a time and a place for pharmaceuticals. Only a fool would say otherwise. Far be it for us to throw the baby out with the bath water! Although cardiologist Dr. Stephen Sinatra, author of *The Sinatra Solution* and other books, is a staunch advocate of supplementation, he is the first to acknowledge that there are certain pharmaceuticals that cannot be replaced by natural products. When such a situation arises, Linda refers her client to a medical doctor.

Doctors who only treat with pharmaceutical drugs have voluntarily painted themselves into a corner in terms of the results they can only occasionally hope to achieve. Linda hears the same theme and variations of the following scenarios over and over again from new clients:

Scenario 1: With a wing and a prayer, the doctor hoped masking the symptoms with drugs over a long enough period of time would tide the patient over until the problem magically cleared up on its own. When this did not happen, the doctor simply ran out of options.

Scenario 2: The doctor told the patient that pharmaceutical drugs were the only hope for recovery and he or she had to stay on the meds forever. The doctor actually believed that the patient had been successfully treated by keeping him or her on a medication for years that merely masked symptoms. However, when the side effects from the drug become worse than the problem it was supposed to treat, the doctor could alter the dosage slightly but other than that was basically out of options. Soon the doctor referred the patient to specialists who gave him or her other drugs to control the problems created by the first drug. In fact, it is common for drug companies to come up with a new drug therapy to treat the side effects of an old drug. And the beat (and the dollars) goes on.

It never ceases to amaze us when we hear clients say that their doctors told them that undesirable side effects of a medication are just the price one has to pay for treating a condition. They should just grin and bear it. They are further conditioned by slick television advertising that promises to quickly treat osteoporosis, impotency, insomnia, or other common ailments with their little pill while also proclaiming the inevitability of side effects. The ads issue warnings so horrible, one wonders why anyone would take such products—*unless they were unaware of safer options.* In our world, side effects, with the exception of the forewarned heavy metal detox, are neither inevitable nor acceptable.

What complicates this scenario is that before the side effects of the drug became unbearable, the patient had a false sense of security that he or she was making real progress when in fact that was not so. Linda points out to clients that a medical slight-of-hand trick is not the same as real healing. Merely buying time and delaying the inevitable consequence of not addressing the origin of the cause does not, in our opinion, constitute healing.

We are not saying that masking symptoms does not have its place. Clearly, there are times where a patient needs to be taken out of pain and suffering. However, both doctor and patient too often think that the temporary relief achieved by taking steroids to calm down inflammatory pain, for example, constitutes real healing. In fact, all that is occurring is that the steroid is chemically deadening the nerves in the inflamed area.

Here are just some of the important causal cofactors of chronic degenerative diseases that Linda consistently finds are generally either ignored by typical lab tests or *not given sufficient weight or credence in assessing the real medical condition. It seems curious to us that these are the same problematic areas where drug therapy is ineffective, nonexistent, or potentially toxic.*

- Fungi

- Parasites

- Genetically inherited miasms

- Improper diet

- Acid-alkaline balance

- Radiation

- Toxicity from heavy metals, inorganic chemicals, drugs, vaccinations, pesticides, electronics, agriculture, food ingredients

- Electromagnetic pollution from cell phones, microwave towers and ovens, power lines, and other sources

The central problem with drugs is that they are generally not designed to detoxify environmental toxins (with the exception of a few rather harsh pharmaceutical chelating agents). Nor do they correct nutritional imbalances, eliminate viruses, and drain toxins out of the brain, the organs, and the lymphatic and endocrine systems. And they are certainly not able to eliminate energetic imbalances or miasms, a concept not even acknowledged in allopathic medicine (see Chapter 8). Drugs do not address energetic imbalances that can only be treated from the perspective of homeopathy, Traditional Chinese Medicine, and Ayurvedic medicine, which are key healing modalities in Linda's medical arsenal.

THE NATURE OF CONTEMPORARY ILLNESS

Perhaps the greatest medical accomplishments of the 20th century were the near eradication of such infectious diseases as tuberculosis, influenza, and pneumonia, which collectively represented the greatest cause of death. When doctors today claim that "miracle drugs" are the main reason that life expectancy is longer, that's both overly simplistic and only partially correct. In the early part of the 20th century, people tended to die at a younger age from these conditions, which were often caused or exacerbated by a lack of sanitation that is of less concern today except in third-world countries. The advent of World War II, coupled with the meteoric rise of the pharmaceutical industry, demanded a public health policy that required quick and easy antibiotic treatment to address the scourge of infectious disease. However, if the ongoing pharmaceutical revolution in healthcare is so wonderful, and is the main reason we are all living longer, why are chronic degenerate diseases like cancer so prevalent today as never before?

At the turn of the 20th century, cancer was relatively rare. Today, it is rampant due to environmental toxins in our air, water, soil, food, workplace, and drugs. In his book *The Alternative Medicine Definitive Guide to Cancer*, researcher Burton Goldberg states: "No other health topic today has the urgency of cancer because no other health condition is escalating as fast. A century ago, 1 in 33 people had cancer; today it is more than 1 in 3 and growing."[1]

Why is there so much cancer today? Our bodies are under a toxic assault as never before in history. This is why Linda has channeled that *the fundamental nature of disease itself has changed*. Diseases stemming from many sources of environmental toxicity have superseded diseases resulting from a lack of sanitation as the leading cause of death. Writing in the same book, Goldberg provides a sobering assessment of the direct or indirect reasons: "In simple fact, we are being slowly poisoned to death. The list of poisons includes pollution, pesticides, carcinogens in our food, air, and water, electromagnetic pollution, tobacco smoke, antibiotics, conventional drugs, hormone therapies, irradiated foods, nuclear radiation, mercury toxicity from dental fillings, diet and nutritional deficiencies, parasites, toxic emotions, x-rays, and more." These poisons are the core reasons behind such emerging diseases as chronic fatigue syndrome, fibromyalgia, endocrinological issues, neurological conditions such as autism, Alzheimer's, and Parkinson's, much cardiovascular disease, and the diabetes and obesity epidemics.

LINDA'S TREATMENT PROTOCOLS: THE INTEGRATION OF MULTIPLE HEALING MODALITIES

Because so much disease today results from man-made environmental toxicity, it is more treacherous and complex to diagnose and treat than at any time in history. So complicated are these issues today that a healer needs all the weapons in the medical arsenal. As a consequence, Linda's approach to treatment with supplements is on the cutting edge of where the field is going. One of the secrets of her success is how she integrates multiple natural healing modalities. Her angelic guides have shaped her appreciation of the strengths and weaknesses of each one. No matter what any healer may say to the contrary, there is one irrefutable fact: *No one healing modality can cure all or even most conditions.*

While different natural healing modalities all have their own distinctive strengths and weaknesses, they can all be integrated into an efficacious whole. Since no two people's biochemistry is exactly the same, it is impossible to generalize and say that every person will respond exactly the same way with any particular remedy. This is a key thesis of ours, and it is certainly one of the reasons for Linda's extraordinary success.

For example, there are certain aspects of healing that homeopathy does better than any other modality in the world. When it comes to clearing out genetically inherited vibrational resonances called miasms, there is simply no equivalent in any other modality. (Miasms are hidden and inherited cofactors in a medical condition that bind in toxins.) Homeopathy is also the only way to clear out a toxin or pathogen that is resonating on an energetic level as opposed to a physical level. Conversely, there are other areas of healing where homeopathy is either useless or of limited value. In certain other cases, it may function alongside herbal or orthomolecular remedies as an adjunct of a larger treatment protocol.

Experience has taught Linda that very few remedies fall under a one-size-fits-all category. There are specific ailments where homeopathy may be an effective treatment option for one person but be ineffective for another. Certain individuals just resonate better with certain types of remedies. When Linda constructs a detoxification program for the liver, for example, she has found that some people do better with an herbal-based program, other people do better with a homeopathic-based protocol, and still others do better with an amino acid like methionine.

Experience has also taught Linda that a beneficial symbiotic relationship can exist between a supplement and a pharmaceutical drug. For example, if a cardiologist proscribes a statin drug, Linda consistently channels that it is beneficial to also take coenzyme Q_{10}, (CoQ_{10}) as it is known in the medical literature that statin drugs often deplete the body of this important nutrient. Likewise, when a doctor prescribes a broad-spectrum antibiotic to kill a bacterial infection, Linda consistently channels that a probiotic should also be taken as a reflex to repopulate beneficial flora in the gut, intestines, and colon that are often destroyed by a proliferation of antibiotics.

Weapons in the Healing Arsenal

The principal natural remedy modalities available to an integrative physician, naturopath, chiropractor, homeopath, acupuncturist, nutritionist, or medical intuitive include:

• Orthomolecular nutrients (vitamins, minerals, trace minerals, amino acids, essential fatty acids, probiotics, enzymes)

• Herbology (Chinese, Ayurveda, European, Amazonian, Native American)

• Homeopathy

• Diet (Anti-Candida Diet, Metabolic Typing, Glycemic Index; see Chapter 12)

• Aromatherapy and essential oils

When addressing a client's issues, Linda constructs a healing game plan that potentially and synergistically utilizes some or all of these natural healing weapons in accordance with their inherent strengths and weaknesses. Although there may be some overlap of function, in general, each of these modalities is designed to accomplish different aspects of the healing process. Any one of these types of natural remedies can accomplish one of three actions:

1. It can cure the condition.

2. It is useless.

3. It is an adjunct or a part of a larger treatment protocol that may include multiple remedies and treatment modalities. This action is the most common.

However, in the real world a significant number of integrative medical doctors or holistic practitioners dispense only a few categories of remedies, each of which have their own inherent strengths and limitations. Here are examples of the strengths and weaknesses of two of the many modalities that Linda works with and how the angels guide her in crafting a treatment program that optimizes a synergy between the various approaches.

Chinese Herbology

A TCM (Traditional Chinese Medicine) practitioner is an acupuncturist who also dispenses Chinese herbs. These healers view health through the lens of meridian and five-element theory. For the last 3,000 years, they have brilliantly cured conditions whose origin is contained within the context of these theories. Unfortunately, we do not find TCM to be particularly effective at detoxifying man-made toxins that are behind so much contemporary illness. Toxicity, as we experience it today, did not exist to nearly the same degree in ancient times. For example, these remedies do not address such looming consequences of toxicity as free-radical proliferation (see Chapter 10).

However, TCM's herbal formulas are brilliant in the supportive role of energetically strengthening, tonifying, calming, or cooling an organ system that is affected by man-made toxicity, which manifests as a syndrome/imbalance from a Chinese perspective. Examples of this include what is called "stagnant liver Qi" or "yin kidney deficiency." The bottom line is that TCM often provides meaningful relief for the patient.

Homeopathy

A classical homeopath utilizes a guidebook called the *Materia Medica* to ask clients a series of probing questions on the overall state of their health. From this, homeopaths are able to deduce the likelihood of finding what is called a constitutional remedy, which can be quite effective and extremely safe. Homeopathy can also eliminate genetically inherited miasms that can be at the root of certain chronic degenerative diseases in a way that no other modality can do. This is a cornerstone of Linda's work and is discussed in detail in Chapter 8.

However, in the real world there are also problems with homeopathy:

• It takes a while for the remedies to work.

• Unless a practitioner does a form of energetic testing (EAV, kinesiology, pendulum), there is still the potential for guesswork in picking the right remedy and potency.

• It may not work as well for detoxification in certain individuals as herbs or orthomolecular nutrients.

• Homeopathy is not taught to any great extent in America so practitioners are few and far between even in major urban areas.

A practitioner does a disservice to the consumer if he or she claims that only one modality is successful in "curing" a wide range of ailments, when in fact the patient's condition may be outside the realm of the core competency of that particular modality. While that practitioner may be able to provide some relief, that is a far cry from real healing.

If one has a serious infection, for example, herbs or homeopathy are simply inadequate. It is time to call out the heavy antibiotic artillery to fend off a marauding infection. Conversely, if an infection can be caught in its early stage, then it is quite possible to get rid of it with herbal, enzymatic, or homeopathic remedies. It is strictly a question of the severity or degree of infection. The advantage to a natural approach, of course, is that a proliferation of antibiotics can lead to fungal disease and other health problems. In addition certain virulent microbial forms or superbugs have mutated into forms that are utterly resistant to antibiotics and have rendered them useless.

The Benefits of Draining the Swamp

Another philosophical difference between pharmaceutical medicine and natural healing methods can be summed up in the following analogy. Suppose you have a swarm of mosquitoes in a swamp. What is the safest way to get rid of them? One approach is to dive-bomb them from the air with a pesticide such as malathion. Sure, you will quickly kill them, but in the process you will also kill everything else that lives in the swamp. The other approach is to drain the swamp. Although this method is slower, over time the mosquitoes will find this an inhospitable place to live and breed and will either die or move elsewhere. In a nutshell, this is why Linda is a confirmed swamp drainer.

The medical analogy to divebombing the swamp with malathion is a doctor who insists on treating minor infections with antibiotics. While an antibiotic will kill a bacterial infection, overprescription of antibiotics can lead to severe fungal disease such as candidiasis. As described in Chapter 5, this may result in various forms of what is referred to as "iatrogenic" or doctor-induced disease that can seriously disrupt the normal functioning of different organ systems. The decision to prescribe antibiotics should be governed by the severity of the infection.

The medical analogy of swamp draining is Linda's detoxification protocols, which beneficially alter the underlying internal ecology of the person suffering from chronic degenerative disease, thereby creating a healthier environment needed for real healing. (This toxic inner ecology is known scientifically as *acidic biological terrain* or *milieu;* the importance of this concept is covered in detail in Chapters 5–7.) Think of your blood as soil. In the same way that amending the soil determines whether it grows beautiful flowers or weeds, the way you amend the "soil" of the blood determines what sort of microbes grow there. Toxicity causes an acidic environment that breeds fungi, parasites, and a host of other undesirable pathogens. Linda's protocols achieve a healing pH balance through dietary modification and the elimination of toxins through various natural detoxification methods and supplements discussed in later chapters. This amending-the-soil concept also enhances immune system function so that future infections may be less severe.

ENERGY MEDICINE: DESIGNED FOR THE 21ST CENTURY

As physicist Werner Heisenberg prophetically stated, the most fruitful developments in human history have come when two (or more) different lines of thought have met.[2] Energy medicine, the newest frontier in the healing arts, often involves the marriage of ancient and more recent healing philosophies and systems. In the case of EAV, this involved advances in electrical engineering and quantum physics integrated with TCM from the East and homeopathy from the West. The common theme of these disparate parts is that, when correctly diagnosed and stimulated, the body has the ability to overcome disease and heal itself.

Although we still believe that EAV is an amazing technology, the need to utilize such equipment became irrelevant with the advent of Linda's channeling gift coupled with Metaphysical Systems Engineering, described in Chapter 3. What makes Linda's diagnostic gift unique is that besides working within the realm of cellular biology and anatomy, she also works in the realm of subtle energies and auric fields outside the allopathic model. While the full extent of her channeling gift defies left-brain categorization, it would be fair to say that part of Metaphysical Systems Engineering is derived from EAV, a diagnostic centerpiece of energy medicine.

In truth, the complexity of medicine in the 21st century requires the integration of diagnostic and treatment protocols from conventional allopathic medicine and energy medicine. The former is akin to the mechanistic approach of Newtonian physics, where the body is viewed as intricate anatomical and biological machinery, analogous to a mechanized clockwork universe. Under this model, a surgeon, like the auto mechanic, can isolate, repair, or replace a defective component so the system will once again function properly. The latter involves a new way of thinking about healing based on the understanding of disease as an expression of information and energy. Related to the Einsteinian perspective of quantum physics, which views human beings as complex networks of energy fields that interface with physical/cellular systems, energy medicine involves the manipulation of subtle forms of energy to positively affect those systems that may be out of balance due to disease states. Rebalancing energy fields may help to regulate cellular physiology.

At the Beneveda Medical Group in Beverly Hills, California, Linda works under the license of Dr. Thom E. Lobe, M.D., who uses cutting-edge energy medicine technologies, ranging from scalar wave technology to advanced Kirlian photography, to help optimize health. (For background on Dr. Lobe and Beneveda Medical Group, see the Preface, www.thehealinggift.com, and www.beneveda.com.) Treatment also involves a wide range of natural supplements that correct imbalances and optimize functioning on a physical/biochemical level. Energy medicine, such as homeopathy, is a carrier of information that corrects and rebalances discordant information. This may be the physics behind the biochemical realities of cellular physiology.

The goal of energy medicine is to heal the whole person. This involves healing the body, the mind, and the spirit. The initial epiphany that Linda and I had in the early years was that this lofty goal was best accomplished through an integration of physical, emotional, and metaphysical information. As Dr. Richard Gerber, M.D., states in his book *Vibrational Medicine*, "The unseen connection between the physical body and the subtle forces of spirit holds the key to understanding the inner relationship between matter and energy . . . and between humanity and God."[3] *Linda's real contribution to the medical arts is the blend of Newtonian physicality and Einsteinian energetics combined with the ancient/new metaphysical frontier of medicine that she accesses through angels and spirits. Linda has gone full circle, traveling back to the future to retrieve a higher source of medical knowledge.*

CHAPTER 3

An Introduction to Metaphysical Systems Engineering^{SM}

The intuitive mind is a sacred gift and the rational mind
is a faithful servant. We have created a society that
honors the servant and has forgotten the gift.
—ALBERT EINSTEIN

TO DESCRIBE THE WIDTH, BREATH, AND DEPTH of what Linda is capable of doing, it is necessary to explain the remarkable blend of scientific, emotional, and metaphysical discoveries that are interconnected in Linda's unique diagnostic and treatment process. She draws from each of these individual components to create an unparalleled level of detail in her diagnosis and treatment. Our angelic guides tell us that Linda must fully explore the totality of the body/ mind/spirit connection in her communication with them to get to the real origin or origins of a physical, emotional, or spiritual issue. That's why we have created three sets of databases pertaining to disease etiology that make up our trademarked diagnostic system called Metaphysical Systems Engineering^{SM}. This consists of three well-organized, very precise databases—a physical database, an emotional database, and a metaphysical database—which allow Linda to receive the maximum amount of detailed information in the shortest amount of time.

The databases, which are our pride and joy, have been constantly expanded and refined since we initially created them in 1994. Their open-ended architecture allows any new medical, emotional, or metaphysical discovery to be added in the future. Our drive to continually expand the databases is a labor of love, borne of the conviction that the databases must include the totality of categories the angels may choose to guide Linda in her work.

If, for example, a specific entry such as a disease etiology, organ structure or function, toxin, remedy, or other pertinent information is not contained in the databases, it is possible that Linda could miss information that is vital to reaching the most complete diagnosis. If the proper entry is in the databases, the chances are extremely high that the angels will lead her to it. That is the primary reason why we continually update the databases and why they can never be too big! The incredibly complicated interweaving of variables behind contemporary illness requires an ongoing commitment to explore, categorize, and integrate the cutting edge of medical, emotional, and spiritual possibilities.

The overall goal of Metaphysical Systems Engineering is to facilitate real and lasting healing for a variety of illnesses, but especially chronic degenerative conditions, instead of superficial treatments that merely mask symptoms or only provide partial or temporary relief. The following steps are needed for Linda to accomplish that:

• Identifying the underlying origin(s) of complaint through a process that is described in Chapter 4, The Physical Databases. This can include critical toxins, pathogens, and imbalances. This may also involve delving into the Emotional and Metaphysical Databases to ascertain emotions and past-life issues that may play a role (Chapters 15 and 18).

• Identifying each of the constituent cofactors in layers and then systematically ranking them in order of priority for either detoxification or correcting an imbalance. Although it is possible that the origin of complaint can be reduced to just one particular toxin or imbalance, it has generally been Linda's experience that most chronic degenerative conditions occur in layers. The idea of establishing a precise priority and sequence of healing is very important because the body can only tolerate clearing a certain number of toxins or imbalances at one time. A detoxification process that goes too rapidly can have unpleasant consequences.

• Identifying the proper types of remedies for detoxification or elimination of an imbalance and establishing a treatment protocol.

LINDA'S UNIQUE DIAGNOSTIC GIFT

Perhaps the most astonishing aspect of Linda's gift, which admittedly is hard for some people to fathom, is that she receives incredibly precise, detailed medical information by hanging her pendulum over words on a printed page.

She channels as she scans with the index finger of her left hand down printed pages of database entries in a specific category while she dangles the pendulum with her right hand. That allows the angels to spin the pendulum to the right in the clockwise direction, indicating a "yes" response, or to the left in the counterclockwise direction, indicating a "no" response. The angels also have a variety of special ways to move the pendulum to communicate responses that are other than yes or no. These signals include such gentle admonitions as "wrong question" or "do not ask that question" or such clarifying comments as "rephrase the question" and *"comme ci, comme ça."*

There is something viscerally astonishing about watching Linda hold the spinning pendulum and shake before your eyes when she receives an important communication from the angelic realms. Even atheists have told me they were awed that something far beyond what they were capable of understanding was happening. *In all the years that I have been blessed to watch Linda do this work, not one person has ever accused her of being a fake or of having received fraudulent information. Something is stirred from deep within people's souls that tells them they are witnessing an authentic miracle.*

Safety Issues

In accordance with the premium we place on the Hippocratic oath, Linda believes that any remedy must pass two pendulum tests with her angelic guides before she can recommend it to her clients.

1. It must be effective.   2. It must be tolerated.

If a remedy is effective but not tolerated, it is unacceptable. Conversely, if a remedy is tolerated but not effective, that is useless. It must simply pass both tests to be considered part of a treatment protocol. Linda's approach constitutes nothing less than an early warning system against the possibility of an allergic reaction or a negative interaction between two or more drugs and/or natural remedies. Her ability to take the guesswork out of potential allergic reactions or drug/supplement interactions dwarfs the capacity of conventional physicians. I imagine that any doctor would love to have a device that could do this.

Scanning the Databases: Linda's "Metaphysical MRI"

I liken what Linda does to being a "metaphysical MRI" for the body, mind, and spirit. A MRI is a device that uses a large magnet, radio waves, and computer to take a clear picture of the inside of the body for the purpose of identifying and precisely locating an abnormality, such as arthritis in the spinal cord. This is really valuable as it answers several important questions:

1. Does arthritis exist in the spinal cord?

2. What is the precise location of arthritis in the spinal cord?

3. What is the degree of severity of joint damage due to the arthritic condition?

An MRI is of no use for the all-important fourth and fifth questions:

4. Why does the person have arthritis?

5. What is the best approach to eliminate arthritis?

Unlike a conventional MRI, *Linda's angelically derived metaphysical MRI relies on information gleaned from the databases based on words instead of images.* The angels guide Linda to the words that identify the name of the disease or syndrome. They also reveal the underlying toxic burdens and other physical, emotional, or spiritual cofactors that are the origin of the illness as well as the best protocols to substantially lessen the condition for that particular individual.

In comparing Linda's gift to an MRI, Linda can determine:

1. The existence of arthritis in the spinal cord.

2. The particular vertebrae where arthritis exists. Linda pinpoints it by scanning a list of vertebrae to determine which one is affected. However, she cannot identify its precise location in three-dimensional space unless she works with plastic models of the spinal cord.

3. The degree of severity of joint damage due to arthritis, which Linda ranks on a relative scale from 1 to 10, with 10 being most severe.

4. Why the person has arthritis. It is important to note that the answers Linda gets may or may not conform to the medical model as understood by conventional allopathic doctors. That is because she may get partial or complete answers related to an underlying disease etiology involving toxicity that are very difficult to detect by conventional testing methods. For example, it is well known in holistic circles that arthritis is often associated with various forms of liver toxicity. This toxicity, in many cases, cannot be measured by a blood liver panel or other standardized test.

In such a case, Linda treats the liver toxicity component of the client's arthritic condition through a detoxification program consisting of a range of supplements that might include herbals, amino acids, homeopathics, and anti-oxidants. For pain management she might channel some anti-inflammatory enzymes or herbal compounds, while also insisting that her client see an orthopedic specialist, chiropractor, or acupuncturist depending on which modality she channels is best.

In some ways, Linda is profoundly more advanced than an MRI, a CT (computed tomography) scan, or any other medical imaging technology. (See "Caveat.") For example, when a woman has a mammogram that comes back with a real positive for breast cancer, it means the cancerous tumor was festering for approximately seven to eight years before it could be picked up by the equipment. In the case of newer thermal image processing equipment, a positive finding means the tumor has been festering for only four to five years.

Caveat

We must categorically and unequivocally state that Linda does not diagnose or treat cancer. However, if during the course of a channeling session the angels inform her that they sense the presence of cancer, she insists the client immediately go to his or her medical doctor for tests to confirm or deny it. What Linda can do for cancer patients is identify the underlying emotional and metaphysical reasons why the patient had to get cancer and the *tikkun* (soul adjustment in Hebrew) associated with it. There is always a spiritual component, sometimes from a past life, which explains why a person has to experience cancer in this lifetime. A person has free will to deal with the meaning of their own mortality—or not.

While it may seem like an astonishing claim, Linda can even detect the presence of a tumor before it actually becomes physical, making her the ultimate early warning system. If she catches the tumor in what in homeopathy is described as being in an energetic or pre-malignant state, she asks the angels if there is an underlying toxic burden associated with the condition. Of course, at this stage the treatment options are far simpler and easier to deal with. However, conventional medicine does not recognize that cancer can first exist in an energetic state. How can Linda be sure she is finding cancer in such an early state before it is physical?

Here is one of several anecdotal stories that reflect a consistent pattern of this miraculous phenomenon. I recall one case several years ago where Linda told a middle-aged client that if he did not pay attention to his prostate and detoxify heavy metals out of his prostate, he would develop prostate cancer within four years. She also urged him to have his doctor do an annual checkup for prostate cancer. The man ignored her advice and never came back. About four and a half years later a mutual friend told us, "Do you remember so and so whom I sent to you four years ago? I just bumped into him and he told me he was being treated for prostate cancer." While Linda's diagnosis was totally accurate, conventional medical thinking—and that of some skeptical clients—does not recognize this energetic paradigm.

Channeling Strategies for Infectious Disease

If Linda is trying to identify a particular, harmful strain of bacteria in the bladder, she does not have to culture a urine sample in a petri dish to see what develops! Rather, she goes to a section in the database containing all known bladder infections and scans this list with her index finger until the angels identify the particular strain of bacteria causing the problem. Linda then determines the virulence of the infection as well as the proper modality needed to treat it.

If Linda channels there is an *E. coli* infection in the bladder, she must first ask her angelic guides if it is physical or energetic. If it is physical, she then uses an arbitrary scale of 1 to 10 to determine the level of virulence of the infection. The degree of virulence determines how it should be treated. If it is a serious infection, then there's no choice but to call out the heavy artillery—antibiotics. Since Linda never deals with pharmaceutical drugs, she suggests the client see Dr. Thom E. Lobe at the Beneveda Medical Group, or his or her regular family doctor, who will run tests and prescribe the appropriate antibiotic. If it is a more minor infection, Linda then goes through the database and channels the specific remedy that best suits that individual. That remedy, which which must be approved by Dr. Lobe, may be herbal, orthomolecular, enzymatic, homeopathic, or some combination thereof. There is also a scenario in homeopathy where a disease state may be caused by an "energetic toxin." This refers to the resonance of a toxin so highly diluted that none of the physical substance remains at levels detectable by a mass spectrometer. Nevertheless, the discordant vibrational energy may have a physical impact on a person's health. In those cases, Linda channels the proper homeopathic remedy that matches and cancels the vibrational resonance.

What the angels have shown Linda—and what is not understood or appreciated in the mainstream medical community—is that even a subclinical amount of a toxin, which is undetectable using current medical technology— may be a major cofactor in an illness or chronic degenerative disease. Three examples come to mind.

1. In Chapter 9, we discuss the difficulty of diagnosing chronic degenerative disease caused by mercury vapors from dental amalgam fillings that have gassed off and burrowed into organ and glandular tissues all over the body and brain. This generally will not show up in a blood, urine, or saliva test unless provoked by a heavy metal chelator, a natural or pharmaceutical product that pulls the poison out of cells often with considerable duress to the individual's physical and emotional health.

2. In Chapter 8, we discuss a concept, little known outside of homeopathic circles, called a genetically inherited miasm, a genetic toxin derived from an infectious disease such as tuberculosis or syphilis, that was experienced by an earlier generation. The presence of this toxin can be tested through a blood test developed by Meckel-Spenglersan GmbH, a small German homeopathic company. (Linda can channel the information without a blood test, although her clients can request the blood test administered by the Beneveda Medical Group.) Treatment involves the transdermal application of the company's proprietary homeopathics. The test can determine the underlying causal factor that sometimes exists behind such chronic degenerative conditions as diabetes, Crohn's disease, and arteriosclerosis. This is not airy-fairy stuff. It was developed by Dr. Carl Spengler, who worked extensively with Dr. Robert Koch, winner of the Nobel Prize in Physiology and Medicine in 1905.

3. A prominent pathologist at a major Los Angeles hospital told me he is often at odds with cardiologists who do not believe that the root cause behind a certain but not insignificant percentage of cardiovascular disease, including atherosclerosis, is undetected and unresolved bacterial infection such as chlamydia lodged in the heart tissues. In fact, in an article entitled "Can Chlamydia Be Stopped?" in the May 2005 issue of *Scientific American*, researchers reported that there might be a link between *C. pneumoniae*, an airborne species of *Chlamydia*, and arteriosclerosis and stroke. Describing the problems associated with this, the article states: "These bugs are wily. Not only do they have varied strategies for evading the body's immune system, they are also notoriously difficult to study in the laboratory."[1] What is interesting is that the angels have guided Linda to find "undetectable" bacteria as a causal factor in heart disease.

BEGINNING THE FIRST SESSION

At the beginning of a channeling session, Linda calls upon the archangels to ask if the first place she should investigate is physical, emotional, or meta-physical issues. Although the majority of clients come to see Linda for physical problems, this is by no means the only type of client she receives. A substantial number of clients also come to her for relationship issues or for other emotional or spiritual guidance. Successful marriages have resulted from her work, as have life-affirming divorces. We have often joked that promoting her gift as a dating service would be far easier and more profitable. However, we are well aware that this is not why Linda has her gift.

Some people who come to see Linda are going through an emotional or spiritual crisis. Even so, the angels might direct Linda to focus on some important health issue that is looming larger than the person realized. We have seen it cut the other way too, although that is rare. The point is *the angels give Linda whatever information the person needs at that time.* The information can range from incredible discoveries that result in meaningful cures to startling life-altering advice meant to elevate consciousness. The answers the angels give may affirm one's deepest hunches or conversely pierce illusions with tough metaphysical love. As one of Linda's first clients, who saw her mainly for emotional and spiritual reasons, so aptly put it, "The thing that's so great about Linda—she tells you just what you don't want to hear."

Assuming the answer is to proceed with matters of physical health, which occurs the majority of the time, the angels direct Linda to begin with the pre-tests, described in Chapter 4. If the answer is no, then Linda generally asks if she needs to go to the Metaphysical Database first (see Chapter 18). If the answer is yes, this could mean one of several things. Maybe one or more of the client's past lives needs to be identified so an unresolved issue from that life can be healed. Perhaps the individual is possessed by an earthbound spirit, which in Hebrew is called a *dybbuk*. Although not a common occurrence, it is, nonetheless, a very real phenomenon that is recognized by almost every culture around the world. Some fascinating case histories discussed in Chapter 18 indicate that this is a subtle process, unlike that shown in *The Exorcist.* Obviously Linda cannot proceed with a health session until the dybbuk is cleared out.

A COMPLEX HEALING GAME PLAN

After scanning the appropriate databases for the angels to identify the issues that must be addressed, Linda prioritizes the various components of the healing game plan in the first session. She also establishes the client's short-term, medium-term, and long-term goals and sets specific milestones for each phase. In subsequent sessions she shepherds the client through the healing journey where he or she experiences a series of what Linda calls "little victories." After reaching these measurable healing milestones, the client starts to feel incrementally but fundamentally better, until real, lasting healing is achieved.

Linda explains to her clients that in the same way it took some time for a medical condition to manifest, it will take time for it to clear up. Patience is required to systematically work through all the layers of detoxification and imbalance. Because each person's biochemistry and capacity to detoxify are different, the angels know that the speed of detoxification varies from person to person and devise the perfect healing protocols for each one.

Over the years different health care practitioners have asked Linda how it is that she can get a client to take a significant number of supplements. These same practitioners say they're lucky to achieve patient compliance for just two or three supplements. Beside the fact that people of consciousness sense the truth and power of angels being channeled through Linda, there are several other explanations.

Linda likens the state of a very sick or chronically diseased individual to a burning building consumed by flames. Her diagnosis is like that of a fire chief who stations firefighters with hoses on the north, east, south, and west flanks of the building so that the fire can be put out most efficiently. Linda calls upon her angelic guides to identify and rank underlying toxic burdens and other biochemical and nutritional imbalances. She then channels the degree of multitasking needed to both peel the layers of the toxic onion and correct imbalances. She cannot overload the client with too many remedies at the same time but must work in phases. In the vast majority of cases involving a chronic degenerative disease, Linda channels a customized alkaline diet which neutralizes the body's pH and helps to buffer the body against the acidic toxic load unleashed during the detoxification process (see Chapter 12). Many cases also require herbal and homeopathic drainage remedies that prep the body for the main detoxification process by first opening the pathways of elimination. Opening the body's sewer system involves:

• Opening up the lymphatic system with drainage remedies, workouts on a mini trampoline, or massage so that toxins will find their way out of the lymphatic system and into various processes of elimination. This is akin to cleaning out the body's sewer system (see Chapter 12).

• Detoxifying the colon, kidneys, and liver through a range of different herbal and homeopathic compounds (see Chapter 12).

Linda also insists that clients get educated about the real nature of their condition. She much prefers that they not passively accept the angelic guidance she channels at face value, but must truly understand the scientific rationale behind the healing game plan. This knowledge is important because it increases the consciousness behind the treatment protocol so that the client is proactive with conviction. The client is now able to ask more meaningful and complex questions of the angels, which is sometimes required in more challenging cases.

Linda cannot possibly do this work alone. That is why, in addition to Dr. Lobe, we have a network of what we consider to be best-of-breed health practitioners—doctors, dentists, acupuncturists, chiropractors, naturopaths, and neurofeedback practitioners in the United States and Europe—whom Linda refers clients to when a healing specialty is needed. Each of these individuals is an amazing healer in his or her own right, and they are willing to work with her because they understand and respect that Linda receives medical information from angels. Linda functions as a medical quarterback to this team of amazing healers and gives them guidance when needed.

Linda believes that there is nothing more disheartening than to spend time and money with a healer and get poor or negligible results. That is why she offers a special service to clients who come to see her at the Beneveda Medical Group, but who do not live in the Los Angeles area. Let's say, for example, Linda channels that a client who lives in New York City needs to see an acupuncturist there. She asks the client to put together a list of five or six acupuncturists and then channels from that list who is the best possible one to treat that patient. This helps the client build his or her own best-of-breed healing team.

PART ONE

Physical Healing

CHAPTER 4

The Physical Databases

The truth will set you free, but first it will make you miserable.
—ATTRIBUTED TO JAMES A. GARFIELD

Everybody, soon or late, sits down to a banquet of consequences.
—ROBERT LOUIS STEVENSON

RESEARCHING AND UPDATING THE DATABASES that Linda channels is a joyous, yet arduous, ongoing task. Since 1994, I have compiled information on disease causation and cure from many sources, including databases of computerized EAV systems, medical textbooks and illustrations, laboratory tests, peer-review journals, and catalogues from supplement companies. I also rely on input from doctors, alternative healers, and lab technicians.

It's enormously challenging to describe Linda's process in a linear fashion due to the complicated health variables that differentiate each client. Each individual's physiology, biochemistry, and pathology bring unique twists and turns on the road to diagnosis and treatment that make her process difficult to standardize. Nonetheless, Linda's complicated detective work, which I have encapsulated in two case studies, is imbued with a certain inner intuitive logic tempered by years of angelic guidance and sound scientific principles.

THE SCOPE OF THE PRE-TEST

One general rule is that Linda always starts by channeling the pre-test shown in Table 4-1, a procedure derived from EAV. The pre-test includes a wide range of topics that provide an overall snapshot of the client's health. The basic profile determines what is worthy of further angelic research during the course of the health reading. The categories describe, in broad strokes, the types of causal factors that have a negative impact on the client's health. The results of the pre-test provide a basic overview of relevant cofactors. This is only the beginning of the search process, albeit an important one. Linda must now drill down to flesh out specific details of each broad category. Given that every client is different, the exact order in which information is revealed may vary.

For example, suppose "hormone deficiency" shows up as a positive in the pre-test. At this point Linda does not know what hormone or hormones are deficient or what organ system or systems this condition could be affecting in a direct or indirect way. It is merely an indication or clue that a hormonal deficiency exists that is worthy of further research. Linda subsequently drills down in the endocrine database (database F) and/or related organ systems to get answers. Now specific core causal factors begin to reveal the true nature of the malaise.

IDENTIFYING THE MOST STRESSED ORGANS AND THEIR CAUSAL FACTORS

As part of the pre-test, Linda asks the angels to rank the Most Stressed Organ, Dominant Focus, and Origin of Complaint in the body. These terms are derived from Vega test protocols:

• **Most Stressed Organ (MSO)** involves identifying the organ, gland, or organ system that is carrying the greatest stress. The stress may be due to any number of factors, including severe toxic, pathogenic, genetic, or emotional conditions. This stress manifests as the highest weakening of organ function and/or the highest degree of inflammation responsible for a chronic condition that can cause functional damage over time.

• **Dominant Focus (DF)** is the predominant underlying health issue in the body. Examples include autoimmune disease, heavy metal toxicity, chronic inflammation, liver cirrhosis (from the hepatic/biliary database), among many possibilities.

• **Origin of Complaint (OC)** involves tracking the DF back to its underlying cause. This could be from a specific environmental toxin, pathogen, genetic issue, or emotion. This manifests itself as the DF in the MSO.

As Linda gathers information, she relies on her angelic guides to tell her where to go next. This may include researching information contained in Physical Databases A–T, which are concerned with organs, glands, and organ sys-

TABLE 4-1. PRE-TEST CONDITIONS

Acid pH diet

Acid pH toxins

Alkaline diet

Alkaline pH

Allergy, airborne

Allergy, autoimmune

Allergy, chemical

Allergy, critical

Allergy, epidermal

Allergy, food

Anabolic excess/deficiency

Autoimmune disease

Biological warfare

Bloating

Brain parasites

Catabolic excess/deficiency

Chakra imbalance

Chemtrails (biological agents)

Circulatory disorder

Chronic fatigue syndrome

Chronic inflammation

Color imbalance

Cyst

Damp heat

Dehydration

Depression

Depression, endogenous

Edema (fluid retention)

Electromagnetic stress

Emotion-activating disease

Emotion-blocking treatment

Emotional hypersensitivity

Energy, left spin

Energy, right spin

Energy-frequency-attracting disease

Energy-frequency-creating pathology

Energy-vacuum-attracting disease

Enzyme deficiency

Enzyme deficiency, cellular

Exhaustion

Fever, acute

Fever, chronic

Fever and chills

Focal disturbance

Free radical/oxidative stress

Fungal proliferation

Gastrointestinal dysbiosis

HAARP, high-frequency energy

Hormone, deficiency/excess

Immune deficiency disease

Infection, bacterial

Infection, bacterial from animal tissue

Infection, energetic

Infection, fungal/yeast/mold

Infection, incubating

Infection, parasite infestation

Infection, rickettsia

Infection, viral

Infection, viral (postviral)

Infection, virus from animal tissue

Malignancy

Malignancy, premalignancy

Malignancy, masked premalignancy

Medical overdose

Meridian imbalance

Metabolic imbalance

Metabolism imbalance, slow

Miasm, acquired

Miasm, genetic

Mineral deficiency

Mineral deficiency, trace minerals

Morphological (abnormally shaped) cells

Nervous system dysfunction

Neurotoxin

Neurotransmitter imbalance

Obstruction

Positively charged cells

Premature aging

Prolapse

Psychological stress

Psychosomatic

Radiation

Regurgitation

Salt overdose

Skin sensitivity

Spiritual, blocking treatment

Stress, emotional

Stress, frequent

Stress, geopathic

Sugar overdose

Syndrome (condition)

TCM syndrome condition

Toxemia, fat

Toxemia, protein

Toxemia, starch

Toxin, chemical

Toxin, dental material

Toxin, environmental

Toxin, food

Toxin, food additive

Toxin, heavy metal:

   Aluminum

   Cadmium sulfate

   Lead

   Mercury

Nickel

Silver

Toxin, hereditary (miasm)

Toxin, residual

Toxin, vaccination

Traumatic injury

Tumor, benign

Tumor, malignant

Unresolved past-life issue

Uric acid toxicity

Physical Databases

A: Body chemistry

B: Cardiovascular

C: Cellular

D: Dental/oral

E: Dermatological

F: Endocrine

G: Gastrointestinal

H: Hematological

I: Hepatic/biliary

J: Immune system

K: Muscle/skeletal

L: Neurological

M: Nutritional/dietary

N: Opthamological

O: Otolaryngologic (ENT)

P: Pain producing

Q: Pulmonary

R: Renal/urological

S: Reproductive

T: Subtle energy systems

U: Remedies

V: Food and diet

Emotional Database

Metaphysical Database

---

tems. Database V, food and diet, is an extensive list of all types of foods and condiments that Linda channels to create a completely customized diet. She utilizes three dietary paradigms in the channeling process: the Anti-Candida Diet,[1] Metabolic Typing,[2] and the Glycemic Index.[3] Database U, Remedies, involves many categories of natural remedies, including vitamins, minerals, amino acids, glandulars, essential fatty acids (EFAs), enzymes, homeopathics, herbal and other plant-based remedies, and flower or gem essences.

Databases A–T share common characteristics; they each have lists of words that relate to particular organ/gland imbalances, structures, and functions. In other ways, they are different. For example, item 6 in this list is unique to the cardiovascular database, which consists of the following sections:

1. Heart imbalances: A list of all potential disease etiology and conditions/syndromes of the heart.

2. Heart pathology: A list of such pathogens as bacteria, viruses, parasites, rickettsia and spirocytes, and fungi.

3. Heart structure and function: A list with illustrations of all the anatomical structures of the heart with descriptions and illustrations of how they function.

4. Blood vessel imbalances: A list of all potential disease etiology and conditions/syndromes of the arteries, veins, and capillaries.

5. Blood vessel structure and function: A list of all the arteries, veins, and capillaries with a description of how they function.

6. An overview of advanced cardiovascular testing protocols containing the latest research on cardiovascular risk factors (from Berkeley HeartLab; www.bhlinc.com).

To show the sheer depth of information that Linda works with, a portion of the cardiovascular database, which is typical of any organ system database, is provided in Appendix A. The Emotional and Metaphysical Databases are also included in the pre-test. Each of these can have a profound impact on physical healing and are discussed later in the book.

An Unexpected Most Stressed Organ

Although it is far more typical for a client to come to see Linda with some preconceived notion about what his or her principal health ailments are, that is by no means always the case. This example showcases one of Linda's most extraordinary gifts: her "early warning detection system" where she is able to detect a health issue well before it physically manifests as a healing crisis.

Cynthia is one of Linda's clients who is highly motivated to achieve a state of glowing health. Cynthia related a classic "Linda story" that cemented her understanding of the uniqueness of Linda's gift. As part of the pre-test workup, Linda channeled that Cynthia's MSO was "dental." Using a special dental chart that identifies the corresponding energetic relationship between the vitality of each tooth and a particular organ system, Linda moved her left index finger over the lower left quadrant of the mouth. Suddenly the pendulum started spinning rapidly to the right, indicating an energetic disturbance. Linda's angelic guides revealed there was something significantly wrong with the bridge located on two molars in the lower left quadrant and Cynthia should immediately get it replaced. Cynthia was obviously disturbed by this advice and could not understand what could conceivably be wrong as she was experiencing no pain or discomfort in that area of her mouth.

Nevertheless, Cynthia set up a visit with a mercury-free, biological dentist (Chapter 12) whose name Linda channeled from a list of such dentists in her area. When the dentist first examined Cynthia's mouth, he declared the bridge looked perfectly fine to him. Who was this person to tell her such rubbish? Had this person even looked into Cynthia's mouth? In a half-joking manner he said he would be perfectly happy to put in a new bridge for approximately $3,000, but in his professional opinion, there was no need for it. Cynthia sheepishly admitted that she had seen a medical intuitive named Linda Freud who was absolutely certain there was some sort of structural problem with the bridge as well as the beginning stages of a bacterial infection in that area. She urged him to take an x-ray to confirm what Linda had gotten.

After examining the x-rays, the dentist shook his head in amazement and announced that the bridge was indeed substandard and defective. Cynthia remembers the dentist saying, "Even a first-year dental school student could see there was something terribly wrong with that bridge." He confirmed that Linda was correct—it had to come out. But because she needed other amalgam removal work, Cynthia decided to attend to that first and postpone removing the bridge until another time. However, a few months later she was back in the dentist's chair as the gums under the bridge had become so inflamed with a raging bacterial infection she could no longer chew food in that area! She never questioned what Linda channeled again.

The Second Phase of the Pre-Test: Baseline Readings of Toxic Loads

After the pre-test is underway, the next step in the diagnostic process involves taking what Linda calls her "baseline readings." These determine the relative level of severity of the underlying toxic burdens revealed in the pre-test. The systemic baseline reading scale on any particular toxin theoretically ranges from 0 to 100 percent and indicates a relative level of saturation of that toxin in the body. A score of 0 percent indicates that the person is completely free of a particular toxin. Of course, 100 percent of a toxin is theoretically impossible, as it would mean the body is completely flooded with a particular toxin. Linda has never measured a score of 100 percent for a particular toxin, as a person with such a score would probably be dead or close to it. However, she has seen some highly toxic people, with scores of 70 percent for a particular toxin.

The systemic baseline reading is the average percentage of a particular toxin across all organs, glands, organ systems, and tissues in the body. For example, if a client's systemic baseline reading for mercury is channeled at 20 percent, this means that mercury is distributed at a 20 percent saturation level on average throughout the body. However, in assessing treatment protocol options, Linda often needs to drill down deeper than this. In order to antici-pate where potential problems may occur during a mercury detox program, Linda takes an organ-specific baseline reading where the excretion of mercury lodged in a particular organ may be problematic. The greatest complications involve the kidneys, liver, endocrine system, heart, and brain.

If, for example, Linda does an organ-specific baseline reading on the kid-neys that shows a 35 percent mercury load, this means that a disproportion-ately higher level of mercury has accumulated in the kidneys and that kidney drainage remedies must first be utilized before a heavy metal detoxification can safely proceed.

Sometimes toxins are revealed in layers much like an onion. Linda must work meticulously much like a detective going layer by layer to discover hard-to-find toxins. For example, Linda may scan the databases for a complete list of toxins or pathogens specifically found in the liver. After she channels that *Streptococcus* bacteria are testing positive in the liver, parasites may sub-sequently be revealed. Linda must assess the level of severity for each under-lying toxin so she can rank and prioritize her healing game plan.

Linda refers to the relative level of toxicity as the "toxic load." She has channeled that the normal, healthy range for the categories of toxins described below is 0 to 5 percent. The higher the load above 5, the more severe the toxic burden. She typically checks the baseline readings of the following categories of toxins during the pre-test:

1. Heavy metal load: An overall composite covering the combined average load of heavy metals including mercury, nickel, lead, aluminum, calcium sul-fate, tin, silver, arsenic, and cadmium (Chapters 9–12). The toxic load of each individual metal is also identified.

2. Fungal/yeast/mold load: Potentially consisting of either a single strain or multiple strains of fungi (Chapters 5–6).

3. Parasite load: Potentially consisting of one or more species of parasites (Chapter 7).

4. Hereditary toxin load: This refers to a genetically inherited miasm, a con-cept derived from homeopathy (see Chapter 8). A miasm is a vibrational res-onance derived from infectious disease (for example, tuberculosis, syphilis, gonorrhea, pneumonia, influenza, and staphylococcal and streptococcal infec-

tions) that was experienced by one's ancestors going back several generations. It does *not* represent the physical form of these diseases. However, it can be the hidden origin of masked or camouflaged symptoms behind many forms of chronic degenerative disease. Most importantly, a miasm can bind in toxins making them difficult to excrete out of the body.

5. Drug toxin load: Usually due to chronic abuse of pharmaceutical or recreational drugs and alcohol. The residue of these drugs may lodge in many places in the body but are commonly found in the liver.

6. Electromagnetic radiation pollution load: From power transmission lines, cell phones, airport radar, microwave towers and ovens, among other sources.

7. Geopathic stress load: From such things as ley lines and radon gas.

8. Chemical toxicity load: From industrial, agricultural, medical, and food additive toxins.

9. Negative emotions: These function like miasms and bind in certain toxins (Chapters 15–16).

Anything above a toxic load of 5 percent indicates the relative severity of any of these environmental toxins or pathogens. Once Linda channels a client's toxic load she is able to rank and prioritize the order of the specific detox protocols needed to eliminate those particular toxins. She then channels if the toxin or pathogen needs to be treated right away, or if it must wait until other layers of the "toxic onion" have first been removed. Sometimes heavy metal toxins are so deeply hidden in bone that they may not show up at all. However, they can leach out during a detox. Because these variables can change over time, Linda must review and update the pre-test at the beginning of every session. Additionally, with mercury toxicity derived from dental amalgams or nickel toxicity due to a crown backed by nickel, these materials must first be removed from the body prior to starting heavy metal detoxification.

Case History: How Linda Uses the Cardiovascular Database

Here is an example showcasing how Linda uses the cardiovascular database to do the detective work needed to set up a healing protocol. This case history is a composite of different scenarios that Linda has experienced and includes references to many issues like miasms and conditions such as fungal, bacterial infections, and mercury toxicity that are discussed in subsequent chapters.

Tony is a 48-year-old executive who experiences an occasional tightness in his chest along with periodic bouts of tachycardia (rapid heart beat), which make him even more nervous. He has stopped exercising because he is afraid he may be overdoing it. His concern stems from the fact that arteriosclerosis and high cholesterol run in his family. Both his father and his uncle died in their 50s from sudden heart attacks.

Tony is determined not to go the way of the men in his family and understands that the same creeping deterioration they experienced is beginning to happen to him. Unlike them, however, he no longer has complete faith in the standard medical system and wants to know what more he can do to reverse the deterioration so that bypass operations and stents do not occur down the road. Two years ago when Tony first suspected he had a problem, he went to a cardiologist who diagnosed that his total cholesterol and low-density lipoprotein (LDL) cholesterol levels were too high. He was put on Lipitor, and over time these levels dropped to the high end of what is considered the normal range. Although this made him feel better emotionally, he was soon to discover that this good news came at a steep price.

After being on Lipitor for a little over a year, Tony noticed that in recent months he had become increasingly forgetful and flustered at work. He felt as though there was "a cloud in his brain" that was causing him to get irritable and short-tempered at work and at home. However, that was not the worst of it. Tony was beginning to slur his words and wondered if he was getting a degenerative neurological condition. He also noticed that he was experiencing a gradual muscle degeneration in his calf muscles and legs. He had no idea why all this was happening and was depressed and scared, so his internist prescribed the antidepressant Paxil. In spite of all this, he was still enthusiastic about Lipitor because his cholesterol levels had come down significantly.

After reading in a men's health magazine about the benefits of taking megadoses of vitamin C for the heart, Tony started taking 5,000 milligrams (mg) a day. About a month later, the frequency and intensity of the tachycardia had increased to an extent that really scared him. He also began to feel a slight arrhythmia (irregular heart beat). It did not occur to him that the vitamin C could be part of the problem so he kept taking it. His cardiologist acknowledged that he indeed had a greater level of tachycardia than before as well as a slight arrhythmia. He recommended that Tony immediately stop all medications and supplements except Lipitor to see if any others were causing the problem. He did not want Tony to stop Lipitor and reminded him of how successful the drug had been at lowering his cholesterol. Over the next month the tachycardia and arrhythmia began to abate and became more sporadic. However, his muscle pains, memory issues, and irritability were getting noticeably worse.

It never occurred to Tony that these symptoms could be connected to Lipitor. His cardiologist expressed such enthusiasm for his reduced cholesterol levels that Tony was a bit afraid to upset the apple cart by dwelling on his new medical problems. In fact, his cardiologist reassured him that side effects of the medication were just a "normal" part of the process. He would just have to learn to live with them if he didn't want to end up like his father and uncle. The cardiologist also suggested that Tony go back to his internist to see why he was having these new problems. Perhaps there were some other drugs that might help him. However, his wife, Terry, who was more intuitive, had never felt quite right about Lipitor, but was afraid to voice her opinion as she knew of no other options. Although he was a bit skeptical at first, Tony reluctantly came to Linda at Terry's insistence, as her health had dramatically improved after working with Linda for six months. As he described his symptoms, Tony began to unravel before the "angel lady," as he called Linda.

Once Linda learned that Tony had been taking Lipitor, Paxil for depression, and 5,000 mg a day of vitamin C, she went directly to the pre-test. Among the items revealed were acid pH, bacteria, drug toxicity, mercury, miasms, and muscle/skeletal issues. Linda channeled that although Lipitor had been successful in lowering his cholesterol level, Tony belonged to a small percentage of people who did not tolerate the drug well. This confirmed his wife's suspicion that Lipitor was the underlying cause of his memory loss, anger management problems, slurring of words, and muscle degeneration in his legs. In addition, Linda channeled that Lipitor had significantly reduced the level of CoQ_{10} in his body—a nutrient beneficial for heart health.[4]

Linda concurred that Tony's obsession with keeping his cholesterol levels down was understandable given his family's health history. The key question that he and his wife had was this: Now that Lipitor had accomplished this goal, was there an alternative approach that could maintain healthy cholesterol levels so that Tony did not have to experience the debilitating side effects from Lipitor?

Linda found it interesting that instead of merely dealing with their question, she was first instructed to focus on a more fundamental issue: *Why did this condition run in Tony's family?* The information on the pre-test provided some clues. Tony's hereditary toxin load (miasms) was 50 percent, an unusu- ally high number (for a detailed discussion of miasms, see Chapter 8). When Linda asked Tony about his family's health history, it became clear that miasms were an important underlying cause. As a boy Tony had heard stories from his Sicilian grandmother on his father's side that her husband had died of a heart attack in his late 50s and left her a widow with three children to raise. He remembered her also saying that her husband's father had died of tuberculosis. Linda then channeled the Polysan colloid miasm database of miasms/ remedies, and two strains of hereditary tuberculosis miasms and a hereditary syphilis miasm tested positive. She channeled that this was the missing link that explained the genetic proclivity for arteriosclerosis and high cholesterol in Tony's family!

After "heart" showed up as the MSO, Linda tested tachycardia and arrhythmia against all known causes and discovered that the dominant focus was bacteria. This prompted her to drill down deeper in a section of the cardiovascular database entitled "heart pathology caused by patho- gens." With pendulum in hand, she proceeded to scan it, confirming that the dominant focus behind the tachycardia and arrhythmia was an energetic *Streptococcus viridans* bacterial infection. This, in turn, had led to the very early stages of mitral valve prolapse (MVP), a common form of valvular dis- ease. Linda's remarkable early warning system provided very good news. Since the condition was not physical, but only in an energetic state, it could easily be treated with homeopathy, and orthomolecular nutrients could be used to strengthen function. However, Linda channeled if this issue was not addressed, it could over time result in a far more serious condition called endocarditis, which could only be treated by Tony's cardiologist.

Linda then channeled that she had to drill down deeper to get the Origin of Complaint behind the energetic *S. viridans* infection in the heart. Linda was led to mercury toxicity as a cofactor behind the infection. She asked Tony if he had any silver amalgam fillings. He replied that he had nine of them. Linda then channeled that when Tony had taken the megadoses of vitamin C, this had chelated some mercury out of his mouth, which found its way to his heart where it contributed to the energetic infection and the early stages of MVP.[5,6] Although taking vitamin C was conceptually a good idea, Tony did not real- ize that it was a potent heavy metal chelator that made him sicker by leaching mercury out of his teeth and into his body.

Most shockingly, Linda channeled that in a rush to get Tony's cholesterol level down, the cardiologist had overlooked a key issue. The mercury toxicity from Tony's old dental amalgams was contributing to the proliferation of free-radical damage (see Chapter 10). This, in turn, was hastening the destructive, oxidative nature of the bad LDL cholesterol that Linda had picked up in the pre-test. Linda channeled that if not corrected, this could bring on more serious cardiovascular disease. Lipitor was simply not designed to address oxidative stress from free radicals or the mercury from Tony's dental amalgams. Since the source of the free radicals and the energetic bacterial infection was mercury that leached from dental amalgam, the removal of the mercury was of real importance for his heart health. Linda explained that although the men's magazine article was correct about the benefits of vitamin C for the heart, it failed to inform Tony that if one had a mouthful of mercury amalgam, the exact opposite was true.

At this point, Tony was beginning to feel a little overwhelmed by the sheer volume of information that had been revealed. He was, for the first time, beginning to get a true picture of the complexity of his health conditions. Linda sought to reassure him that, with the information she would give him, his doctor might be open to a more integrative approach. The key question he posed to Linda was this: Other than dietary modifications, what could be done in the short term to support healthy cholesterol management if his doctor allowed him to wean off of Lipitor? Linda told Tony there were nutritional supplements that offered synergistic benefits to assist dietary modification. These could help him maintain healthy cholesterol levels within normal range as well as strengthen overall heart function. Linda went to the remedy database and channeled suggestions for a more comprehensive nutritional approach that would also prevent further oxidation of LDL cholesterol and improve the endothelial lining of arterial walls. Linda asked Tony to ask his cardiologist to consider such nutrients as niacin, pomegranate extract, fish oil, CoQ10, L-arginine, taurine, magnesium, and red yeast rice extract as well as extracts of traditional Ayervedic remedies such as Indian gooseberry fruit and curcumin.

Tony was dumbfounded to learn that Lipitor is a patented synthetic molecule that is a modified version of a natural compound found in red yeast rice extract. This is nature's original statin drug.[7,8] Statins work by inhibiting a key liver enzyme from producing cholesterol.

Tony's obsession with the numbers in his cholesterol tests indicated that he did not really comprehend the full nature of his cardiovascular disease. To further clarify, Linda urged him to give his cardiologist a printout she had prepared from peer-reviewed journals and medical books that provided a brief crash course on the negative repercussions of mercury toxicity on heart disease. This included its effects on cholesterol, free radicals, arteriosclerosis, inflammation, adenosine triphosphate (ATP) production, and hypertension (see Chapter 10). She also provided reprints on cholesterol management from the book *Disease Prevention and Treatment* and an article entitled "Lower Cholesterol Safely: Nutritional Interventions for Healthy Lipids." (Both of these are available on www.lef.org.) As Linda began to channel and organize information from these sources along with her database, a game plan was beginning to emerge. The basics of that program were that Tony would:

1. Continue to work with his cardiologist. Since his LDL cholesterol levels were no longer in what his cardiologist considered a danger zone, Tony would show him the series of peer-reviewed clinical studies documenting the viability of a natural supplement approach coupled with specific dietary suggestions that Linda had given him. With his doctor's permission, Tony would start a program to slowly wean off Lipitor based on a precise program that Linda channeled and replace it with a combination of natural remedies that managed and maintained healthy cholesterol levels, strengthened heart function, and combated free radicals. The cardiologist would monitor Tony on a monthly basis, and as long as his cholesterol levels did not go up, he would stay on the program with his cardiologist's consent. Tony would also get his doctor's permission to proceed with dental amalgam removal by a mercury-free, biological dentist.

2. Wean off Paxil under his doctor's supervision and replace it with flower/gem essences, orthomolecular nutrients, and meditation techniques, all of which were channeled by Linda (see Chapter 15).

3. Go on a rigorous alkaline and high-fiber diet that Linda channeled for him.

4. Take homeopathic remedies to get rid of the energetic form of *S. viridans*.

5. Begin a program of sequentially removing the genetically inherited miasms that Linda channeled.

6. Start to open up his lymphatic duct system with a homeopathic drainage remedy in preparation for a heavy metal detoxification program.

Tony walked out of his session with information overload. Although he acknowledged the correlations between what the cardiologist had told him and what Linda had confirmed, there were many newly revealed aspects of his condition. However, Tony now understood why his wife had urged him to see Linda, and he was eager to embrace the treatment plan she channeled. He called Linda the next day to tell her he had found a website called www.medications.com and read testimonials from people on Lipitor who had experienced symptoms very similar to his own. He was stunned to discover that Lipitor was the fifth highest ranked drug on that website in terms of the number of complaints of side effects. He no longer felt so alone.

After faithfully following the complete program for a few months, Tony reported that the tachycardia and arrhythmias had stopped, and he was feeling confident enough to begin some steady but gentle physical exercise. His irritability, memory loss, slurring of words, and muscle degeneration in his legs had also completely disappeared. Best of all, his cholesterol levels had stabilized at normal levels. The whole process took approximately nine months of dedicated work on Tony's part. The results spoke for themselves: Tony was ecstatic.

Caveat

The information and products we have discussed here are solely to support health and not intended to diagnose, treat, prevent, or cure any disease, and they should not be used as a substitute for diagnosis and treatment by your personal physician.

CHAPTER 5

Fungal Disease:
The Modern Consequence
of Environmental Toxicity

Beware of false knowledge; it is more dangerous than ignorance.
—GEORGE BERNARD SHAW

A CRITICAL ASPECT OF LINDA'S PRACTICE involves detoxifying clients who have multiple hard-to-diagnose chronic degenerative conditions caused by environmental toxins that are often ignored or misunderstood by most allopathic physicians. The number one complaint she hears from her clients is that they are exhausted and depleted. It is no accident that the number one *effect* of toxicity that Linda channels is fungal disease. Not surprisingly, it's also an area of diagnosis that was usually overlooked by their practitioners. For example, when clients with chronic fatigue syndrome (CFS) come to see Linda, they are amazed to find out that some form of fungal/yeast/mold proliferation is a significant part of why they are feeling so depleted. For our purposes, the terms "fungus," "yeast," and "mold" will be used interchangeably even though there are distinct differences among them.

When Linda and I were tested by Drs. Dorfmann and Haefeli in the early 1990s, they determined that the severe CFS we suffered from was due in part to advanced fungal disease. We realized then that our European practitioners were far more advanced in diagnosing and treat fungal infections with natural methods. They recommended that we study the work of Dr. Günther Enderlein (1872–1968), the German microbiologist who developed a series of brilliant homeopathic remedies, which Linda now uses to treat all fungal conditions. Dr. Enderlein asserted that modern allopathic medicine failed to recognize the full extent of fungal disease and its hidden relationship with many chronic degenerative conditions. (His approach is discussed in Chapter 6.)

Our research into the true nature of fungal disease has evolved considerably since then. We have come to realize that unless a practitioner has experience with natural remedies, they tend to view conditions such as vaginal yeast infection (vaginitis), oral fungus (thrush), skin fungus (eczema), jock itch (male candidiasis), or toenail fungus as isolated, localized health issues, not symptomatic of a deeper malaise. As a result, they are unlikely to know much about the devastating effects of fungal/yeast overgrowth called candidiasis that can exist in multiple locations throughout the body.

FUNGAL/YEAST OVERGROWTH

Fungi and yeasts produce harmful toxins (mycotoxins) and enzymes (exoenzymes) that kill or disable their food sources such as beneficial flora, so that nutrients cannot be assimilated. Consequently, such mycotoxins as gliotoxin, aflatoxin, and acetaldehyde can severely weaken the immune system. Gliotoxin, produced by certain species of yeasts—*Candida albicans* and *Aspergillus niger*—inactivates a number of vital cellular enzymes, promotes free-radical damage, and kills vital cells including macrophages, T lymphocytes, and hepatocytes (liver cells). Aflatoxin is a carcinogen considered so potent that it was weaponized by Saddam Hussein's scientists as part of his arsenal of biological weapons. Acetaldehyde, derived from alcohol that is produced by the yeast and released when the yeast is killed, is also a potential carcinogen that can cause dermatitis, allergic reactions, chemical sensitivities, headaches, and digestive problems. According to www.fungusfocus.com, "It should be no surprise, then, that fungal and yeast infections are frequently associated with 'mysterious' illnesses such as CFS and arthritis. The fungus is injecting its host (you) with toxins to dissolve and digest you. Even if the infection is localized, the toxic enzymes are transported by the bloodstream throughout the body."[1]

Candida albicans normally exists at very low levels in the body. However, toxicity pushes the body into a disease state through an overgrowth of candida known as candidiasis. A scourge of modern society, candidiasis is frequently present whenever there is some form of heavy metal, electromagnetic pollution, radiation, chemical, or drug toxin. In addition, alcohol abuse, recreational drug use, smoking, unsafe sexual practices, unhealthy dietary decisions, and even negative emotions are also prime sources of this type of fungal disease.

Candidiasis is not a systemic yeast infection in the true sense of the word. An overgrowth of candida in the intestines called gastrointestinal dysbiosis, for example, does not mean that the fungus is growing wildly unchecked throughout all the other organs (although it most definitely can exist in multiple locations and organs). Rather, systemic in this case means that the effects of toxins produced by the overgrowth of the fungus are absorbed into the bloodstream with far-reaching consequences throughout the body. Unfortunately, because the overuse of certain drugs, particularly antibiotics, is among the leading causes of candidiasis, many allopathic physicians are uncertain of what to do and the drug companies appear in no hurry to act.

As a result, too few doctors connect the dots between the symptoms of fungal disease and a clear diagnosis of candidiasis. This lack of awareness explains why a significant number of allopathic doctors do not acknowledge the complex relationship between environmental toxicity and poor lifestyle decisions—which are *often the true, festering cause of the patient's illness.* This limitation explains why people who have suffered for years with candidiasis and/or CFS are turning to integrative physicians or holistic practitioners in increasing numbers.

THE LINK BETWEEN CHRONIC FATIGUE SYNDROME AND FUNGAL DISEASE

What in broad strokes is referred to as CFS is one of the most common complaints among Linda's chronically ill clients. So debilitating is this condition that it is sometimes referred to as "the flu that never ends." While it is generally agreed that a compromised immune system is the central feature of this mysterious syndrome, what does that actually mean? In his book *Chronic Fatigue, Fibromyalgia, and Environmental Illness,* author Burton Goldberg writes of a truism that we have consistently found in our research into chronic degenerative diseases: "One of the hallmarks of alternative medicine thinking and practice is that there is rarely, or never, a single cause of any illness; diseases are developed out of multiple converging imbalances and deficiencies."[2]

It was originally believed that Epstein-Barr virus (EBV) was the cause of CFS. However, when medical researchers at the Centers for Disease Control and Prevention (CDC) and the National Institutes of Health (NIH) attempted to standardize the definition of CFS they were surprised to find that many people with CFS do not exhibit high EBV antibody levels as previously believed.

While there is no one exact cause of CFS, Linda has channeled that a component of candidiasis or some other fungal disease is almost always present. Clearly, the two most common causes of pathogenic fungal overgrowth are the indiscriminate overprescription of antibiotics and chronic leakage of mercury from dental amalgams. In more severe cases, other potential primary or secondary cofactors that cause or further exacerbate the condition are listed in Table 5-1.

Physicians too often forget that antibiotics such as penicillin are forms of fungi. Rather than treating a mild to moderate bacterial infection with different types of natural antibacterials (such as oregano and olive leaf extracts, colloidal silver, grapefruit seed extract, turmeric, homeopathy), allopathic doctors' training often precludes them from considering anything other than antibiotics. When doctors prescribe repeated rounds of antibiotics, they risk causing candidiasis, which causes a chain reaction, blocking the absorption of vital nutrients and further breaking down the immune system. Linda has frequently heard from clients that the prevailing view of their physicians was that the side effect of candidiasis was a necessary evil that the patient must

TABLE 5-1. POTENTIAL COFACTORS IN CHRONIC FATIGUE SYNDROME

PATHOGENS	TOXINS	LIFESTYLE FACTORS
Fungi	Chemical toxicity	Acid pH diet
3 most common forms:	Fluoride, pesticides, and many others too numerous to mention	Excessive alcohol, chocolate, coffee, colas, dairy, meat, and deep-fried, fermented, and processed foods
Aspergillus niger	**Drug toxins**	
Candida albicans	Chemotherapy	
Mucor racemosus	Prolonged course of birth control pills	**Anaerobic environment**
Other strains of fungi		
Parasites	Prolonged use of anti-inflammatory steroid drugs	Lack of oxygen
Cestoda: many forms of tapeworms	Recreational drugs	**Negative emotions/ stress**
Nematodes: many forms of worms	Repeated or prolonged course of antibiotics	**Smoking**
Protozoa: many forms of amoebas	**Heavy metal toxicity from multiple environmental sources**	**Unsafe sexual practices**
Trematoda: many forms of flukes		
Mycoplasma bacteria	Aluminum, cadmium, lead, mercury, nickel,	
Lyme disease	**Radiation/electromagnetic pollution**	
Viruses		
Coxsackievirus	Cell phones	
Cytomegalovirus	ELF waves	
Epstein-Barr virus	Microwave towers/ovens	
Herpesvirus	Power lines	
Mononucleosis	Radar	

stoically endure. The same consequences hold true for non-steroidal anti-inflammatory steroidal drugs (NSAIDs) and chemotherapy, which tend to suppress or kill healthy intestinal flora, creating an environment that allows fungi, parasites, and harmful bacteria to proliferate. This, in turn, leads to a weakening of the immune system, which promotes many forms of chronic degenerative disease, including chronic fatigue syndrome.

Linda finds that her CFS clients often suffer from a variety of digestive and intestinal conditions that result from chronic dysbiosis. Overgrowth of unfriendly bacteria, protozoa, or *Candida albicans* yeast, coupled with the depletion of friendly bacteria, causes breaks to develop in the intestinal lining. This "leaky gut" condition allows partially digested food macromolecules to leak into the blood, causing the intestinal wall to become inflamed where it then begins to erode. That, in turn, promotes multiple food allergies, autoimmune disease, ulcers, appendicitis, malabsorption of nutrients, and Crohn's disease. The stage is set for fungal infections such as candida as well as parasites to invade other organs.

THE MANY EFFECTS OF FUNGAL/YEAST-CONNECTED ILLNESS

In addition to the medical issues, there are a spate of health conditions where a fungal/yeast cofactor may be overlooked. Therefore, if you feel chronically "sick all over," your doctor/healer may have overlooked candidiasis, gastrointestinal dysbiosis, or some other form of yeast-connected illness. Here are the health symptoms that most frequently occur in individuals who later test positive for some form of yeast-connected illness.

• Recurrent vaginal and urinary tract infections, prostatitis, allergies, food allergies, jock itch, athlete's foot, bronchitis, and arthritis.

• Feeling "spaced out" with brain fog or problems with concentration, memory, depression, or insomnia.

• Feelings of fatigue and exhaustion (chronic fatigue syndrome). Fungus/yeast-related illness is now recognized as a cofactor linked to childhood conditions of autism and attention deficit/hyperactivity disorder (ADD or ADHD).

• Recurrent gastrointestinal issues such as irritable bowel syndrome, gas, leaky gut syndrome, dysbiosis, constipation, diarrhea, bloating, abdominal and intestinal cramps, or heartburn.

• Hormonal disturbances, including premenstrual syndrome, menstrual irregularities, low sex drive, sugar cravings.

- Extreme sensitivities to chemicals and odors such as tobacco smoke, perfume, and colognes.

- Unusually dry skin, eczema, rashes, itching, and rectal itching.

A Typical Case

Here's a typical example of a client suffering from obvious fungal disease; she's a composite of numerous clients Linda has seen. Anne is a 32-year-old college-educated woman suffering from chronic vaginal yeast infections, digestive problems related to candidiasis, and what her doctor had rightly called chronic fatigue syndrome. However, even though he had affixed a name to her general malaise, he was unable to provide any long-lasting relief from her multiple symptoms. After a few years of this very frustrating and expensive process, a friend suggested that Anne see Linda. Although Anne was initially skeptical, she was also clear that she had reached the end of the line with her current doctor's standard allopathic medical approach.

Here's a brief overview of Anne's medical history and symptoms: Anne had, as she explained to Linda, lived her life "in the fast lane" during her twenties and was now paying an enormous price for it. Anne frequently felt exhausted and had little energy. Her chronic vaginal yeast infections were repeatedly treated with Monistat, an anti-fungal cream. However, when the condition reoccurred, her doctor decided to give her something stronger and prescribed Diflucan, an oral broad-spectrum anti-fungal. Although this temporarily got rid of the problem, her energy and life force continued to be zapped. A few months later the yeast infection returned again—this time with a vengeance.

Anne had been on birth control pills for over ten years. She was also the unwitting victim of a former boyfriend who gave her a sexually transmitted disease (STD), which was treated with antibiotics that further inflamed her yeast infection. Her periodic bladder infections and streptococcus infections were also treated with antibiotics.

Anne's medical problems contributed to the eventual breakup with her boyfriend, which, in turn, fueled negative feelings of worthlessness and despair. For relief from her bad luck with men, she turned to the same addictive comforts that had previously served her well in her twenties without health consequences. These included smoking pot, an increase in casual drinking, and a penchant for sweets and junk food.

This time, however, it was different. Anne began to put on weight, and her menses were becoming irregular. She soon experienced bloating, nausea, and stomachaches. Her doctor suggested taking Mylanta and, when that proved insufficient, prescribed a stronger antacid. Anne no longer enjoyed her demanding job as a legal secretary and wondered if she would ever get married and have babies. Most recently, her doctor had given her a prescription for Prozac and had recommended she see a psychiatrist. In effect, the doctor gave up.

Angelic Detective Work Reveals a Higher Level of Medical Truth

When Linda went through the pre-test, she was not surprised to find a venerable litany of cofactors affecting Anne. Anne was stunned and told Linda that her doctor had never suggested any of these items was part of her problem. They included:

Acid pH diet	Fungal proliferation	Nickel
Acid pH toxins	Gastrointestinal	Parasites
Brain parasites	dysbiosis	Psychological stress
Drug overdose	Heavy metals	Sugar overdose
Electromagnetic	Mercury	Uric acid buildup
pollution	Miasms	
Enzyme deficiency	Mineral deficiency	

After the pre-test, Linda drilled down into these various categories, which revealed additional layers of information. Here is a brief summary of Linda's assessment of Anne's overall health. (Many of the subjects discussed here are covered in subsequent chapters.)

Anne had seven old, deteriorating silver amalgam fillings in her teeth. The leakage of mercury amalgam vapors caused the terrain of her blood to turn highly acidic. In addition, the nickel backing on an old crown was also leaking, further exacerbating her heavy metal burden. Linda channeled that the mercury vapors had leached into various tissues, organs, and glands in her body, wreaking havoc in various ways.

The combination of mercury leaching from her fillings, drug toxins, and poor diet upset the applecart of her inner ecology. With so much acid and toxicity her body had become a breeding ground for fungi, molds, harmful bacteria, and parasites, all of which are known to thrive in an acidic terrain (see Chapters 6, 7, 10, and 12). Linda channeled that Anne was suffering from two different species of fungi—*Candida albicans* and *Aspergillus niger*—as well as parasite liver flukes and a low-level *E. coli* infection in her bladder. Her liver tested as the most stressed organ, which was caused by various drug toxins including Diflucan.

The byproducts of acidosis caused the proliferation of harmful bacteria which overwhelmed her beneficial flora, further weakening Anne's immune system. Healthy flora are vital to breaking down cellulose and preventing fermentation and putrefaction in the small intestines. So when beneficial flora are missing, a terrain change occurs that paves the way for a form of fungal disease called gastrointestinal dysbiosis.

Anne was also producing insufficient levels of hydrochloric acid and other digestive enzymes needed to assist in breaking down food. The resulting unhealthy intestinal mucosa effectively blocked the assimilation of beneficial minerals and metabolic products while allowing heavy metals to pass through. These metals, in turn, blocked normal oxidative processes and promoted free radicals. Even though Anne was becoming overweight, she was literally starved for beneficial vitamins and minerals, which could not permeate the dysbiosis lining her gastrointestinal tract.

Mercury and candida had leached into her kidneys and bladder and were certainly cofactors in the chronic infections in those areas. In fact, Linda channeled that mercury had spawned a general increase in free radicals throughout her system, which impacted her overall immune system and further exacerbated her chronic fatigue syndrome. Mercury had also leached into her thyroid and was a cofactor in the slowdown of her metabolic function and in creating a hypothyroid condition. In addition, mercury vapors had broken through her blood-brain barrier and were a cofactor in her mood swings, depression, and insomnia.

Other sources of toxicity contributed to the acid soup in her blood. These included marijuana, alcohol, birth control pills, and her highly acidic diet, loaded with too much sugar, coffee, meat, greasy cooking oils, trans fats, toxic food additives, and other horrors of overly processed food.

Linda explained to Anne that she indeed had fairly serious health issues for a woman in her early thirties, and her condition was certainly not psychosomatic. Linda channeled that it would be advisable to work with her doctor to wean off Prozac and replace it with amino acids and flower essences. Now it was time for a dose of medicinal "tough love." If she was truly sick and tired of being sick and tired, then she first had to have a major attitude adjustment that consisted of loving and nurturing herself. Part of accomplishing this goal entailed making the necessary proactive dietary and lifestyle changes needed to restore her inner ecology, detox the environmental poisons and candidiasis out of her body, and transform her negative emotions. If she was lazy about taking the remedies, sticking to an admittedly restrictive, customized anti-candida diet that Linda channeled, or gave in to her self-destructive habits, her health would never improve. Linda would provide very precise channeled guidance, but Anne had to make a real commitment to her health.

Problems with the Allopathic Model for Treating Candidiasis

Let us now examine the reasons why Anne's doctor had very little success in treating her multiple health problems. The primary flaws in the pharmaceutical approach her doctor used were:

• The inability to recognize that toxicity was the *real source* of Anne's problem. The doctor never once suggested that mercury amalgams, marijuana, alcohol, and birth control pills could be contributing factors to her multiple conditions. Perhaps he had no training in detoxification protocols. Anne had asked him about a book a friend had recommended called *The Yeast Connection* by Dr. William Crook, M.D., and her doctor dismissed it as a "fad," not supported by "real science." As far as he was concerned, no particular lifestyle changes were necessary, only drugs.

• The inability to consider a proactive approach to compensate for the well-known side effects of the antibiotics and birth control pills he had prescribed. How difficult would it have been for the doctor to advise Anne to take a potent probiotic to repopulate the beneficial flora destroyed in the bacterial "war of the worlds" so commonly associated with these drugs? Though her candidiasis had festered for months, the doctor's reactive method of fungal drug treatment only started when the problem reached a crisis. In addition, the doctor failed to recognize that prolonged history of drug therapy often makes the organisms resistant to the drug.

• The inability to recognize that Anne's vaginal yeast infection was not a localized phenomenon, but was also affecting her gastrointestinal tract and other organs. Monistat only worked on the vaginal infestation of candidiasis and did not address the problem in a systemic manner. While Diflucan did kill the fungus throughout her body, repeated usage of the drug had a toxic effect on her liver (hepatotoxicity). The doctor also did not take into account the need to eliminate the dead fungal/yeast organisms by the body's immune system, lymphatic system, and excretory organs. No wonder that after taking Diflucan, Anne suffered nausea and exhaustion—the pangs of what is called "fungal die-off" or Herxheimer reaction. Her medications that killed yeast caused a flu-like response that occurred as yeast cells died. Their mycotoxins and exoenzymes were expelled and then absorbed in her bloodstream. *As a result the fungus always returned because the true origins of the pathogens—heavy metal toxicity, antibiotics, birth control pills, an acidic diet and biological terrain, and negative emotions—were not being addressed.*

• The inability to recognize that leakage from old mercury amalgam fillings constituted a toxic burden that contributed to the acidic terrain of Anne's blood and bodily fluids. The doctor simply had no point of reference to understand that without changing her inner ecology through biological dentistry (see Chapter 12), diet, lifestyle changes, and supplements, it was almost impossible to achieve long-lasting healing results. The localized approach of only treating with Monistat as well as the broad-spectrum approach of Diflucan are metaphors for the medical model described in Chapter 2: the mosquito-infested swamp is dive-bombed by malathion instead of drained.

• The inability to recognize that sugar, breads, and fermented and acid-forming foods were the equivalent of pouring gas on the fire and that a highly alkalized diet is an absolute necessity in restoring the inner ecology to health.

THE DISCONNECT BETWEEN MAINSTREAM AND ALTERNATIVE APPROACHES IN DIAGNOSING FUNGAL DISEASE

We are not singling this particular doctor out for criticism. He is no better or worse than other doctors whose practice is based solely on the pharmaceutical model. It just that when it comes to treating candidiasis and chronic fatigue syndrome, the pharmaceutical approach is of limited value because of its one-dimensional nature. It does not address the principal biological reasons why Anne could not heal—toxicity and an acidic milieu. The thought process behind the pharmaceutical model goes no further than this—kill the fungus, plain and simple.

How can it be that the vast majority of pharmaceutically oriented doctors whose patients eventually turn to Linda are unable to successfully diagnose or treat the origins of fungal disease? Given that doctors are highly intelligent, highly educated people, where does the disconnect come from? There are several reasons for this.

• The majority of allopathic physicians do not attribute any of their patients' symptoms to candidiasis. This is why they are unable to treat the symptoms caused by it. That is also why the prominent University of California immunologist Dr. Alan Levin, M.D., estimates that one out of three people is adversely affected by candida.[3]

• Allopathic doctors who only treat infections with antibiotics and who only recommend birth control pills for their female clients invariably find that a significant percentage of those patients end up with the form of candidiasis known as vaginitis. One can only conclude that they operate under a belief system where side effects, such as candidiasis, are acceptable. According to a 2005 article by Carol Wilson in *Advanced Nursing Practice*, "Yeast infections affect 75 percent of American women during their reproductive years, and 40 to 50 percent of these women will endure recurrent episodes. . . ."[4] Linda is amazed at how few physicians even recommend something as simple and innocuous as beneficial probiotics (see Chapters 12 and 13) as a defense against candidiasis from antibiotics and birth control pills. It's common knowledge among most alternative practitioners that probiotics restore beneficial flora, promote the proper pH, and strengthen the immune system, all of which help control vaginitis.

• Allopathic doctors are generally not trained to diagnose the environmental origins of fungal disease, only to pharmaceutically treat the condition. They are simply unaware of the fact that the existence of fungi is usually symptomatic of a deeper malaise. The principal method of testing for fungi at traditional medical laboratories involves blood, urine, and stool tests, each of which has real limitations that make it difficult to understand what candida is really doing to the body. A blood antibody test is of limited value since a person with a highly compromised immune system no longer produces enough antibodies. A urine test is only applicable for localized infections. A stool test shows the presence of candida but does not demonstrate the immune system's reaction to it. In addition, none of these tests is concerned with issues of biological terrain. These are just some of the reasons why European experts such as Dr. Thomas Rau, M.D., medical director of the Paracelsus Clinic in Switzerland, believe that darkfield live blood cell analysis, a microscope approach not well understood in America, is necessary for practitioners to have a more complete picture of what is really going on.

AN ALTERNATIVE APPROACH TO DIAGNOSING FUNGAL DISEASE

Dr. Rau generally subscribes to the medical philosophies of Dr. Günther Enderlein, a brilliant German researcher who made the greatest contributions to the study of fungal forms through a biological construct he called pleomorphism, discussed in the next chapter. Dr. Enderlein devoted his career to the study of live blood through a microscopic universe that revealed an entirely new paradigm in microbiology. He utilized a darkfield microscope with a light condenser that illuminated objects from the side as opposed to a brightfield microscope that shined light directly through the sample. (See "The Diagnostic Advantages of Darkfield Microscopy.") The brightfield light can overwhelm the eye and tends to wash out objects seen with a darkfield scope. Fine microscopic structures are now visible to the human eye with a darkfield microscope that otherwise might be lost in the sea of light that normally flows through the eyepiece of a brightfield scope. The latest version of darkfield technology allows minute microscopic objects to be magnified up to 1,000 times and projected onto a video monitor. This lets the patient observe the results of this analysis, which glow against a black background (see www .biomedx.com).

The Diagnostic Advantages of Darkfield Microscopy

In an article from the Semmelweis-Institut in Germany entitled "The Value of Darkfield Microscopy," Dr. Rau writes, "Darkfield microscope investigation of living blood gives early reliable insights into tendencies of many different types of illnesses. It has proved itself over a number of years as a reliable and essential means of establishing a diagnosis and is an integral part of the doctor's assessment of the patient's regulatory ability. In this way of looking at biological holistic medicine, illness is not regarded as a phenomenon of an isolated disorder of an organ but as a disorder of a dynamic process of regulation which involves the whole organism . . . Like time-lapse photography, [darkfield microscopic investigation] can display the rate of tendency of the blood and its cells to degenerate better than any other test."[5]

A drop of fresh blood placed under a darkfield microscope provides valuable information needed to gauge overall health and the state of the immune system. It also reveals anomalies in the blood that relate to deficiencies in nutrients, dysfunctional bodily systems, and toxins in the body, specifically:

- The level of acid affecting the biological terrain that promotes the development of harmful microbes, including fungi, yeasts, molds, bacteria, viruses, and parasites.
- Possible vitamin, mineral, and trace mineral deficiencies.
- A lack of oxygen.
- The inability of the body to digest animal protein.
- The level of heavy metal toxicity.
- Indications of dysbiosis.
- Factors related to a predisposition to cardiovascular disease, kidney disease, and cancer.

I recall that in 1990, at the height of my illness, I read articles translated from German in *Explore* magazine about the incredible diagnostic virtues of darkfield live blood cell analysis and the work of Dr. Enderlein regarding chronic fatigue syndrome and heavy metal toxicity. It seemed logical to us that darkfield analysis might provide answers to these issues. Although we had done plenty of blood tests, no doctor had seriously suggested fungal disease as a cofactor in our illness. Prior to leaving for Germany in 1992 with Linda, I had searched in vain, unable to find anyone doing darkfield analysis of fungal forms in Los Angeles. Nobody at a large conventional laboratory associated with a prestigious local hospital had ever heard of darkfield live blood cell analysis, let alone the theory of pleomorphism. When I asked our doctors and lab technicians what they knew about the relationship of chronic fatigue syndrome to fungal forms like *Candida albicans* and *Aspergillus niger*, my question was greeted with a deafening silence.

Upon further research, we were stunned to find out that the government does not, in any meaningful way, endorse darkfield live blood cell analysis. Although it has been standard practice in Europe for almost 100 years, this technology is still considered "experimental" by our government bureaucracy. To be accepted, experimental protocols must be followed that include costly legal and business expenses needed to set up an Institutional Review Board (IRB) and receive special certification from CLIA (Clinical Laboratory Improvement Amendments). Obviously, meeting these requirements is beyond the reach of most practitioners. What this means to the American consumer is that our government health care system, for mysterious reasons, has decided it is best to make it difficult for alternative American health practitioners to have access to the same sophisticated diagnostic technology that their European counterparts have used for almost 100 years. In a manner similar to EAV, another key tool in the diagnostic process of German Biological Medicine has essentially been held hostage by bureaucratic meddling in the scientific process of discovery.

CHAPTER 6

Pleomorphism:
The Lost Chapter of Biology

All truths are easy to understand once they have been discovered;
the point is to discover them.
—GALILEO GALILEI

TO UNDERSTAND LINDA'S APPROACH to treating chronic degenerative disease involving all types of fungal infection and certain types of bacterial infections, it is necessary to undertake a brief historical review of scientific discoveries in microbiology that began in France in the 1800s and evolved in Germany with the theory of pleomorphism in the early 1900s. Only then can we appreciate how these brilliant theories and remedies were unfortunately relegated to the fringes of medicine. Pleomorphism challenges conventional medical thinking and standard methods used to treat illnesses associated with microbes. It strikes at the very core of basic medical belief—that germs cause disease.

At the outset, we must make clear that we are not referring to the transmission of acute infectious diseases from obvious external sources. These differ *significantly* from the development of chronic illnesses with no obvious cause. Pleomorphism claims these types of chronic conditions are caused by microbes in body fluids. Therefore, this discussion excludes sexually transmitted diseases (STDs), ingesting infected food and liquids (dysentery, typhus), nonsterile surgery or injections (hepatitis, HIV/AIDS), and infections from infected animals (malaria, rabies) and known airborne transmission (colds, flu, mumps, measles, tuberculosis, among others). As we know, health care practitioners treat people with contagious diseases without getting ill themselves. We offer a detailed explanation of why this occurs.

Our intention is to spur renewed interest in a valuable approach that slipped through the cracks in treating chronic disease caused by microbes. The urgency to do so is underscored by the fact that more people in the United

States now die from the mostly hospital-acquired staph infection (MRSA, methicillin resistant *Staphylococcus aureus*) than from AIDS![1] In an article in the February 2009 issue of *The New England Journal of Medicine* entitled "Antibiotic-Resistant Bugs in the 21st Century: A Clinical Super-Challenge," researchers at the University of Texas Medical School in Houston warn that people are dying from "superbugs" because our antibiotic arsenal has run dry, leaving the world without sufficient weapons to fight ever-changing bacteria.[2]

To set the stage, Dr. Kirk Slagel, N.M.D., M.Ed., Sanum therapy instructor for Biomed International, offers an analogy between pleomorphism and a normal process that occurs in nature where microbes facilitate breaking down debris into organic matter. "When a living organism is less healthy, it is more susceptible to opportunistic infections. Bacteria and fungi tend to increase in type and quantity and inhabit this organism more easily. Eventually, if the organism succumbs and dies, these microbiological components of nature break down the organism into basic organic matter. This organic matter is used as material for further growth of other life forms.

"The interesting point is when the macroorganism is less healthy or dying, there is an increase in opportunistic microorganisms such as bacteria and fungi only as long as there is material on which they may exist. Once the macroorganism has either returned to health or has died and is in the final stage of decaying organic matter, *the bacteria and fungi disappear. And this is where the mystery lies. Where do the increased number of bacteria and fungi come from and where do they go once the organism has decayed?*"[3]

Although we consider this process normal for the natural world, we think quite differently when it comes to illness, death, and our relationship with the microbe. This is due to the pharmaceutical axiom—the microbe always causes illness, which can only be treated with an antibiotic. The only goal is the eradication of harmful pathogens. However, this way of thinking short-circuits a basic medical debate: When illness develops, which came first, the microbe or the altered biological terrain that allowed the microbe to breed? Where does the microbe come from? The origin of these basic, unresolved questions dates back over 150 years!

HOW THE THEORY OF PLEOMORPHISM
WAS DISCARDED BY MAINSTREAM MEDICINE

In *Sick and Tired*, author Robert O. Young, Ph.D., reveals the sordid history of how theories that culminated in pleomorphism got lost in the shuffle of 20th century medical thought. He states that it "revolves around an all-too-common historical occurrence—the rejection of wisdom or scientific discovery in favor of a more popular, convenient, or politically desirable system."[4] As the teachings of Socrates and Galileo so aptly demonstrate, this is hardly the first time in the history of science that higher truths have been intentionally disregarded. Nor is it probably the last.

To understand how these higher medical truths which have influenced Linda's approach to treating chronic degenerative conditions were conveniently swept under the rug, we must review this lost chapter of biology. It involves three medical researchers: Claude Bernard, Antoine Béchamp, and Günther Enderlein, who all suffered the same fate as they struggled against scientific and economic prejudices to explain their discoveries.

In the mid-1800s French physiologist Claude Bernard (1813–1878) developed his theories of biological terrain. Antoine Béchamp, a professor at French universities in Montpellier, Strasbourg, and Lille (1816–1908), subsequently expanded on this in his theory of microzymas, a direct contrarian point of view to the germ theory of chemist and businessman Louis Pasteur (1822–1895). Pasteur's shrewd ability at public relations steamrolled over the complicated and esoteric Bernard/Béchamp approach, causing his germ theory of disease to become the dominant force in microbiology and pharmaceutical medicine. Günther Enderlein (1872–1968), a German microbiologist and zoologist, used the Bernard/Béchamp theories to further develop the theory of pleomorphism. This proved to be the springboard that launched his brilliant homeopathic remedies.

The origin of the controversy goes back to a series of acrimonious debates between Louis Pasteur and Antoine Béchamp, which threatened the status quo of the burgeoning pharmaceutical industry. *The importance of Pasteur's triumph over Béchamp in shaping the future direction of medicine cannot be underestimated. It determines how we think about the origin and cure of disease as well as how billions of dollars are spent annually on scientific research and are reaped in pharmaceutical profits.* However, prior to delving into this historical/medical/public relations' debacle, we must first explore the essential concept of biological terrain contributed by Claude Bernard.

Claude Bernard and Biological Terrain

In Chapter 2 we introduced biological terrain as a core concept in Linda's philosophy of healing and detoxification protocols. The following analogy bears repeating: Suppose you have a swarm of mosquitoes in a swamp. The two ways to eliminate it are to dive-bomb the swamp with a pesticide like malathion that kills everything or drain the swamp. Then, the mosquitoes have no place to breed and die off. Understanding pleomorphism involves an awareness of how an acidic milieu breeds unhealthy pathogenic forms. This approach to the origin of illness is often at odds with conventional medicine.

Claude Bernard understood that much disease was primarily related to the body's underlying milieu, not to germs or pathogens. He originated a new understanding of the relationship between the biological terrain and the microbe. He believed that an unhealthy milieu led to an accumulation of toxins at the cellular level. He observed that the biological terrain undergoes various changes due to an imbalanced diet, stress, and internal and external toxins. These changes lead to disease by creating systemic weakness, which decreases the body's ability to function. The changes accumulate in the fluid and tissues around the cells and alter their natural pH balance, causing them to become more acidic. This promotes the growth and development of opportunistic microbes like bacteria and fungi, which Bernard believed arose from this altered milieu. Some microbial forms such as candida are normally present but can proliferate under acidic conditions. This is akin to the normal process in nature where debris accumulates and microbes facilitate breaking it down into organic matter.

Pasteur Versus Béchamp: How Science Wilted under the Pressure of Salesmanship and Economics

Although Pasteur was a distinguished chemist, he had no degree in the life sciences. Nevertheless, he realized his grandiose scientific aspirations by virtue of being a successful business entrepreneur and banker (see Figure 6-1). In contrast, Béchamp was a distinguished doctor, research scientist, and teacher with advanced degrees in medicine, pharmacy, chemistry, and physics (see Figure 6-2). Considered one of the brightest scientists of the 19th century, Béchamp attained so many scientific achievements that when he died, it took eight pages in a scientific journal to list them all!

In her book *Béchamp or Pasteur? A Lost Chapter in the History of Biology*, Ethel Douglas Hume claims that Pasteur "repeatedly plagiarized Béchamp's work, distorted it, and submitted it to the French Academy of Science as his own!"[5] Apparently, the source of Pasteur's rivalry with Béchamp stemmed from the fact that Béchamp did research that saved the French silk industry from devastation by silkworms, even though Pasteur had been commissioned by the industry to solve it! The personal and professional jealousy that arose

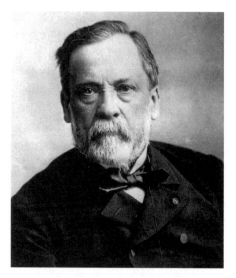

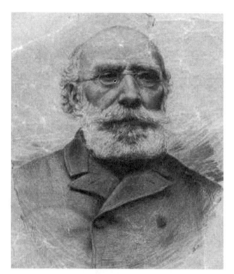

Figure 6-1. Louis Pasteur.   Figure 6-2. Antoine Béchamp.
Used with permission of Getty Images.
Photographer: Popperfoto. Collection: Popperfoto.

from this soon blossomed into hatred. Pasteur's personal vendetta to discredit and destroy Béchamp might only be an interesting historical footnote if not for the fact that it set the stage for the battle over the germ theory of disease—the very foundation of modern medicine! Béchamp responded by calling Pasteur's theory "monstrous." The war was on.

Refusing to acknowledge the relevance of biological terrain, Pasteur subscribed to the idea that microbes always maintained the same fixed form, monomorphism (mono = one, morphism = forms), as opposed to the concept of microbes changing forms, pleomorphism (pleo = many, morphism = forms). He believed that microbes, which somehow came from external sources and invaded the body, were the principal cause of infectious disease. Yet he never provided any real information about the origin of the actual germs. Sickness, he believed, was due to chance. It was the job of medicine to defend humanity against fate by declaring war against microbes.

To his credit, Pasteur was the first to recommend that milk should be heated to kill germs through his process of pasteurization. This technology brought him considerable wealth and influence that allowed him to focus on other financially rewarding opportunities in medicine. French government public health policy now focused on a cure for infectious diseases. Using often unethical methods, Pasteur focused on developing vaccines for the pharmaceutical industry.[6]

Meanwhile, Béchamp researched the nature of fermentation, a process involving chemical reactions that split complex compounds into simple substances in the absence of oxygen. He believed this process led to an increase in the pathological microorganisms associated with disease. Béchamp observed that molds, which are fungoid growths that break down organic matter, were formed by a collection of tiny fermented granulations. He isolated and named them microzymas. Béchamp believed that these granulations, which are smaller than single-cell organisms, could, under certain conditions, evolve into single-cell bacteria. Therefore, cells could no longer be regarded as the basic units of life. Even more astonishing, these microzymas were indestructible as all Béchamp's efforts to kill them failed.

Béchamp's theory of microzymas states that the microzyma is an independent living element capable of multiplying. Microzymas exist within cells, the fluid between cells, the blood, and the lymph. They function as a builder of organisms at the inception of the life process and a facilitator of decay within the death process. According to Dr. Young, "Béchamp saw the life process as a continual cellular breakdown by microzymian fermentation—even in a healthy body."[7] However, when the biological terrain is in an unhealthy state of acidosis, according to Béchamp, a fermentation process involving either alcohol or lactic acid is accelerated. The microzymas become disturbed and change their form and function, evolving into newly developed microscopic forms: bacteria, yeasts, fungi, and molds! Young also notes that "they reflect the disease and produce the symptoms."[8]

In his masterwork *The Blood* (1908), Béchamp wrote: "I am able to assert that the microzyma is at the commencement of all [biological] organization. Since microzymas in dead bacteria are also living, it follows that they are also the living end of all organizations, living beings of a special category without analogue.... [Microzymas] carry in themselves the elements essential for life, or for disease, for destruction and for death. . . . Our cells, as can constantly be observed, are being continuously destroyed by means of a fermentation very analogous to that which follows death."[9] An interesting aside is that Béchamp's concept of microzymas coincides nicely with the biblical commentary that "from dust you are made and to dust you shall return" (Genesis 3:19).

An example of how radically different the theories of Pasteur and Béchamp are is how each man explained the souring process that happens quickly when fresh milk is not refrigerated. Béchamp taught that milk is a living nutritive medium containing germs when it comes out of the cow. Shortly after a cow is milked, the milk contains a few thousand germs, which are quickly transformed into bacteria. An hour later that number has multiplied to tens of thousands. Several hours later there are hundreds of thousands. It is through a natural metabolic process that these bacteria are able to cause fermentation of milk.

Pasteur had a completely contrarian view. He taught that in its natural state, milk is completely germ-free, and germs from the outer world are transported via currents in the air into the milk. When the milk goes sour, it is because germs, principally bacteria, have crept into the milk. Because Pasteur masterfully promoted his pasteurization process, both industry and the public blindly accepted his explanation about why it worked.

Dr. Young observes: "Pasteur made his theories seem correct by promoting the practice of injecting animals...[using] preparations made from the diseased tissues of previously sick animals, thus making the injected ones sick. This gave the appearance that a germ caused a disease, when in fact these preparations were extremely poisonous. This is not a scientific procedure, but simply demonstrates the fact that you can make someone sick by poisoning his or her blood. The attentive reader will see the errors here: First, Pasteur was confusing disease with its symptoms. Second, the method of injection can by no means be said to duplicate a natural 'infection.' Based on his theory of microzymas, Béchamp warned emphatically against such direct and artificial invasion of the blood."[10] In the final analysis, the problem of what theory to believe can be summed up with the old adage: Within every lie there is some truth; otherwise no one would believe it.

Pasteur maintained that only unchanging and external germs in the air were the cause of disease. While Béchamp never denied that certain diseases such as influenza occurred this way, he steadfastly held to the view that these airborne forms were not the only way that disease could occur and that the body literally "grows its own" under adverse milieu conditions.

Pasteur's real genius was a flare for self-promotion and public relations. Béchamp's devotion to scientific integrity proved no match for his nemesis. No matter how flawed his ideas, Pasteur's pervasive influence and salesmanship were economically in step with the burgeoning pharmaceutical industry. Béchamp's approach to biological terrain management that achieved wellness through slower acting natural methods fell out of favor. Little concern was paid to the diet and lifestyle of the patient, while surgeries and expensive drugs with often serious side effects were advanced as the only way to cure all manner of disease.

However, it appears that Pasteur must have carried guilt in his heart that both Bernard and Béchamp were correct. It has been reliably documented that on Pasteur's deathbed in 1895, he recanted, declaring, *"Claude Bernard was right . . . The microbe is nothing, the terrain is everything."*[11] However, by this time the die was cast. There was no going back for his followers in the scientific establishment or in the pharmaceutical companies. Thus, the monomorphic viewpoint prevailed over the pleomorphic.[12]

Pasteur's dominance set the direction of almost all subsequent microbial research. It is obvious that there have been great advantages with modern antibiotics that have saved countless lives in times of war and peace. However, since the microbes are now outsmarting the antibiotics, a growing number of researchers believe that the antibiotics' model is a dead end for future research. We are at a crossroads where a fresh approach must be found. The time is ripe for a reexamination of pleomorphism.

The Next Chapter: Enderlein and Pleomorphism

In Pasteur's monomorphism, a microbial species is rigidly fixed in its structure and function. For example, a staphylococcal organism is always a staphylococcal organism. In pleomorphism, Dr. Günther Enderlein came to the completely opposite conclusion: microbial species are not fixed but are stages in the growth cycle of different life forms (see Figure 6-3). His darkfield microscope research (see Chapter 5) revealed that the origins and cycles of microorganisms can abruptly change from a harmless and benign form to a virulent pathogen. Dr. Enderlein's research greatly expanded upon Bernard's and Béchamp's concept that microbes go through cycles where they advance and ultimately decline in pathogenicity based on the biological terrain. (Pathogenicity is the ability of an organism to produce an infectious disease in another organism. It's often used interchangeably with the term "virulence" to describe the degree of damage done by a pathogen, which is any infectious agent such as bacteria, fungi, viruses, or parasites that cause disease.)

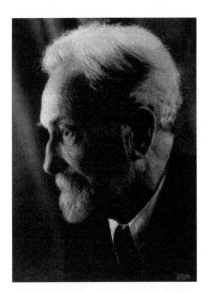

Figure 6-3. Dr. Günther Enderlein.

In his landmark book *Bacteria Cyclogeny* (1925), Dr. Enderlein revealed his main discoveries from research on typhus in 1916. His central thesis was that a primal microbial form that he called an endobiont exists within every red blood cell (erythrocyte) of humans and all mammals. The endobiont is a tiny biological unit of life from which other microorganisms emanate. It is subject to a variation in form through changes in the biological terrain. Dr. Enderlein called the basic visible stage a "protit," which was conceptually similar to Béchamp's microzyma. Dr. Enderlein believed that all diseases were related to the evolution and pathogenic development of the primordial endobiont into parasitic growth forms. These forms have their own metabolism with their own toxic metabolites, such as D-lactic acid, which in turn can poison the terrain of the host organism.

Dr. Enderlein coined the term "cyclogeny" (cyklos = circle; genos = birth) to describe the evolution of the endobiont through a complete cycle that occurs when the biological terrain warrants it. The higher the endobiont rises through its development cycle, the more toxic it becomes. The process starts when an overly acidic terrain causes the harmless early-stage protits to begin an upward development cycle that evolves into higher disease-causing forms that include bacteria, fungi, and molds.

Dr. Enderlein believed that a high consumption of animal fats, proteins, and refined sugars triggers the harmless protits' upward development cycle into higher toxic microbial forms. These induce an anaerobic environment, which causes the fermentation process described by Béchamp. This, in turn, produces harmful lactic acids and oils that poison the body. Linda likens this process to a person having an internal mini-brewery producing lactic acid and yeast.

Persistent fermentation saturates the body with acid. This acid excess is then deposited in different body tissues, upsetting the normal acid-alkaline balance, which contributes to many forms of chronic degenerative disease, ranging from arthritis to ulcers.[13] Dr. Enderlein also identified other toxic cofactors responsible for the acidic degradation of the terrain, including heavy metals, radiation, and certain pharmaceutical drugs as well as other chemical substances in the environment. In order to shift an acidic terrain toward a more healing environment, Linda recommends a highly alkaline diet, rich in leafy greens, for clients with advanced levels of fungal disease.

Dr. Enderlein noted that the highly toxic microbes may revert back to the original harmless protit phase in one and/or two therapeutic ways:

1. There is a shift toward an alkaline terrain through diet and lifestyle modification.

2. The person uses specialized homeopathic remedies discussed later in this chapter.

According to Dr. Enderlein, two types of primordial endobionts become fungi: *Mucor racemosus* and *Aspergillus niger*. Dr. Enderlein used these fungal forms to create the foundational medicines in his repertoire of homeopathic remedies (see discussion below).

We are aware that the idea that one species of pathogen under certain adverse terrain conditions can change into another species—bacterium into yeast, yeast to fungus, fungus to mold—will strike many microbiologists as medical heresy! Although further research is needed to prove whether Dr. Enderlein's radical explanation is correct, *we agree and do not support this aspect of the theory*. We are, however, convinced that other, less-controversial aspects of his theories on degenerative diseases are correct. We know toxicity creates an acidic milieu that becomes the breeding ground for many different types of pathogens including harmful bacteria, fungi, parasites, and viruses. It is important to remember that the bulk of Dr. Enderlein's theories were formulated before the discovery of DNA and other modern, universally accepted methods of cell analysis. Yet, the experience of internationally respected doctors such as Dr. Thomas Rau, as well as Linda's astonishing level of clinical success, attests that an incredibly effective, safe healing process is occurring, even if we do not understand all the mechanisms behind it. While the dispute rages on over Dr. Enderlein's theories, Linda remains unwilling to throw the baby out with the bathwater.

HOW LINDA TREATS FUNGAL AND BACTERIAL DISEASE WITH GERMAN BIOLOGICAL MEDICINE

Two small German companies, Sanum-Kehlbeck and SanPharma, manufacture incredibly effective homeopathic products based on the work of Dr. Enderlein, which are distributed in America. In our opinion, the track record of these remedies, backed by clinical studies in healing candidiasis and other fungal disorders, is unmatched in terms of efficacy and safety. At the end of the day, nobody knows exactly why these remedies developed by Dr. Enderlein work. *We just know that they work beautifully*. Since Linda's focus is healing, her most obvious concerns are issues of safety and efficacy. We are unaware of any practitioners whose patients have ever had any harmful side effects from these remedies.

Dr. Enderlein's premise was that his homeopathic fungal remedies worked by supplying the body with beneficial protits. This promoted a degradation response between these protits and the higher pathogenic forms, reverting them back to lower, harmless forms that normally exist. Dr. Haefeli claimed they assisted antibodies produced by the immune system.[14] Thus, the body's natural defenses are supported and restored, promoting gentle self healing. According to the *Isopathic/Homeopathic Materia Medica*, these remedies work by normalizing "the equilibrium between the endobiont and the organism."

Under the guidance and direction of Dr. Thom Lobe, Linda has treated specific types of fungal and minor bacterial infections with either Sanum or SanPharma products, along with an alkalized anti-fungal diet and other detoxification protocols, with great success. The reduction and elimination of fungal forms is a key, ongoing component of almost all detoxification programs that Linda designs. Only occasionally does she find the need to augment with other natural products such as grapefruit seed extract, caprylic acid, pau d'arco, enzyme blends, aged garlic, and colloidal silver in conjunction with the pleomorphic remedies. However, probiotics are almost always needed to replenish beneficial flora, which have been radically diminished by candida.

Virtually all the clients Linda sees who have chronic fatigue syndrome and/or heavy metal toxicity have a significant level of fungal proliferation. Although Linda quite regularly treats *Candida albicans*, other forms of fungi are equally dangerous. The most prevalent are *Mucor racemoses, Aspergillus niger,* and *Penicillium chrysogenum,* which in their remedy form are used clinically to support the treatment of the following conditions:

• *Candida albicans* occurs naturally in the intestines without causing any damage. However, when the immune system is weakened from antibiotic overuse or chronic mercury amalgam leakage or other heavy metal exposure, candida spreads throughout the intestines and penetrates into other organs. The immune system is compromised due to acidosis and toxemia, resulting in a myriad of symptoms. Candida can cause such conditions as gas, bloating, food allergies, brain fog, memory issues, headaches, vaginitis, prostatitis, respiratory infections, skin infections, athlete's foot, earaches, gingivitis, sinusitis, and endocrine imbalances with blood sugar dysregulation.

• *Mucor racemoses* affects blood viscosity and red/white blood cells. It is often found in many diseases of the cardiovascular and circulatory systems. The formation of many blood clots falls within its life cycle. As a result, in its remedy form, the *Mucor racemoses* fungus helps to dismantle coagulation, increase oxygen, and open up blocked passageways. Linda contends that people who consume an overabundance of animal protein tend to develop this fungal form. She says, "Too much meat or dairy feed *Mucor racemoses.*"

• *Aspergillus niger* is usually associated with diseases affecting connective tissue, the respiratory system, skin, digestive organs, and tuberculosis miasms (Chapter 8). These include such conditions as asthma, bronchial infection, eczema, and arthritis, as well as prostate, urological, and genital infections. This fungal form often settles in the lymphatic system and the joints.

• *Penicillium chrysogenum* is a fungus often associated with bacterial inflammation. As a remedy, it is known to support the treatment of streptococci, staphylococci, and other bacterial infections. These bacteria are often associated with acute infections including earaches, dental issues, respiratory infections, strep throat, scarlet fever, rheumatic fever, urinary tract infections, and pus-causing diseases.

An Interesting Adjunct to Antibiotics

The Sanum-Kehlbeck Company manufactures Sanukehl remedies, a line of complementary homeopathic products that are highly useful following treatment with antibiotics prescribed by a medical doctor. They make the conventional process of using antibiotics safer and more efficacious.

It is well known that certain microbial forms of bacteria and fungi produce toxic proteins called antigens. In order to protect themselves from their own toxins, these microbes produce polysaccharides (large complex carbohydrate molecules), which can be thought of as antigen absorbers that bind themselves to toxic protein antigens, rendering them harmless to the microbe. However, in people with compromised immune systems, these toxins can remain after a pathogen has been eliminated by antibiotics. These toxins can become irritants causing inflammatory processes or reoccurring symptoms. Unless eliminated, they can eventually become cofactors in various chronic degenerative conditions.

Sanukehl remedies contain haptens, partial nontoxic antigens derived from polysaccharides of certain bacteria or fungi. By itself, a hapten is incapable of producing an immune response. However, by attaching itself to a larger toxic protein antigen that has remained in the body, it becomes a complete antigen called an epitope, which is recognized by the immune system. This stimulates a cellular immune response by activating T-lymphocytes, which then completely eliminate these bacterial toxins.[15]

CHAPTER 7

Parasites: Stealth Marauders of Disease

The healer's job has always been to release something not
understood, to remove obstructions . . . between the sick patient
and the force of life driving obscurely toward wholeness.
—ROBERT O. BECKER

ALTHOUGH THE CENTERS FOR DISEASE Control and Prevention (CDC) acknowledge the reality of parasite infestation, the CDC does not see fit to include it in the section on their website entitled "Top 20 at CDC.gov." This is amazing considering that Linda detects some level of parasite infestation in at least 40 percent of her clients! She commonly finds parasite disease in people suffering from such environmental toxins as heavy metals, chemicals, electromagnetic pollution, drugs, and/or chronic fatigue syndrome (CFS).

How widespread are intestinal parasites in America? According to medical researcher Ann Louise Gittleman, M.S., C.N.S, "At least 48 states have fought measurable outbreaks. And a study in *The American Journal of Tropical Medicine and Hygiene* found that 32 percent of a nationally representative sample of 2,896 people tested positive for infections."[1] Even the CDC's most recent statistics bear out the notion that parasite infestation has reached epidemic proportions in the United States today:

• "*Trichomonas* is the most common parasitic infection in the United States, accounting for an estimated 7.4 million cases per year.

• "*Giardia* and *Cryptosporidium* are estimated to cause 2 million and 300,000 infections annually in the United States, respectively. Cryptosporidiosis is the most frequent cause of recreational water-related disease outbreaks in the United States, causing multiple outbreaks each year.

• "There are an estimated 1.5 million new *Toxoplasma* infections and 400 to 4,000 cases of congenital toxoplasmosis in the United States each year; 1.26 million persons in this country have ocular involvement due to toxoplasmosis; and toxoplasmosis is the third leading cause of deaths due to food-borne illnesses (375+ deaths)."[2]

The sources of parasites range from agricultural runoff, outdated water-treatment systems, imported food, sexually transmitted disease, international travel, and overuse of antibiotics. These factors have dramatically increased our exposure and susceptibility to these microscopic invaders. For instance, parasites could come from an influx of *Giardia lamblia* found in dairy cow manure in upstate New York that winds its way through agricultural runoff into tributaries of the Hudson River that flows down to New York City. It could affect the surfer in Malibu through runoff from storm drains. It may be in the crop of strawberries coming from Mexico. It may be at your local sushi restaurant. It may be from your sexual partner.

Dr. Omar M. Amin, Ph.D., a professor of parasitology at Arizona State University and founder of the Parasitology Center Inc., is a recognized international authority with more than 130 major publications and books on parasitology. Here is what he says about the pandemic proportions of parasite infestation in the United States today: "If you think that, in the United States, we are safe from such third-world infections, then you are greatly misinformed. Some estimate that about 50 million American children are infected with worm parasites, only a small portion of which are detected and reported. This is particularly worrisome when one recognizes that microscopic, single-celled protozoans make up about 90 percent of all parasitic infections in the United States, according to the CDC. If existing parasitic infections are evenly distributed, there would be more than enough parasites for every living person to have one."[3]

A common misconception exists among both physicians and the general public that parasite infestations principally occur in tropical third-world countries where poor hygiene practices and malnutrition are commonplace. The lack of awareness of the risk factors associated with parasites has made them a silent epidemic. As Ann Louise Gittleman writes in her excellent guide for the layperson entitled *Guess What Came to Dinner?* "American doctors and other health professionals have had so little training with parasitic diseases that they are not alert to clinical symptoms . . . The physician's lack of suspicion and concurrent underdiagnosis has left the public totally unaware of the scope of the parasite problem . . . Estimates suggest that by the year 2025 more than half our planet's 8.3 billion inhabitants will be infected with a parasitic disease. No longer solely a third-world problem, virtually every type of exotic parasitic disease has been found on our shores."[4]

Everyone—physicians and patients alike—needs to know the full range of chronic health problems that can result from this epidemic. Parasite infections compromise our immune system, digestive tract, lungs, liver, brain, and heart as well as other organ systems. They can cause chronic fatigue, leaky gut syndrome, dysbiosis (imbalance of the intestinal bacteria), irritable bowel syndrome, diarrhea, fibromyalgia, sleeping disorders, ulcerative colitis, allergies, sexually transmitted diseases, and many other diseases. Some forms of parasites are detected in blood, urine, or feces. Other forms of amoebas like *Giardia lamblia* are transmitted in cyst form and can exist in that larval stage for up to six months under fingernails, in the brain, spinal cord, eyes, heart, bones, or skin. More than fifty types of parasites can infect organs and tissues in the body.

WHAT PARASITES DO IN THE BODY

Gittleman describes the many ways that parasites can wreak serious hidden havoc in the body:

• "Parasites destroy cells in the body faster than cells can be regenerated, thereby creating an imbalance that results in ulceration, perforation, or anemia.

• "They produce toxic substances that are harmful to the body. In cases of chronic infection, the body's immune response can be pushed into overdrive, producing elevated levels of eosinophils. These are specialized white blood cells that normally combat any microscopic pathogen, but when their level is elevated, they themselves can cause tissue damage that results in pain and inflammation.

• "The presence of parasites irritates the tissues of the body, inducing an inflammatory reaction on the part of the host.

• "Some parasites invade the body by penetrating the skin, producing dermatitis. During their developmental stage, other parasites perforate and damage the intestinal lining.

• "The size and/or weight of parasitic cysts, particularly if they are located in the brain, spinal cord, eye, heart, or bones, produces pressure effects on these organs. Obstruction particularly of the intestine and pancreatic and bile ducts can also occur.

• "The presence of parasites depresses immune system functioning while activating the immune system response. This can eventually lead to immune system dysfunction."[5]

Hulda Clark, the author of the controversial book *A Cure for All Cancers*, contends that there is a link between parasite disease and certain forms of cancer. When Linda asked her angelic guides if parasite infestation can be a precursor to cancer, she was told that this is one of many potential triggers that can promote cancer in the body. That's why it is expeditious to treat parasite infestations quickly.

HOW LINDA ANALYZES PARASITE DISEASE

Here's how Linda uses Metaphysical Systems Engineering to drill down to get very detailed levels of information. If Linda finds parasites in a client's pre-test, several questions now arise:

• What is the location of the parasite infestation in the body? After scanning the extended anatomy section with her pendulum, Linda channels the infestation is in the liver.

• What is the severity of the parasite infestation? Linda takes a baseline measurement and determines the parasite load is at 35 percent. This is a fairly serious degree of infestation that demands immediate treatment.

Linda now turns to the Parasite Analysis Chart shown in Table 7-1 (see page 96) and writes the word "Liver" in the space for "Organ in circuit." This psychically alerts the angels to focus specifically on all information concerning parasites in the liver. By now the client is getting concerned. After all, his family physician never mentioned anything about parasites. Although the client is in poor health, his bowel movements are normal. How could he possibly have parasites?

Linda goes through the chart and determines, for example, that the client has liver flukes, a type of trematoda called *Clonorchis sinensis*. She then goes to "Causal Factors" and channels the words "fish" and "raw food." Before she can say anymore, the client, suspecting the worst, blurts out, "Don't tell me it's from sushi! I eat it at least twice a week at this trendy sushi bar in Beverly Hills. It's one of my favorite foods." Linda then relays the bad news; the culprit is indeed sushi. When the client wants to know which of his symptoms are due to parasites, Linda reveals: "That's why you're anemic and feel tired all the time. Your liver issues, in turn, are affecting your gastrointestinal tract and colon."

LINDA'S ADDITIONAL OBSERVATIONS ON PARASITE DISEASE

If the client seeks verification of her findings, Linda recommends that a doctor order a lab-purged stool test for parasite infestation like that from Genova Diagnostics. While the Genova Diagnostics test is accurate in determining the presence of parasites in the digestive tract, intestine, and colon, it may be of only limited value in determining whether parasite infestation exists in the liver, brain, or elsewhere in the body. Linda may also channel other tests involving blood, saliva, urine, CT scan, biopsy, and cultures.

Acute parasite infestation can be successfully treated by antibiotics. If the degree of severity is as high as the previous example, there is no choice but to call for antibiotics. In such cases, Linda will immediately refer the client to a medical doctor who, after conducting the appropriate tests, can prescribe Flagyl or something similar. However, sometimes Flagyl causes severe side effects. According to the *Physicians Desktop Reference*, this may include seizures, abdominal cramps, constipation, diarrhea, headache, loss of appetite, nausea, upset stomach, vomiting, irritation or discharge from the vagina, and numbness or tingling in the arms, legs, hands, and feet.

Obviously, it's preferable to treat this condition naturally, if possible. If Linda channels that parasites can be successfully treated by something other than antibiotics, she will channel the best remedy to facilitate a cure for that client from a list of herbal and homeopathic remedies. Linda has had an incredible success rate using this approach. She also believes that detoxification and dietary alkalization are important in helping to abate parasite proliferation. Although parasites may enter the body in a myriad of different ways, they thrive in the same acidic biological terrain that causes the proliferation of fungi. This is why Linda refers to the pair as "traveling buddies." The underlying milieu of acidosis of the blood is the same biological pre - requisite needed for both parasites and fungi to thrive in different parts of the body.

TABLE 7-1. PARASITE ANALYSIS CHART
Organ in Circuit:

SYMPTOMS

Abdominal distention	Diarrhea	Liver enlarged	Eczema
Abdominal pain	Dysentery	Lymphatic swelling	Hives/rash
Allergy	Fever	Mucus	Itchy dermatitis
Anemia	Gas and bloating	Muscle aches	Papular lesions
Asthma	GI distress	Myocarditis	Sores
Bloody stools	Granuloma	Nervousness	Swellings
Chills	Headache	Orbital edema	Sleep disturbance
Chronic fatigue	Immune dysfunction	Penis discharge	Spleen enlarged
Constipation	Irritable bowel	Pneumonia	Teeth grinding
Convulsions	syndrome	Prostatic secretion	Vaginal discharge
Corneal ulcers	Joint pain	Skin conditions	Weight loss
Cough	Kidney/bladder swelling	Cutaneous ulcers	

CAUSAL FACTORS

Animals	Housefly	Food preparation	Sexual contact
Birds	Mosquito	Fruits	Swimming
Cats	Sand fly	Pork	Travel
Dogs	Other	Poultry	Water contamination
Farm animals	Wild animals	Raw food	Workplace issues
Cattle	Animal waste	Restaurant	Agriculture
Horse	Antibiotics	Vegetables	Daycare centers
Poultry	Food	Heavy metal toxins	Immigrants
Swine	Beef	Immunosuppressive	Meat packing
Other	Berries	drug	Military
Insects	Eggs	Poor hygiene habits	Other
Flea	Fish	Sewage leaks	

COMMON SPECIES OF PARASITES/DISEASES

Protozoa (Amoeba)	*Cyclospora*	*Trypanosoma*	Flagellate diarrhea
Acanthamoeba	*cayetanensis*	*gambiense*	*Giardia lamblia*
Balantidium coli	*Dientamoeba fragilis*	*Trypanosoma*	Intestinal amebiasis
Blastocystis hominis	*Entamoeba coli*	*rhodesiense*	*Entamoeba histolytica*
Cryptosporidium muris	*Entamoeba hartmanni*	Amebic hepatitis	*Endolimax nana*
Cryptosporidium	African sleeping	Amebic liver abscess	Interstitial brain
parvum	sickness	*Entamoeba histolytica*	pneumonia

COMMON SPECIES OF PARASITES/DISEASES (continued)			
Naegleria sp.	**Cestoda**	*Mansonella ozzardi*	Trichinella
Leishmania	Beef tapeworm	*Mansonella perstans*	*Trichinella spiralis*
braziliensis	*Taenia saginata*	*Mansonella*	
Leishmania donovani	Dog tapeworm	*streptocerca*	**Trematoda**
Leishmania tropica	*Dipylidium caninum*	*Onchocerca volvulus*	Blood fluke
Malaria	Fish tapeworm	*Wuchereria bancrofti*	*Schistosoma*
Plasmodium	*Diphyllobothrium*	Fish Roundworm	*haematobium*
falciparum	*latum*	Anisakine larvae	*Schistosoma*
Plasmodium malariae	Pork tapeworm	Hookworm	*japonicum*
Plasmodium ovale	*Taenia solium*	*Necator americanus*	*Schistosoma mansoni*
Plasmodium vivax		*Ancylostoma*	Intestinal fluke
Pneumonia (parasitic)	**Nematoda**	*duodenale*	*Fasciolopsis buski*
Pneumocystis carinii	Dog heartworm	Pinworm	Liver fluke
Rheumatoid arthritis	*Dirofilaria immitis*	*Enterobius*	*Clonorchis sinensis*
Giardia lamblia	Dog/ cat roundworm	*vermicularis*	Oriental lung fluke
Toxoplasmosis	*Toxocara canis*	Roundworm	*Paragonimus*
Toxoplasma gondii	*Toxocara cati*	*Ascaris lumbricoides*	*westermani*
Trichomonas	Filaria	Strongyloides	Sheep liver fluke
Trichomonas	*Brugia malayi*	*Strongyloides*	*Fasciola hepatica*
vaginalis	*Loa loa*	*stercoralis*	

Testimonial: Maria's dramatic weight loss

Maria had trained to be a ballet dancer and had been actively doing Pilates for many years. Her workout program consisted of doing Pilates three days a week and weight training two days a week, with frequent jogging and use of a rebounder. She worked as a hydrocolon therapist and always prided herself on having a high awareness of what constituted a healthy diet and lifestyle.

In her early forties, Maria unexpectedly experienced a rapid weight gain—17 unwanted pounds!—as well as chronic fatigue, chronic kidney/ bladder infections with blood in her urine, frequent urination, and brain fog— all for no apparent reason. (See "Are Parasites Making You Fat?") Maria had not changed her lifestyle or experienced menopause. She had been in a happy, committed, long-term relationship and was unaware of any emotional reason that would contribute to her condition, which was now making her depressed and lowering her energy and motivation.

Still Maria was not a quitter and suspected that she might have a thyroid problem. She decided to be proactive and sought out a medical specialist in Beverly Hills who had been recommended to her. After completing a battery of tests, she was confounded when the tests, which included a thyroid panel, came back negative. She stayed under the doctor's care for a year, during which he prescribed various supplements and rounds of antibiotics to treat her chronic infections. However, her condition continued to deteriorate.

During this time Maria decided to revamp her exercise routine and hired a high-priced personal trainer who put her on a five-day-a-week workout. She was put on a fairly restrictive diet of 1,200 to 1,500 calories a day, which consisted of healthy vegetable and fruit salads, a little fish, no sugar, and water or herbal tea. As a further discipline, her trainer insisted that Maria meticulously journal every time she ate or exercised. After six weeks of this rigorous routine, Maria had lost only one pound! Her personal trainer and doctor were dumbfounded. She decided to try a whole new approach and sought out Linda's services.

When Linda ran the pre-test on Maria, it showed "bladder" as the first MSO and "neurological" as the second MSO. No surprise there. However, they were to prove secondary, because they, along with the weight gain problems, shared a common and undetectable cause—major parasite infestation (*Balantidium coli* and *Cryptosporidium muris*). Apparently Maria's doctor had not thought of this possibility and had not ordered a stool sample test. Even if he had, there is no guarantee that the infestation would have shown up. Maria had not complained of colon or gastrointestinal problems, and a stool test could hardly be expected to detect parasites in the bladder and the brain. Other contributing factors included acid pH toxins, a high level of fungi and gastrointestinal dysbiosis, a significant number of miasms, and heavy metal toxicity, even though Maria had had her amalgam fillings removed several years earlier. Linda immediately put her on the appropriate program to address her multiple issues, many of which could be traced to parasite proliferation.

After going on Linda's program, Maria wrote us: "Within 16 days I dropped 16 pounds and two dress sizes without exercise or any extraordinary effort with calorie control! By the 25th day I had more energy than I knew what to do with. Shortly after that, the cycle of kidney/bladder infections, blood in the urine, and frequent urination had ended. I was clear minded and felt like I was in high school again. Linda Freud gave me the key to my healing."

Are Parasites Making You Fat?

Along with a toxic and sluggish thyroid, Linda considers parasite infestation to be one of the great hidden factors in people who have real problems losing weight. In an article entitled "Are Parasites Making You Fat?" Ann Louise Gittleman reveals a hidden link between people who are overweight and parasite disease:

- **Parasites block the absorption of nutrients.** "Parasites inflame the membrane that lines the digestive tract, hindering the absorption of vitamins, minerals, fats, and other nutrients that balance hormones, stabilize blood sugar, and boost metabolism, notes Dr. Elson Haas, M.D., director of California's Preventive Medical Center of Marin."

- **Parasites trigger yeast overgrowth.** "Parasites hinder the growth of beneficial bacteria in the gut, creating an environment that allows yeast to flourish. 'And since yeast are fermenting organisms, they cause gas, bloat, and pain,' says Carolyn Dean, M.D., N.D., coauthor of *The Complete Natural Medicine Guide to Women's Health* (Robert Rose, 2005). 'Yeast overgrowth also activates the immune system, triggering allergic reactions that suppress the thyroid gland and cause unstable blood sugar.'"

- **Parasites acidify body systems.** "A natural byproduct of parasites is acid, which can damage organs, breakdown muscle tissue, and cause the central nervous system to become sluggish. Ironically, the body's self-preservation system can make the problem worse: 'The body responds by shuttling acid into fat cells and slowing metabolic rate so more protective fat can be stored,' explains clinical researcher Robert O. Young, Ph.D., coauthor of *The pH Miracle for Weight Loss* (Warner Wellness, 2007). 'This is the body's way of getting acids out of circulation, but it makes losing weight virtually impossible.'"

- **Parasites make organs sluggish.** "Parasites can emit indole catabolites and other toxins that the liver and kidneys have to work hard to excrete. 'These organs can quickly become sluggish, leading to fatigue, irritability, and weight gain,' cautions Dr. Dean."[6]

CHAPTER 8

Miasms: The Invisible Enemy in Chronic Disease

Every truth passes through three stages before it is recognized.
In the first it is ridiculed, in the second it is opposed,
in the third it is regarded as self-evident.
—ARTHUR SCHOPENHAUER

WHEN "HEREDITARY TOXIN," "ACQUIRED MIASM," or "genetic miasm" shows up on a client's pre-test, Linda immediately knows that the angels have given her a very important clue in determining critical underlying cofactors in the client's disease profile. She then goes to the section of the database entitled "miasm" to continue her investigative research. Linda has channeled that miasms exist in virtually all of her clients. Yet, the vast majority of Western medical professionals are completely unaware of these hidden, subtle energies that profoundly affect our health.

Miasms are vibrational resonances that constitute a deep susceptibility or predisposition to specific disease states. Samuel Hahnemann (1755–1843), a German physician known as the father of homeopathy, called these predispositions "chronic miasms" and found that they pass in various ways from person to person. He believed they often constitute the original cause behind most chronic degenerative disease. The word *miasm* in German means "an obstacle to cure." Hahnemann believed that unless this obstacle to cure was properly dealt with, a complete cure was difficult to obtain.

Miasms can be thought of as "masked infections" that consist of vibrational resonances containing symptoms associated with an infectious disease inherited from one's ancestors or from an infection acquired during one's lifetime. These resonances, however, do not transfer the original infectious disease itself, but only the symptoms in a masked or unrecognizable form. Linda uses an interesting visual analogy to describe miasms: "Think of your health problem as a clogged drain pipe under your bathroom sink. Although there will probably be other debris on top of it, unless you remove the hair at the bottom of the sink—the miasms—the water from the faucet cannot flow through."

According to homeopathy, the body acts as a holistic storage device on both the cellular and emotional level. In the same way that an athlete can train his or her muscle memory to retain a specific physical motion or a musician can train his or her muscle memory to perform a specific passage of music, once an electrochemical coding for cellular or emotional memories becomes deeply entrenched, it is very difficult to remove. Using this train of thought as an analogy, we can more fully appreciate that Samuel Hahnemann's incredibly brilliant but highly esoteric theory of miasms is a major contribution to medical science.

The angels have also revealed to Linda—and her years of practical experience with clients confirm—that it is difficult to construct a complete health picture of an individual without understanding chronic miasms. They are often the root cause behind certain difficult-to-diagnose chronic degenerative conditions as well as various types of chronic disease that run in families. For example, research has shown that the core genetic cause of type 2 diabetes in a family may be an inherited tuberculosis miasm! (See Polysan remedy T in Table 8-1 on pages 111–112.)

A MEDICAL VISIONARY'S DISCOVERY

Hahnemann's first principal discovery was that the treatment of disease should occur by means of natural substances that produce symptoms similar to the disease being treated, which he called "the law of similars." He acknowledged that utilizing these substances could greatly aggravate the condition as well as produce other side effects. He therefore developed a system of diluting the substance to the point where taking the diluted substance made the symptoms disappear. Today, we understand that a natural substance can be diluted to such an extent that it is no longer considered a physical substance but becomes a vibrational resonance. Hahnemann called this process of dilution into different potencies *dynamization*.

Hahnemann published his next, and most controversial, theory of chronic miasms in various editions of his classic text, *The Chronic Diseases*, in the early 1800s. He revealed that "the nature of chronic miasmatic disease is slow and insidious in its onset and gradual in its progression. These negative transformations gradually increase until they bring on complex pathologies that eventually are a major cause of premature old age and death. The chronic miasms are the effects of infections that are not self-limiting and which cause considerable damage to the immune system, the vital force, and the constitution."

Hahnemann noticed that while some patients were seemingly cured by medicines and other treatments, they still remained vulnerable to particular categories of ailments. While these categories appeared to be unrelated, Hahnemann was able to trace the origin of the symptoms back to a common root—a symptom shared with the "cured" disease. These observations led to his theory of miasms as subtle, potential forces that create particular disease characteristics. These concepts became a cornerstone of Hahnemann's homeopathic philosophy. Perceiving the miasmatic basis of disease enables the healer and the patient to understand the very foundation behind many weaknesses in the body.

GENERAL CHARACTERISTICS OF MIASMS

In a four-part article in *Homeopathy Today* entitled "The Thought Behind the Action," professor and homeopath Ann Jerome (formerly Croce), Ph.D., RS Hom (NA), director and faculty member of the Academy of Classical Homeopathy, expounds on Hahnemann's theories: "The first principle to understand is that miasms are not an isolated affliction. They are the fundamental susceptibility in all living things."[1] Here is a summary of the general characteristics of miasms:

• The action of miasms is destructive. They are the aspect of our being that makes us weak and vulnerable to both contagious and indigenous diseases. They deplete our energy and our strength to resist the physical and mental challenges of life.

• Miasms are named for our ancestors' diseases from which they originated. There are two types of miasms: chronic and acute. A chronic miasm manifests by repeatedly attacking a person over time through such conditions as asthma, arthritis, and depression. Acute miasms are divided into two categories: (1) a condition such as influenza that can reoccur in various strains or (2) childhood diseases such as chicken pox, measles, or mumps that only occur once in a lifetime. These diseases can create subsequent conditions that may be activated by a wide range of stressors such as emotional problems, suppressed immune system, and toxicity. Hahnemann traced them to such infectious diseases as tuberculosis, syphilis, and gonorrhea that are derived from one's ancestors or acquired by the patient. However, chronic miasms only share a loose connection to the original disease in that they contain only some of the characteristics or symptoms of the original condition. These symptoms appear in a masked or unrecognizable form. They are not the disease itself.

• Chronic miasms form part of each individual's genetic makeup and lie dormant indefinitely or can be in varying stages of activation, ranging from partly opened to fully active. Most people inherit several miasms, but over the course of a lifetime a person may also acquire additional miasms through infectious disease.

• When chronic miasms are dormant, their characteristics remain but their power is reduced. When miasms are active, they cause imbalance, susceptibility, and disease.

• Miasms also contain patterns of emotional expressions. Certain negative emotional states are consistently found in people with certain miasms. They are also responsible for certain transgenerational negative emotional states that run in families.

• Miasms do not necessarily predict a specific disease. However, a statistically significant number of case histories since the early 1800s, along with corroborating microscopic blood evidence by Dr. Carl Spengler (discussed later in this chapter), strongly suggest a cause-and-effect relationship between a patient's current symptoms and the condition of the ancestor who originally acquired that condition.

• The same forces that tend to create health or disease also affect a miasm's degree of power. Good nutrition and a healthy lifestyle weaken miasmatic influence. Stress and environmental toxicity strengthen its influence. The good news is that the proper homeopathic treatment can either eliminate a miasm or render it dormant.

• Multiple miasms are generally, but not always, addressed one at a time in layers. As one miasm is brought under control, another may arise and create new symptoms and ailments.

Hahnemann's Four Ways of Acquiring Miasms

Hahnemann described four ways that miasms may be acquired:

1. **Genetically inherited miasms.** Long before the discovery of DNA and genetically inherited diseases, Hahnemann noted that certain illnesses tended to run in certain families. Moreover, he observed that even if family mem-

bers' diseases did not exactly mimic each other, they shared similar characteristics and patterns. This led Hahnemann to conclude that the primary way
people acquired miasms was from their parents. Since siblings usually inherit
many of the same miasms, they have a similar potential for getting a particular illness or symptom. However, each sibling has other characteristics and
experiences that affect which miasm is active. Therefore, even though the
underlying miasmatic burden is often quite similar, each family member may
experience a different individual destiny in his or her health history.

This predisposition to a disease pattern can produce a variety of apparently unrelated conditions that may go back several generations. If, for example, a person's great-great-grandfather had syphilis, that person could
experience any number of skin disorders as a result of his or her ancestor's
disease. One of the services that Linda offers to couples who are planning to
conceive a child is that she works with the husband and wife to eliminate each
partner's underlying miasmatic burdens. She has channeled that this radically
reduces the likelihood that their future offspring will inherit them. What a
marvelous present to offer a child!

2. **Miasms acquired from disease.** An acquired miasm is a resonance of an
infectious disease that is principally derived from either tuberculosis or sexually transmitted diseases such as syphilis or gonorrhea (see Table 8-2 on
page 114). This resonance remains in the body long after the condition has
been cured. According to Professor Jerome, a miasm from these "resolved"
conditions can result in a subsequent disease derived from the aforemen-
tioned conditions. A miasm can express itself in many aspects of a person's
life. For example, the core cause of a common debilitating condition such as
asthma may be a result of a genetic or acquired miasm. To determine this, a
homeopath must be skilled in subtle medical detective work. Many probing
questions must be asked of the patient to understand the individual symptoms as these may determine which particular miasm is active. Asthma that
becomes worse in cold, damp weather may be a different miasm than asthma
that becomes worse from overexertion.

3. **Miasms from mismanagement of disease.** In Hahnemann's era, syphilis
and gonorrhea were commonplace. The prevailing allopathic treatments of
the day suppressed the infection that over time frequently resulted in a new
miasm, though it appeared that the person had ostensibly been cured. Professor Jerome comments: Hahnemann "observed that survivors of gonorrhea
commonly returned for treatment of rheumatic problems and other inflam-
mations within a few years after being treated for the disease. He postulated

that gonorrhea and its suppression had created a new vulnerability in them, a new Achilles' heel, a new miasm."[2] There is currently discussion within the homeopathic community that vaccinations may also trigger miasms leading to such conditions as autism.

4. **Miasms from individual transmission of a previous disease/miasm.** Hahnemann observed that wives of men who contracted gonorrhea sought treatment for similar ailments even though they had not contracted gonorrhea itself. That strongly suggests that the miasm may be transmitted from one person in close proximity to another. To support this, Hahnemann subsequently observed that the children of such couples also ended up developing the same health problems. It's since been discovered that miasms can also be transmitted by blood transfusions.

Hahnemann's Three Categories of Miasms

Although other researchers later identified other miasmatic forms like tuberculosis and cancer, Hahnemann identified three original miasms, which he named *psora, syphilis,* and *sycosis,* and the patterns of physical and emotional expressions related to them.

1. *Psora.* Hahnemann identified psora as the primary, universal miasm that creates the susceptibility to other miasms and diseases. He referred to it as the miasm of lack and weakness, and it is characterized by conditions of the bowels and the skin. Psora is an internal disorder that externalizes—for example, asthmatics who suffer with eczema. Hahnemann's list of medical conditions includes a wide range of dermatological problems as well as asthma, pleurisy, stomach ulcers, swollen glands, cataracts, diabetes, tuberculosis, and epilepsy. Physical symptoms may include dry, itchy skin, burning sensations in the hands and feet, digestive troubles, being cold, defective bone development, hyperactivity, allergies, and problems of the liver, lungs, heart, and circulatory system. The emotional profile of psora is people who have poor self-image and often do not finish what they start. They tend to be timid, fearful, indifferent, overly sensitive, restless, easily fatigued, or depressed.

2. *Syphilis.* The syphilitic miasm affects many people, though only a small percentage have actually suffered from syphilis. While syphilis was fairly common in Hahnemann's time, today the syphilitic miasm is primarily acquired by heredity. Hahnemann referred to the syphilitic miasm as the

miasm of destruction. It is related to many diseases of the nervous system as well as psychological disorders, including alcoholism, depression, suicidal impulses, and insanity. It is also associated with heart, blood, and skeletal conditions as well as blindness and deafness.

3. *Sycosis.* Like the syphilitic miasm, sycosis is acquired mainly by heredity and often accompanies psora. The original infectious disease behind this miasm is gonorrhea. Sycosis is responsible for many sexual and urinary disorders, afflictions of the joints and the mucous membranes, and those conditions worsened by damp weather and sea air. Arthritis and rheumatism, asthma, bronchitis, cystitis, and warts are said to be partly or mainly sycotic.

What Activates a Miasm

In the article "The Itch That Cannot Be Scratched: Understanding Eczema and Psoriasis for a Practitioner," Brian Knight, director of the Health Arts College of Melbourne, Australia, had these insightful thoughts about what activates miasms: "Miasms lie dormant in a person's genetic makeup until a pre-encoded trigger is activated by the occurrence of something contraindicated to that individual's maintenance of well-being. These triggers are most commonly a trauma or intervention of some kind that affects the person's physical, mental and/or emotional status.

"Prime triggers are invasive assaults on the immune system like immunizations and ingested substances that stress the body. Drugs, like antibiotics or corticoids, are also one of the biggest triggers for miasms. Using the metaphor of a jack-in-the-box, the miasm lies contained and dormant inside its box of genetic encoding, primed and ready on its highly tensioned spring, until something triggers the catch; like an unnecessary and unwelcomed jab from a hypodermic needle assaulting a new born baby's immune system with a [hepatitis] B inoculation, for instance. This invasive assault triggers the catch, freeing the miasm to leap out of its containment and make an often dramatic appearance in the person's life, by way of a physical ailment, or in the case of the newborn, possibly even death."[3]

OUR INTRODUCTION TO MIASMS

Subsequent generations of homeopaths in Europe expanded Hahnemann's list by declaring that tuberculosis and cancer were also miasmatic. Linda's ability to identify masked tuberculosis and recommend the precise homeopathic remedies has had a profoundly beneficial impact on many of her clients. In fact, she credits it as part of the reason for her tremendous success. However, our discovery of this healing treasure trove came about in a spiritually serendipitous manner, with future repercussions that were unimaginable at the time.

In the fall of 1992, I went to Germany again, this time with Linda, who was also quite ill, in search of cutting-edge detoxification protocols to help alleviate our considerable health problems. We visited Dr. Helmut Schimmel, M.D., inventor of the Vegatest method, who recommended that we both take a blood test to determine if one of the underlying cofactors in our complicated conditions was miasms. We had never heard of this, but were willing to proceed based on our confidence in Dr. Schimmel. Little did we know how valuable this would prove for us.

Dr. Schimmel explained that miasms could go back several generations and could involve various strains of tuberculosis, syphilis, pneumonia, malaria, influenza, and staphylococcal and streptococcal infections. To test for this, he recommended homeopathic remedies called Spenglersan colloids that detect and identify chronic inherited miasms. These are nontoxic, highly purified, immune blood derivatives, which he described as therapeutic agents that double as both diagnostic tests and treatment protocols.

Spenglersan colloids are described by the German manufacturer, Meckel-Spenglersan GmbH, as "homeopathic, microbiological immune modulators produced from antigens and antitoxins of frequent infections raised to a [homeopathic] potency of D9, which are rubbed into the skin." When the liniment-colloids are applied to such sensitive areas as the inside of the elbow, the thigh, or the stomach, " . . . their effect is one that dissolves bacilli and binds up toxins. They free the diseased organism of their so-called 'inherited and endogenic toxins.' " Linda concurs with the company literature, which goes on to say, "The fact that they have had great success in treating illnesses that resisted every other therapy shows that Spengler was on the right track."[4]

Dr. Schimmel explained that these colloids had been developed by the Swiss tuberculosis researcher Dr. Carl Spengler, whom he described as "possibly the most advanced researcher into tuberculosis and other infectious diseases in the 20th century."[5] When I expressed puzzlement about why neither Linda nor I, nor anyone we knew in America, had ever heard of either Dr. Spengler or these products, Dr. Schimmel patiently explained that the research and thought process behind these products was out of sync with the pharmaceutical approach that dominates medicine in America, thus relegating it to the fringes of medicine in this country.

The remedies are popular with European doctors who take a more integrative approach to healing a wide range of conditions. For example, Dr. Konrad Werthmann, an Austrian gastroenterologist with more than thirty years of experience with Spenglersan colloids, believes that these remedies have profound implications as hidden cofactors for all sorts of digestive, intestinal, and colon issues. For example, he believes there is a strong relationship between a large consumption of milk and irritation and inflammation of the intestinal mucosa that lead to leaky gut syndrome. He attributes this relationship to the consistent test results he gets on patients who test positive for *Mycobacterium tuberculosis typus bovinus* antibodies, which react with primary antigens from milk. He believes this form of tuberculosis miasm is ultimately responsible for leaky gut syndrome.[6]

Spengler's Research Scientifically Validates the Existence of Miasms

Though many readers may be willing to accept Linda's diagnosis of miasms without knowing the scientific basis for them, others may be skeptical about their existence, since miasms are not part of allopathic medicine practiced in the United States. Here is a very brief history of the scientific basis for miasms.

In the 19th and early part of the 20th century, clinical tuberculosis was the leading cause of death throughout Europe and America. An intensive research effort was underway that resulted in important medical breakthroughs in treatment of this disease. Heinrich Hermann Robert Koch (1843–1910), the world-renowned German bacteriologist, isolated *Mycobacterium tuberculosis* with a sophisticated microscope and staining technique he developed (see Figure 8-1). In 1905, he received the Nobel Prize in physiology or medicine for his investigations and discoveries in relation to tuberculosis. He soon thereafter started working with Swiss tuberculosis researcher Dr. Carl Spengler (1860–1937; see Figure 8-2). Together they isolated two additional microbes: *Mycobacterium tuberculosis humanus brevis* (Koch type) and *humanus longus* (Spengler type).

While working closely with his father Dr. Alexander Spengler (1827–1901), director of the Davos Tuber-

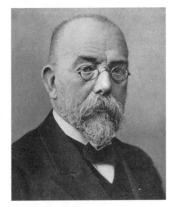

Figure 8-1. Robert Koch.

culinic Sanatorium in Davos, Switzerland, Dr. Carl Spengler developed the first microbial antigenic colloids in the late 1800s as a treatment for tuberculosis. However,

Spengler came to realize that they were, in fact, quite effective in treating many other chronic degenerative conditions that ostensibly *did not have any relationship to tuberculosis.* After years of arduous research involving thousands of cases of tuberculosis at

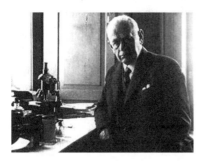

his father's sanatorium, he came to two very important conclusions: (1) Tuberculosis in its miasmatic form was a major root cause of many chronic degenerative conditions. (2) Almost all infections considered to be purely tubercular were actually based on combined infections.[7]

Dr. Spengler was one of the first researchers to recognize that, in addition to its easily recognizable forms, tuberculosis appears at least as often in hidden form, which is very difficult to

Figure 8-2. Dr. Carl Spengler.

identify.[8] Dr. Spengler's hypothesis was that tuberculosis was not merely a disease of the lungs, but when *Mycobacterium tuberculosis* combined with other microbes, it could be found in many different places in the body, including the internal organs, skin, and bones. He identified that it existed as a "camouflaged systemic illness" of the stomach, intestine, liver, gallbladder, pancreas, heart, and glands with internal secretions. He noted that tuberculosis also exists in the guise of very different infectious diseases such as influenza, certain types of pneumonia, and rheumatism.[9]

Dr. Spengler believed that many chronic disorders were, in reality, masked infections of tuberculosis that were hereditarily passed on to offspring. According to him, "the sources of these illnesses were tuberculosis toxicoses, luetic (syphilis), and [other] toxic inherited diseases that extend over several generations."[10] In fact, the remarkable success of his Spenglersan colloids strengthened his conviction that an inherited or acquired infectious disease is part of the combined disease phenomenon that is the underlying cause behind a significant percentage of chronic degenerative diseases.

In an article entitled "The Tubercular Constitution as a Common Cause of Chronic Diseases and Its Treatment with Naturopathic Regulation Therapy," German scientist and author Dr. Peter Schneider describes a revolutionary aspect of Dr. Spengler's blood work that seems to verify Hahnemann's revolutionary supposition about the genetic nature of miasms. "Spengler's work was focused on the different morphology of strains of various mycobacteria and with the close relationship between tubercle bacteria and the pathogenic agent of syphilis, whose bacterial form is found in mixed cultures from tuberculosis patients. Spengler showed [by way of microscopy] that the presence of the syphilis pathogen could be demonstrated within the cells of an organism in an ultra-small and primitive variety—*even when an infection by this pathogen had never occurred during the individual's lifetime.*

"It was assumed that the general spread of 'inherited' syphilis stems from the beginning of the 16th century, when a whole population was infected with a syphilis pandemic 'imported' [to Europe] from America. Anyone who did not die of this infectious disease at that time retained a residual toxicity in the body that was passed on through generations and, according to Spengler, would later show up as an 'inherited virus.' "11

Dr. Spengler maintained that pathogenic microbes disrupt the binding of oxygen to hemoglobin on red blood cells (erythrocytes) through a fermentation process. The microbes attack the erythrocytes, which then become the carriers of inherited toxins, toxins made by the body, and toxins from the environment. According to *Materia Medica:* "These specific inherited allergens are transferred from the mother's blood onto the child and may burden the descendants over several generations."12

Diagnosing Miasms Using Spenglersan Colloids

The diagnostic test for miasms consists of adding a drop of blood to a small portion of each of the Spenglersan colloids and observing the intensity of the bacterial antigen-antibody reaction. Aggulation or clumping of the blood indicates a reaction between specific antigens and antibodies due to an inherited or former infectious disease. The degree of aggulation is measured by one of four levels—strong positive, moderately positive, mildly positive, no response. The test shows the practitioner which miasms exist, their level of severity, and the appropriate colloids to use.

When Linda and my blood tests came back positive for several of the colloids (Figure 8-3), I immediately understood the significance of this discovery and was grateful that yet another piece of my amazingly complicated health puzzle had been deciphered. Dr. Schimmel told us that he had had remarkable success curing a range of difficult chronic degenerative disorders with Spenglersan colloids *when nothing else had worked.*

After some research, we were delighted to find that a Canadian company, Biomed International (www.biomedicine.com), had recently started distributing the remarkable Spenglersan colloids in America under the brand name of Polysan colloids.

Linda does not need to use Dr. Spengler's blood test because she is able to channel the same information using Table 8-1. The table shows the relationships among the types of chronic illnesses, the infectious miasmatic agents, and the specific Polysan colloids. These remedies have worked wonders for Linda's clients. Readers who have a chronic condition whose root cause has not been determined through traditional lab tests may want to see if they can find a health care professional who is open to identifying miasms through this blood test.

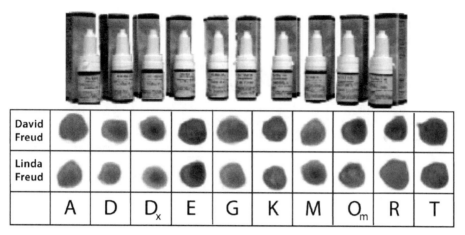

David Freud									
Linda Freud									
A	D	D_x	E	G	K	M	O_m	R	T

Figure 8-3. David and Linda's blood tests from 1992 show varying degrees of aggulation which corellate with the severity of inherited toxins. The tests without any darkened colorations are negative; those with darkened colorations are positive to varying degrees. The toxins that correspond to the letters are listed in Table 8-1.

TABLE 8-1. DETECTION OF HIDDEN DISEASE DUE TO MIASMS USING POLYSAN REMEDIES

Types of Chronic Illnesses	Composition of Miasms	Polysan Remedy
Aging, arteriosclerosis, hypertension, incontinence, polyuria, senility, urinary flow obstruction	1. Mycobacterium tuberculosis typus brevis 2. Mycobacterium tuberculosis typus bovinus	A
Dental focus (cause of infection) and infection	1. Streptococcus lacticus 2. Streptococcus pyogenes 3. Streptococcus haemolyticus 4. Streptococcus viridans 5. Staphylococcus albus 6. Staphylococcus pharynges 7. Staphylococcus aureus 8. Diplococcus lanceolatus 9. Mycobacterium tuberculosis typus bovinus	D
Other dental and oral infections	1. Streptococcus lanceolatus 2. Staphylococcus aureus	Dx
Prostate conditions, joint disorders, insomnia, memory problems, neurasthenia, inflammation	1. Luetic antigens (syphilis)	E

TYPES OF CHRONIC ILLNESSES	COMPOSITION OF MIASMS	POLYSAN REMEDY
Respiratory symptoms of virus, pulmonary disorders, colds, flu, angina, inflammation	1. *Bacterial pneumoniae* 2. *Virus influenza Spengler* 3. *Bacillus influenza Pfeiffer*	G
Asthma, allergies, hay fever, circulatory disturbances, cystitis, colic, thromboses	1. *Streptococcus lanceolatus* 2. *Staphylococcus aureus* 3. *Diplococcus pneumoniae*	K
Fever, malaria, chills	1. *Plasmodium malaria* 2. *Plasmodium falciparum* *These are forms of protozoa (parasites)*	M
Benign and malignant neoplasms, warts, moles, circulatory disturbances, vascular disease	1. *Streptococcus lacticus* 2. *Streptococcus pyogenes* 3. *Streptococcus haemolyticus* 4. *Streptococcus viridans*	Om
Pain associated with rheumatism, gout, arthritis, tuberculosis, neuralgia, lupus uric acid buildup	1. *Mycobacterium tuberculosis humanus brevis* 2. *Mycobacterium tuberculosis humanus bovinus* 3. *Streptococcus pyogenes*	R
Tuberculosis, diabetes, headache, cognitive memory, arthritis, rheumatism pain, lupus, disease symptoms for lungs, skin, kidneys, intestines, lymphatics	1. *Mycobacterium tuberculosis typus humanus* 2. *Mycobacteium tuberculosis typus brevis* 3. *Mycobacterium tuberculosis typus bovinus* 4. *Diplococcus pneumoniae* 5. *Streptococcus mucosus*	T

WHAT DIFFERENTIATES LINDA'S UNIQUE APPROACH TO MIASMS

The diagnosis of miasms is primarily the domain of homeopathic physicians, although a few integrative medical doctors and naturopaths have now added it to their diagnostic repertoire. The most common approach a homeopath uses to diagnose miasms involves intense powers of observation and questioning. With this information, a good practitioner can deduce which miasmatic remedies are needed to lift the malady. Many practitioners, however, struggle just to get bits and pieces of information, as the diagnostic process takes years of dedication to master. The problem with this approach is that it may not address other essential aspects of the overall healing process.

Some practitioners may also use the Polysan colloids blood test to determine the presence of multiple miasms. Certainly using the blood test is more definitive than relying only on the powers of observation, but there are still limitations because the Polysan colloids do not cover the totality of miasmatic possibilities. Though the test may show that the need for one remedy may be stronger than for another, that fact alone does not determine the optimal sequencing order of miasmatic detoxification protocols, which is essential in eliminating miasms.

I cannot stress enough that what separates Linda from other health care practitioners we know of is that she receives all her information from archangels and angels. Certainly, there are brilliant homeopaths and other practitioners who have devoted their professional lives to the study of miasms. However brilliant they are, however astute are their powers of observation and deductive reasoning, they are simply no match for the angelic horsepower Linda can access. Archangel Raphael does not need to consult either manuals or blood tests to know which Polysan colloids or other homeopathics are needed to peel the "miasmatic onion" in the correct order. *He just knows.* Raphael identifies the changing patterns of energy and information through what Linda calls "metaphysical antivirus software" for the body, mind, and spirit. Such is the power of archangels.

After "hereditary toxin" and/or "acquired infectious toxin" appear on the client's pre-test, Linda goes to the chart in the database, shown in Table 8-2, and scans with the pendulum to see if any of the remedies made from extreme dilutions of these infectious diseases show up in active or miasmatic form. She then cross-references this against Table 8-1. If the pendulum indicates a miasmatic infection resonance in Table 8-2 that is not in Table 8-1, she channels the specific homeopathic resonance needed to clear out the miasm.

Knowing the proper sequence of treating multiple miasms is quite important, as the following statement from the *Journal of Online Homeopathy* attests: "If the homeopath does not know the layers of the miasms in their proper order, he or she will not know what to look for in the future, so that some dramatic complication may just 'pop' out of the vital force as if it came out of nowhere."[13]

Archangel Raphael doesn't worry about such things. As a result, we are unaware of any other practitioner who can analyze multiple miasmatic burdens to the extent that Linda can do it. This involves:

• Ranking and prioritizing the layers of the miasmatic onion.

• Determining the precise homeopathic dilution of a particular energetic toxin or pathogen that needs to be cleared in order to eliminate a particular characteristic of the disease profile.

TABLE 8-2. PARTIAL LIST OF PRINCIPAL MIASMS

Bacillinum	Streptococcus viridans Card
Carcinosinum	Syphilinum
Luesinum	Toxoplasmosis
Lymphogranuloma	Tuberculinum marmoreck
Medorrhinum	Tuberculinum
Psorinum	Tuberculinum avis
Sarcominum	Tuberculinum bovinum
Scirrhinum	Tuberculinum Burnett
Streptococcinum	Tuberculinum Denys
Streptococcinum B haemolyticus	Tuberculinum Kent
Streptococcus faecalis	Tuberculinum Koch
Streptococcus haemolyticus	Tuberculinum residuum
Streptococcus pneumoniae	Tuberculinum Rosenbach
Streptococcus pyogenes	Tuberculinum Spengler
Streptococcus rheumaticus	Tuberculinum testiculatum
Streptococcus scarlatina	Variolinum
Streptococcus viridans	

What this means is that Linda's diagnostic capability is analogous to using a calculator to solve an advanced mathematical problem rather than an abacus. The angels simply tell Linda what miasms a person has, the proper sequential order needed to detoxify them, and what homeopathic potency of a particular remedy is needed to do the job. *No guesswork is involved. It is perhaps this aspect of her diagnostic gift, more than any other, along with her ability to diagnose "undiagnosable" toxicity, which separates her from any other practitioner whom we are aware of. This allows her to heal or significantly improve difficult conditions.*

As I have watched Linda develop her psychic abilities over the years, I never tire of watching her do the sequencing of genetically inherited miasms. She is doing diagnostics on such a high level that it's like watching Arthur Rubenstein play Chopin, John Coltrane play jazz, Michael Jordan play basketball, or Tiger Woods play golf. We are unaware of any other methodology currently available, other than angelic communication, for attaining such levels of detail. This is not meant, in any way, to put Linda on a pedestal. *Quite the con-*

trary. It is necessary for Linda to remain humble in order to be a pure vessel through which to receive this information.

MIASMS AND CHRONIC DEGENERATIVE DISEASE

What we have learned about the relationship between miasms and chronic degenerative disease is nothing less than a medical breakthrough:

1. There is a direct link between the severity of chronic degenerative diseases and the number of genetically inherited or acquired miasms a person has. The most chronically ill people whom Linda has worked with were always the ones who exhibited the greatest number of miasms.

2. There is more environmental illness today due to man-made toxicity than at any other time in human history. Never before has such a deluge of pollutants affected the very air we breathe, the water we drink, and the food we eat. Now there are new classifications of illness that never existed before. In addition, toxic dental materials such as amalgams and mercury in vaccinations mean that a majority of Americans are now affected by the scourge of heavy metal toxicity, although they don't know it.

3. *There are many miasms that also bind in environmental toxins so the body cannot excrete them in a normal way.* Linda likens this to trying to rip out something that is bound in by magnets, glue, or Velcro. Clearly, one of the most important pieces of information the angels have revealed is the necessity of clearing out multiple miasms *prior* to commencing a heavy metal detox. The way Linda describes the process speaks volumes: "When the layer of 'magnets and glue' are eliminated and then a natural heavy-metal chelator is introduced to detoxify mercury, the mercury simply 'slides out' of the body instead of being ripped out."

When toxins such as mercury are bound in, they negatively impact the biological terrain of the blood and other bodily fluids by creating acidosis (hyperacidity). This, in turn, sets up a breeding ground in the body for fungal proliferation, parasite infestation, and bacterial and viral infection. This changes the terrain of the digestive and intestinal tract, causing dysbiosis, which, among other things, inhibits the absorption of vital nutrients through the lining of the intestines. The subsequent fungal, parasitic, viral, and bacterial outbreaks that fester in an acidic terrain are the principal precursors of much chronic degenerative disease in the world. This scenario is often the physical trigger for a significant amount of cancer.

4. Linda has channeled that there are certain cause-and-effect relationships between miasms and some common degenerative conditions that occur later in life. For example:

• A significant percentage of medical conditions, including type 2 diabetes, asthma, leaky gut syndrome, and arteriosclerosis that runs in families, can be traced to an unresolved vibrational resonance of an inherited tuberculosis miasm.

• A significant percentage of enlarged prostate (benign prostatic hyperplasia, or BPH) in middle-aged men can be traced to an unresolved vibrational residue of mumps.

• A significant percentage of osteoporosis can be traced to tetanus from a DPT shot (diphtheria/pertussis/tetanus) received as a child or from a tetanus booster later in life. Linda has channeled that a majority of her clients (though by no means all) safely process the diphtheria and pertussis components of the vaccination without problem. However, tetanus can have a major negative impact on bones.

• A significant percentage of Crohn's disease, leaky gut syndrome, and irritable bowel syndrome is associated with *Mycobacterium* from dairy products that cause an inflammatory response in the intestines. This confirms the hypothesis of Dr. Konrad Werthmann as described earlier in this chapter.

• A significant percentage of childhood neurological conditions ranging from attention deficit/hyperactivity disorder (ADD/ADHD) to autism can be traced to an unresolved relationship between thimerosal, a mercury preservative in vaccines, and various miasms that bind mercury in the brain. This makes it very difficult to excrete mercury through conventional heavy-metal detoxification protocols.

Scientific Study Validates Connection between ADHD and Miasms

Homeopathic physicians have long known that the tuberculosis miasm is one of the main causes of symptoms related to attention-deficit hyperactivity disorder (ADHD). This fact was corroborated by a 2002 South African study published in the *Journal of Tropical Pediatrics* entitled "Tuberculosis Meningitis and Attention Deficit Hyperactivity Disorder in Children." The purpose of the study was to investigate the prevalence of ADHD in children who recovered from tuberculosis meningitis (TBM). During this study, all 21 subjects in the TBM group were given thorough clinical-neurological examinations, and parents and teachers of each of the 21 subjects in the TBM group and each of the 21 subjects in the control group completed questionnaires. All 21 TBM group subjects displayed symptoms of ADHD. They were significantly more hyperactive, aggressive, and compulsive, with more pronounced levels of attention deficit, than members of the control group. Researchers concluded that "ADHD is a common, long-term complication of TBM."[14]

Implications of this study reveal the need for additional research regarding the dramatic link between miasms and the "cured" tuberculosis condition in children, all of whom subsequently became afflicted by ADHD. From a homeopathic perspective, this ADHD is the leftover effect of TBM disease.

TOWARD AN INTEGRATION OF GENETICS AND MIASMS

Those who remain skeptical of the theory of chronic miasms should consider the following logic: The primary cause of death for centuries was infectious disease, including tuberculosis, influenza, pneumonia, syphilis, typhoid, and malaria. The causes of these diseases were bacterial, viral, or parasitic organisms. Hahnemann and others who followed him theorized that miasms carry the vibrational resonances of those diseases from generation to generation. If Spengler's blood work protocols are understood correctly, then the theory of inherited vibrational resonances from infectious disease combined with the homeopathic understanding of miasms has real scientific merit.

While DNA is a proven genetic marker for a predispoition to various diseases including cancer, establishing the existence of miasms through bloodwork or energetic means is a highly useful, complementary approach that predates the discovery of DNA. In *Alternative Medicine: The Definitive Guide*, author Burton Goldberg writes: "Hahnemann's concept of miasms accurately prefigures today's description of oncogenes . . . Onogenes are believed to transform normal cells into cancer cells . . . This inherited genetic mutation represents a *molecular residue* from a previous generation. [Conversely,] a miasm represents an *energy residue* of an illness from a previous generation . . . In recent years, homeopaths have added a cancer miasm to Hahnemann's original three."[15] They have observed that miasma show a broadly focused predisposition to cancer in general, whereas oncogenes are coded for specific types of cancer.[16]

Linda has channeled that more meaningful cures for cancer will come about when there is an integration of the concepts discussed in this book—

homeopathic miasms, biological terrain, pH, fungi, parasites—with the modern-day study of genetics and oncogenes. She has also channeled that there are almost always underlying metaphysical, spiritual, and emotional blockages behind cancer. That is because cancer provides the ultimate opportunity for the soul to address the issues around one's own mortality—or not. Ultimately, our Creator has a multitude of different spiritual, emotional, and physical triggers at His disposal in the body that can provoke cancer. When the trigger is pulled, it results in chromosomal mutations that ultimately result in cancer.

Linda channels that what is not yet understood or appreciated is where modern genetic research intersects with the study of miasms. Linda is available to collaborate with sincere and open-minded geneticists who wish to work toward a complex integration of understanding in this field.

CHAPTER 9

Mercury: The Thousand-Headed Monster of Chronic Degenerative Diseases

The right to search for truth implies also a duty. One must not conceal any part of what one has recognized to be true.
—ALBERT EINSTEIN

THE ANGELS HAVE REVEALED TO US that the most widely underappreciated and misunderstood factor behind much chronic degenerative disease is heavy metal toxicity that poisons the body. Of these metals, unquestionably, the worst perpetrator is mercury, which can be derived from a wide variety of sources, including dental amalgams, root canals, fish, vaccinations, thermometers, thermostats, medical waste, or industrial accidents. So serious are the health implications from this particular heavy metal and so central is it to Linda's work that it's necessary to devote four chapters to the problem—this overview, how mercury affects the body (Chapter 10), how mercury affects the brain (Chapter 11), and how Linda treats chronic mercury poisoning (Chapter 12). Since each person's biochemistry is a little bit different, it is fair to say that mercury poisoning also affects each person who suffers from it in a unique way. That's what makes it so difficult to pin down as a causal factor and why Linda refers to it as "the thousand-headed monster of chronic degenerative diseases."

After plutonium, mercury is considered by toxicologists to be one of the most poisonous naturally occurring substances in the world. It is considerably more toxic than lead, cadmium, or arsenic.[1] So toxic is mercury to human health that the U.S. Centers for Disease Control and Prevention (CDC) acknowledge that *no safe level* has ever been determined.[2,3,4] This is why it is so carefully regulated by the Environmental Protection Agency (EPA), the Occupational Safety and Health Administration (OSHA), and other regulatory agencies.

The deadliness of high levels of mercury in the environment is well documented. Perhaps the most famous case of mercury poisoning is the widespread devastation that occurred in Minamata Bay, Japan, when the Chisso factory dumped 100 tons of mercury into the bay between 1932 and 1968. The mercury was used to manufacture acetic acid, a chemical compound used to make vinyl chloride for floor tiles and artificial leather. A study of the disaster later revealed that over 5,000 people in the surrounding area suffered horrific physical and neurological damage from severe mercury toxicity, and more than 1,000 people died.

One of the most severe mass poisonings in history occurred in the early 1970s in Iraq when nearly 95,000 tons of seed grains treated with a methyl mercury-based fungicide were accidentally baked into bread for human consumption. More than 50,000 people were poisoned and over 5,000 died. Many were hospitalized for weeks before methyl mercury poisoning was correctly diagnosed.

Although accidents like this are both tragic and inexcusable, that is not the primary focus of our discussion. Clearly, the effects of acute mercury poisoning such as these disasters, along with other common mishaps such as swallowing the contents of a mercury thermometer or eating mercury-contaminated fish, are obvious and acknowledged health hazards. To its credit and as a result of increased media and consumer awareness, gov - ernment and industry have in recent years made significant strides in reducing or eliminating mercury components in products ranging from thermometers, thermostats, automobiles, paint, and batteries to medical waste. Apple Computer is aggressively marketing the fact that its computers are now mercury-free. This is why it is so astonishing that despite the World Health Organization's report in 1991 declaring that *the predominant source of human exposure to mercury was from dental amalgam,* the use of mercury amalgam is still perfectly legal in much of the world.[5] How can this possibly be? Unfortunately, and as surreal as this may sound, we do not yet live in an enlightened enough society that values scientific certainty over economic, political, and legal realities of life.

Certainly one of the goals of presenting this information in such detail is to increase public awareness to such an extent that this saddest of chapters in the health of over *200 million unsuspecting American citizens*[6] (and much of the rest of the world, for that matter) can finally be brought to an end. The point is that no one would voluntarily submit to having mercury amalgams placed in their mouths if they truly understood what many leading researchers believe is a "toxic time bomb."

THE INSIDIOUS NATURE OF CHRONIC EXPOSURE
TO MERCURY FROM DENTAL AMALGAM

The principal difference between environmental disasters and dental amalgams is that the former is an example of *acute* poisoning while the latter represents the effects of *subacute chronic exposure* of lower levels of mercury over time. This process is called *micromercurialism* and is separate and distinct from acute mercury poisoning. However, because a myriad of different symptoms triggered by chronic exposure are misdiagnosed and therefore remain untreated, the horrific physical and emotional damage done to untold millions of people from mercury found in dental amalgam is a far more insidious and widespread problem than any other form of mercury toxicity.

A "silver filling" is not a true alloy. It is an unstable mixture made from approximately 50 percent liquid mercury with the remaining 50 percent composed of silver along with smaller amounts of zinc, tin, and copper. The central claim of the American Dental Association (ADA) and other pro-amalgam proponents is that mercury is rendered molecularly inert when it is combined with silver to form amalgam. However, they fail to acknowledge that mercury escapes continuously over the life of the filling in the form of vapor, ions, and abraded particles.[7] As a filling begins to corrode, it releases small yet measurable amounts of mercury vapors (up to 15 micrograms of mercury per day) through mechanical wear and evaporation. Even worse, every time you chew, have a hot drink, or brush your teeth, the amount of mercury released is dramatically increased.[8] It is estimated that an average individual with eight amalgam fillings absorbs up to 120 micrograms of mercury every day.[9] Another source states that such an individual has the equivalent of 6 grams of mercury in his or her body, a concentration sufficient to shut down a school chemistry lab or send a toxic clean-up crew to a lake.[10]

Mercury is easily released from an amalgam in the form of mercury vapor. Bacteria in the oral cavity change this vapor into an even more dangerous form called methyl mercury. On average, 80 percent of the mercury vapor inhaled into the lungs is then absorbed into the bloodstream,[11] reaching brain tissue within one blood circulation cycle.[12] The severe toxicity of methyl mercury is attributed to its ability to pierce any cell membrane in the body and cross all barriers, even the placenta and blood-brain barrier.[13] When this form of mercury crosses the blood-brain barrier, it causes many different types of neurological problems and brain function disturbances described in Chapter 11. When it crosses the placenta, it can inhibit brain development of the fetus and create cerebral palsy or psychomotor retardation in the latter stages of development.[14]

Putting the Danger of Other Common Sources of Mercury Toxicity into Perspective

In light of the World Health Organization's report, which also states that the daily absorption of all forms of mercury in fish and seafood is only 2.3 micrograms[15], it continues to amazes us that the Food and Drug Administration (FDA) focuses most of its research dollars on the dangers posed by mercury in fish rather than on the far greater dangers posed by dental amalgam fillings. While their concerns over fish do have merit, it is a complete distortion of the truth to say that the buildup of mercury in human tissues comes primarily from eating fish. As Dr. Russell L. Blaylock, M.D., wryly points out in his book *Health and Nutrition Secrets*, "*In truth, we get almost seven times more mercury from dental amalgams as from fish and other seafood.*"[16]

What can be said with certainty is that larger fish of any species are also older fish that have had more time to accumulate toxins like mercury. Therefore, although Linda channels that the FDA's list of fish that pregnant women and children should avoid (swordfish, shark, tilefish, and king mackerel) is correct, she also believes it is preferable for everyone to eat smaller and younger fish of any given species. Admittedly, it is difficult for the consumer to determine whether a fish is younger and smaller or large and older. Thankfully, the issue of mercury toxicity from fish does not occur in the Freud household. Linda merely places the pendulum over fish at our local fish market or that are listed on restaurant menus to determine if we should buy it. After all these years, I still gaze in wonderment when she does this.

The next most obvious danger of mercury poisoning comes from vaccines that contain a mercury preservative called thimerosal. Linda has channeled that the alarming increase in the number of children suffering from what is clearly an epidemic of such childhood neurological conditions as autism, Asperger's disorder, and ADD/ADHD is often due to thimerosal that is difficult to excrete out of brain tissue (Chapter 11).

THE POLITICS OF DENTAL AMALGAM

Americans currently receive over seventy million amalgam fillings a year[17], and dentistry is now the second largest user of mercury in the United States.[18] That is economic reason enough for the American Dental Association, the powerful trade organization for American dentistry, to have politically stonewalled and scientifically misrepresented the dangers of mercury fillings for almost the last 150 years. The current stall tactics of the ADA seem more like an attempt to forestall a wave of class-action lawsuits, which in recent years have been filed by numerous consumer groups, as well as groundbreaking legislative proposals in Congress that threaten the dental status quo.

An overwhelming body of scientific evidence found in hundreds of peer-reviewed studies conducted in countries around the globe links many types of chronic degenerative disease to low levels of heavy metal toxicity derived from dental amalgam. Yet, dental amalgam for the most part still technically enjoys the legal protection of the FDA and the ADA as well as the economic and political might of the dental amalgam industry.[19] However, due to a public outcry from consumer groups, concerned scientists, and members of Congress, the battle to eliminate deadly mercury amalgam goes on. To keep abreast of the latest developments in the amalgam war, see www.toxicteeth.org, the website of Consumers for Dental Choice (CDC), an advocacy group in Washington, D.C.

The lie that the ADA has steadfastly perpetuated since its inception is this: Mercury is made virtually harmless when it combines with other metals used to produce amalgam. In doing so, the ADA has performed an enormous disservice to the health of an unsuspecting public as well as their own trusting constituency! The ADA has conveniently ignored the results of extensive autopsy studies conducted in Sweden in 1989 that showed the pituitary glands of dentists held 800 times more mercury than did the glands in people who were not in the field of dentistry![20] This is not surprising as dentists inhale harmful levels of mercury vapors when they put in or drill out mercury fillings. In their book *Uninformed Consent,* authors Hal Huggins and Thomas Levy speculate that "if emotions are centered in the pituitary and thyroid glands, massive exposure to mercury vapors eight hours a day just might help explain why, as a profession, dentists rank highest in suicide."[21]

Perhaps more meaningful than any scientific evidence or ethical standard needed to push for the demise of amalgam in America is the old adage "follow the money." In 2007, Bank of America Securities issued a report to Dentsply, the second largest manufacturer of amalgam, urging them to make a "business decision" to phase out of the amalgam business due to risks from a negative regulatory environment and negative publicity.[22]

Consumers for Dental Choice states: "The FDA lags behind at least a dozen nations by failing even to give warnings of mercury exposure or to protect children and fetuses from this unnecessary use of mercury . . . Mercury fillings are now absolutely unnecessary. One-third of dentists never use mercury fillings in any patient. Mercury amalgam is [now] merely a convenience for the dentist—the domain for the factory-line dentist, the lazy dentist, and the dentist unwilling to learn. Their protector: the American Dental Association, which has two expired patents on mercury amalgam and pay-for-play contracts with amalgam manufacturers."[23] Linda refers to these factory-line, lazy dentists as "auto mechanics in your mouth who have no awareness of the toxic materials they use."

The question that a typical reader will surely ask after reading our admitted diatribe against mercury fillings is that if they are so dangerous, how could the FDA and the ADA, in all good conscience, possibly allow their continued use? To adequately explain this sordid state of affairs, we cannot divorce a medical discussion of the dangers of mercury fillings from the political and economic realities of public health policy in America. As we open this can of worms, we must start at the beginning.

A Brief History of the American Dental Association and the Amalgam Wars

According to Dr. Blaylock, in *Health and Nutrition Secrets*, "Mercury was already known to be a danger to human health when amalgams were first introduced into the United States over 150 years ago . . . The American Society of Dental Surgeons, the first dental society in the United States, attempted to put a stop to it by requiring that its member sign a pledge that stated 'It is my opinion and firm conviction that any amalgam whatsoever is unfit for the plugging (filling) of teeth.' "[24]

However, in spite of the ban, mercury amalgams began to be used because *they were so much cheaper* than gold or true silver fillings. So many dentists were removed from the society because of amalgam violations that the society itself finally collapsed by 1850. Profits from using the new amalgams were just too great to resist. As a result, the ousted members (those who cheated on their written oath purely for financial gain) formed their own society in 1859 called the American Dental Association.

A second amalgam war was provoked in the 1920s by Professor Alfred E. Stock, a leading chemist at the Kaiser Wilhelm Institute in Germany. After suffering adverse effects from mercury in his laboratory, he surmised that many potential health problems might arise from mercury amalgam fillings. His groundbreaking research was published in the leading medical journals of his day, but the outbreak of World War II caused his work to fade into obscurity.

We are currently in the advanced stages of the third and hopefully final amalgam war where the scientific evidence is truly overwhelming. It is highlighted by more modern methods of detecting trace amounts of mercury vapor using mass spectrophotometry, the Jerome mercury vapor analyzer, and real-time photographic evidence described in this and the next chapter. Leading the fight for good science is the International Academy of Oral Medicine & Toxicology (IAOMT), an organization made up of concerned dentists, physicians, and medical researchers committed to promoting safe dental materials and procedures. They have produced an informative video about the dangers of mercury entitled "The Smoking Tooth." Posted on Linda's website (www.thehealinggift.com), the video provides shocking visual evidence that irrefutably rebuts the safety claims made by proponents of amalgam.

Other Countries Ban or Partially Ban Mercury Fillings

Every health-conscious American should ask the FDA and ADA to explain why they do not acknowledge the same scientific facts that are clearly understood in other parts of the world. As of 2008, Sweden, Norway, Denmark, and Austria have completely banned the use of dental amalgam for everyone. England, Germany, Canada, Australia, New Zealand, and Japan have imposed partial bans, which vary from country to country. The restrictions may include pregnant women, people with kidney disease, and children.[25,26] This means that if an American is visiting Stockholm, Oslo, Copenhagen, Vienna, London, Munich, Montreal, Sydney, Auckland, and Tokyo and has a toothache, the odds of him or her being able to find a dentist who would fill the cavity with silver amalgam are probably slim indeed. Differences also extend to dental school curriculum in other countries. In Japan, for example, the technique of making silver amalgam fillings and placing them in the mouth is no longer taught in Japanese dental schools.[27] In contrast, it's still standard operating procedure to teach American dental students how to work with this poison.

Surely, this must give pause for thought. What is it that the ministries of health and dental associations in all these countries understand that the FDA and ADA do not? Linda has a rather acerbic way of describing these discrepancies in toxic awareness: "The guys making the Mercedes and Volvos don't think that amalgam is too good for you. Only the guys making the Chevys seem to think that it still has real merit." When she says this to a client, it subliminally speaks volumes, and the message is understood.

Most European countries are also far more evolved in their environmental regulatory outlook regarding dental mercury. Due to the high level of mercury released from dental offices, almost all European countries require amalgam separators in dental offices. Presently, in America only eight states and a few cities require dentists to install amalgam separators in their offices. This constitutes nothing less than gross neglect. As part of the Sierra Club's

2002 Mercury Policy Project, it released a report claiming that U.S. dentists used forty metric tons of mercury for dental amalgam, making that the largest source of mercury in our wastewater treatment plants.[28]

Mercury and other toxic chemicals are also accumulating in fish and wildlife at dangerous levels. The number of lakes in the United States with warnings not to eat fish and wildlife has been growing rapidly and has reached over 50,000 (20 percent of all U.S. significant lakes), along with 7 percent of all U.S. river miles, all the Great Lakes, and many coastal bays and estuaries.[29] These obvious environmental and medical reasons prompted Erik Solheim, Norwegian Minister of the Environment, to state in 2008 that part of the reason for the ban on dental amalgam in his country is the risk it causes to the environment. "Mercury is among the most dangerous of environmental toxins. Satisfactory alternatives to mercury in [dental] products are available and it is therefore fitting to introduce a ban."[30]

IDENTIFYING THE CORE ISSUE: A PROBLEM OF DIAGNOSIS

The problem of achieving a definitive diagnosis of mercury poisoning is compounded by the fact that chronic mercury poisoning from silver amalgam fillings is an insidious condition because the poison can literally burrow into the deepest cellular recesses of virtually any organ or brain tissue. It can lurk in the glands of the endocrine system, cling to heart muscles, saturate nerve endings and neurons (brain cells), and invade bones and fatty tissues. That makes it very difficult to detect as well as detoxify.

What complicates matters is that mercury entering the body through this chronic leaching process does not circulate freely in the bloodstream or urine, thus making it almost impossible to diagnose through traditional methods. Conventional testing methods involving blood, urine, and saliva cannot adequately detect mercury because these are not places where mercury accumulates. Nor do these tests reveal levels of mercury stored in tissues. Because mercury resides in tissues, it has to be "chelated," or brought out by means of a chelating agent, *in order to measure it*—unless you are Linda or a competent EAV practitioner. Only a urine test might reveal what is being excreted, but without the chelation process to force mercury out of tissues that would generally be nil. As a result, most traditional laboratory testing protocols for mercury are misleading and often meaningless. This and the fact that chronic leakage of mercury from dental amalgam is not discussed in medical schools are the principal reasons why it is usually overlooked by the mainstream medical community as the cause of so much chronic disease.

To make the case that mercury accumulates in organ, gland, and brain tissues, two studies—one on sheep and one on monkeys—were conducted by a team from the University of Calgary headed by Dr. Murray Vimy, D.D.S., and Dr. Fritz Lorscheider, Ph.D. Their work, published in the prestigious *FASEB Journal*, showed that radioactively labeled mercury released from amalgam fillings placed in the teeth of these animals appeared in their kidneys, intestinal walls, and brain within twenty-nine days.[31]

Methyl mercury vapor exhibits unusual characteristics. It is unable to be absorbed into water, but it can dissolve into lipids. It does not bind with oxygen but instead is transferred directly into tissues. As described in the next chapter, mercury has a high affinity for sulfur compounds and attaches to the sulfhydryl group inside the cell, which helps to facilitate its journey throughout the body. In *Mercury Poisoning from Dental Amalgams: A Hazard to the Human Brain*, Swedish researcher Dr. Patrick Stortebecker, M.D., Ph.D., describes in detail how mercury vapor is first released from dental amalgams through various entrances (oronasal cavity, lungs, and saliva) and then circulated through various pathways of transport (lymphatics, blood, nerves, and cerebral-spinal fluid) to the brain, organs, tissues, and bones.[32]

Certainly one of the most common causal cofactors of chronic degenerative disease that Linda finds in her practice is mercury poisoning derived from amalgam fillings. Even clients who come to Linda after having their mercury fillings removed are stunned to discover that *the damage has already been done. The mercury has leached into multiple areas of the body and brain where it has wreaked havoc in a variety of ghastly ways.*

Linda channels the presence of mercury by going to the Physical Databases where she scans a list of every organ, gland, bone, tissue, artery, or vein in the body or brain with her pendulum and index finger. She notes each entry where the pendulum spins to the right, indicating a location where mercury has lodged. Invariably, she has found that the organ, gland, or system with the greatest level of mercury is usually the MSO from the pre-test.

How Other Practitioners Test for Mercury Toxicity

For the rest of the world (with the exception of competent EAV practitioners and healers using Dr. Dietrich Klinghardt's Autonomic Response Testing method[33]), the most accurate method of testing for mercury in the body is using a chelating drug that binds to metal in what is called the Provoked Urine Challenge. Two samples of urine are taken—one before administration of the drug and one after. In the test, a pharmaceutical chelating agent such as DMSA (meso-2, 3-dimercaptosuccinic acid) or DMPS (dimercaptopropanesulfanate) is administered that binds to and removes mercury, lead, and arsenic out of the tissues where it has formed stable complexes with these metals. They are then excreted out of the body through urine. The two samples are sent to a CLIA-certified laboratory such as Doctor's Data, Inc. or MetaMetrix, which analyzes the urine utilizing a state-of-the-art mass spectrometer which detects trace amounts of mercury measured in parts per million. Test results are provided as a numeric value plotted on a bar graph indicating that the level of mercury is within normal range, elevated, or very elevated. Unlike Linda, it cannot tell where the mercury is located—just that it exists somewhere in the body. (See "Large-Scale Lab Study Proves Dental Amalgam Affects Mercury Body Burden.")

The problem with a DMSA or DMPS challenge, however, is that these drugs have the potential to damage the kidneys or liver in people who turn out to have really high levels of mercury. That's because heavy metals such as mercury, cadmium, and lead are potent nephrotoxins which can markedly decrease renal function, resulting in decreased efficiency of filtration that is essential to normal kidney function. That is critical during any sort of chelation therapy, where increased mobilization of these toxic metals requires an elevated demand on renal clearance. If the kidneys are functioning poorly prior to chelation therapy, an increased mercury burden often leads to kidney damage. This is why we highly recommend that your doctor or other health care professional conduct a thorough assessment of renal function. This is best achieved by a creatinine clearance test, which will help the practitioner determine safe and appropriate levels of the chelating agent.

Linda recommends that anyone who suspects he or she may have mercury toxicity should take a Provoked Urine Challenge given by a doctor who is trained and experienced in safely administering the test and is recommended by the American College for Advancement in Medicine (ACAM). This not-for-profit association is dedicated to educating physicians and other health care professionals on the latest findings and procedures in integrative and alternative medicine.

Large-Scale Lab Study Proves Dental Amalgam Affects Mercury Body Burden

In the November 2008 issue of the prestigious *Townsend Letter for Doctors & Patients,* there was an article entitled "Mercury Testing and Treatment" by Dr. Bruce M. Dooley, M.D., from New Zealand that described the results of the first large-scale study utilizing the Provoked Urine Challenge that had recently been conducted in America. I also spoke by telephone with Dr. Dooley, who provided the following information:

"In 2008, I participated as a keynote speaker in a conference in Los Angeles entitled Extreme Health Makeover. The attendees, who included a significant number of health care professionals, heard the latest information on how to achieve optimal wellness. As a result of this conference, we were able to collect and process the urine of over 1,000 individuals who currently had amalgam fillings using oral DMPS-provoked two-hour urine mercury tests. These were performed at the independent lab, Doctor's Data. To my knowledge, this is the first time this large a group has ever been studied, and we are now trying to grasp the health implications to United States, Canada, and other Westernized populations which have mercury dental amalgams.

"The outcome of this conjoined mass testing frankly astonished me and others familiar with mercury. Consistently, we found that 75 percent of the group tested in the red zone or very elevated with 20 percent in the elevated yellow zone. *Thus, we can say with confidence that 95 percent of the population will display a significant tissue burden of mercury. When these data are extrapolated to the entire population, the numbers are staggering.*"[34]

The significance of this large-scale study is that it scientifically validated a body of knowledge that Linda and I learned the hard way, from our own medical histories as well as through arduous research. This much is clear: Older mercury fillings—at least those fillings that have been gassing off mercury vapors in an adult's mouth since childhood—are almost certain to lead to some form(s) of chronic degenerative disease and/or neurological condition(s) later in life.

THE MANY MEDICAL CONDITIONS CREATED BY MERCURY TOXICITY

The sheer number of medical conditions associated with leakage from dental amalgam and other sources of mercury toxicity is truly astonishing to us. Mercury can be either the primary cause or a secondary cofactor behind so much chronic disease. That is why Dr. Dietrich Klinghardt, M.D., Ph.D., a pioneer in mercury detoxification, has correctly characterized it as "the mother of all toxins."[35] Table 9-1 contains a comprehensive list of physiological symptoms compiled from several highly reputable sources listed in the Suggested Readings and Resources. A list of neurological and psychological symptoms appears in Chapter 11. It is hoped that both lists will be real eye-openers for the sufferers of these conditions. In addition, we hope they will inform the many sincere medical doctors of various subspecialties, who seek additional new approaches to not only alleviating symptoms but actually eliminating the underlying toxic burden that often is the real cause of chronic disease.

TABLE 9-1. PHYSIOLOGICAL SYMPTOMS OF MERCURY POISONING

Cardiovascular System

Abnormal blood pressure, high or low

Anemia

Angina

Arrhythmia

Arteriosclerosis

Elevated cholesterol

Elevated homocysteine

Elevated triglycerides

Heart attack

Heart murmur

Pressure/pain in chest

Tachycardia

Digestive System

Bloating

Colitis

Constipation

Diarrhea

Diverticulitis

Food sensitivities, milk and eggs

Heartburn

Irritable bowel syndrome

Loss of appetite

Stomach cramps

Ulcers

Ear, Nose, Throat, and Teeth

Bad breath

Bleeding gums

Bone loss around teeth

Burning sensation in mouth

Enlarged salivary glands

Gingivitis

Glaucoma

Hearing loss

Increased flow of saliva

Leukoplakia

Loosening of teeth

Loss of teeth

Metallic taste in mouth

Mouth ulcers

Periodontal (gum) disease

Sinusitis

Sore throat and persistent cough

Stomatitis

Swollen tongue

Tinnitus

Ulceration of oral mucosa

Endocrine System

Adrenal fatigue

Chronic low body temperature

Cold hands and feet

Decreased sexual drive

Diabetes

Enlarged prostate (BPH) with frequent urination, especially at night

Erectile dysfunction

Estrogen imbalance

Hypothalamus-pituitary-adrenal axis imbalance

Hypoglycemia

Hypothyroidism

Testosterone imbalance

Weight loss issues

Immune System

Allergies

Anemia

Antibiotic resistance

Autoimmune disorders

Amyotrophic lateral sclerosis (ALS)

Arthritis

Hypothyroidism

Lupus erythematosus (LE)

Multiple sclerosis (MS)

Scleroderma

Cancer

Leukemia

Chronic fatigue syndrome

Chronic infections

Bacterial and mycobacterial

Candida and other fungal/yeast

Parasite infestation

Viral infections such as Epstein-Barr, mononucleosis, pneumonitis

Susceptibility to flu, colds, etc.

Swollen glands

Kidney Disease

Edema

Bladder infection

Inhibited kidney filtration

Kidney infection

Kidney stones

Nephritis

Painful urination

Liver Disease

Blocked methylation, phases
  I & II

Liver detoxification pathways

Pain Producing

Arthritis

Osteoporosis

Pain in joints

Slow healing

Reproductive System

Birth defects in offspring

Infertility

Sterility

Respiratory System

Asthma

Bronchial spasms

Skin

Acne

Dermatitis/eczema

Excessive itching

Excessive sweating

Night sweats

Rashes

Rough skin

Skin flushes

CHAPTER 10

How the Monster Rears Its Head

*How often do you get the chance to improve
the lives of a billion people?*
—Dr. Hal Huggins, a pioneer mercury-free dentist
at the 1996 launch of Consumers for Dental Choice

Research studies have proven that unstable amalgam fillings produce methyl mercury vapors that leach over time into many body tissues, organs, and the brain. They disrupt and impair many core biochemical and metabolic processes throughout the body and brain, making mercury from dental amalgam the "mother of all toxins." Mercury has proven to be cytotoxic (toxic to cells), neurotoxic, immunotoxic, reproductive toxic, and endocrine disrupting.[1] In order to understand the role mercury plays in specific disease etiology, we must first understand how mercury causes severe biochemical and metabolic damage on a *cellular level* that is behind so much chronic degenerative disease.

MERCURY NEGATIVELY IMPACTS CORE BIOCHEMICAL PROCESSES

Our bodies contain a complex network of antioxidants, amino acids, metabolites, and enzymes that work together to prevent oxidative damage to proteins, DNA, and lipids. Mercury greatly increases free-radical production within the cell and lipid peroxidation, a degenerative oxidative process, in the cell membrane. Much of the damage done by mercury results from free-radical damage to many parts of the cell, including the mitochondria, nucleus, cytoplasm, and microsomes.[2] Playing havoc with the cell's electrons is particularly dangerous since electrons are the glue that holds molecules together. Here's a brief overview of how free radicals and lipid peroxidation work.

- **Free radicals.** A free radical is any atom or molecule that contains an odd number of electrons, including a single unpaired electron in its outermost shell. Free radicals are an unavoidable, destructive byproduct of normal metabolism. Mercury and other heavy metals, however, increase their destructiveness. The widely accepted free-radical theory of aging postulates that our slide into decrepitude is the result of irreversible damage done to these biomolecules that gain or lose a single electron, converting them into unstable, highly reactive, toxic free radicals. Oxygen free radicals called reactive oxygen species (ROS) are the main agents of this destruction. These dangerous chemical compounds possess a voracious appetite for electrons and lipid peroxides. Electrons are ripped away from tissues, proteins, DNA, and the fatty acids in cell membranes, leaving a trail of destruction in their wake—akin to the rust that accumulates on an old car.

- **Lipid peroxidation.** This degenerative oxidative process occurs in lipids (unsaturated fatty acids) within cell membranes. It can affect such lipids as phospholipids, glycolipids, and different forms of cholesterol. Mercury disturbs fatty acid metabolism when free radicals steal electrons from these lipids in cell membranes. This results in a chain reaction that spreads oxidative damage throughout the cell, forming unstable fatty-acid free radicals that lead to another generation of ROS.

Mercury significantly accelerates the level of free-radical proliferation that can deplete, inhibit, or modify antioxidants and other substances, including ATP (adenosine triphosphate), glutathione (GSH), superoxide dismutase (SOD), zinc, selenium, calcium, vitamins A and C, as well as important amino acids, hormones, and enzymes. The destructive force of scavenging free radicals damages or destroys numerous cellular functions, affecting such basic tasks as the ability to complete an enzymatic reaction, synthesize a protein, transport oxygen across a cell membrane, or otherwise promote healthy organ function. A consequence of inadequate antioxidant protection, oxidative stress causes the molecule to become unglued, denatured, and damaged. This drain of electron energy negatively affects the body's ability to detoxify. This, in turn, promotes the inflammatory process of oxidation, which does irreparable damage to cells, tissues, and the immune system.

To fight the effects of free radicals and lipid peroxidation, Linda advocates providing strong antioxidants, which can be thought of as anti-inflammatory reinforcements. These are obtained through supplements including vitamins, minerals, proteins, amino acids, and enzymes. Although Linda likes antioxidants such as vitamins C and E, for a mercury toxic client she is more likely to channel a more potent variety such as alpha lipoic acid (ALA), curcumin extract, liposomal glutathione, methionine, selenium, n-acetyl cysteine (NAC), ecklonia cava extract, and, on occasion, high-quality dark chocolate (naturally sweetened with agave).

The Biochemical Nightmare of Mercury on Our Cellular Building Blocks

Amino acids are the principal building blocks of all proteins and enzymes. Sulfur is also present in all proteins and many enzymes. Sulfhydryls (also called thiols) are cells composed of a sulfur atom and a hydrogen atom. They are important because they determine the structure and function of proteins and enzymes. However, the mercury atom or molecule has a high affinity for sulfur that causes them to bind to any molecule with a sulfur or sulfur-hydrogen combination. So when mercury from amalgam binds to sulfhydryls, it diminishes or destroys the structure and function of sulfur, blocking and interfering with the normal binding process of sulfhydryls, called sulphur oxidation. In addition, mercury binds to the protein structure itself, making it potentially toxic. *Because sulfur is present in so many amino acids, proteins, enzymes, hormones, nerve tissues, and red blood cells, all these building blocks of the body are subject to attack by mercury toxins.* The damage unfolds on the cellular level in the following ways.

Cellular Disaster 1: Amino acids. The primary sulfur-containing amino acids in the body are cysteine, methionine, and taurine. Whenever mercury binds to these amino acids or their metabolites, it depletes and/or inhibits their availability to perform their normal metabolic function. Mercury blocks the conversion of precursor amino acids into sulfates, taurine, glutathione, vitamin B_{12}, and folic acid. This results in a weakened immune system and increased oxidative stress, which has a profoundly negative effect on many organ systems. It also elevates levels of homocysteine, a high-risk factor in cardiovascular disease and neuropsychiatric disorders.

An integral part of Linda's process of rectifying the damage done to the body and the brain by mercury involves replenishing depleted amino acids and enzymes that are also antioxidants. She channels those organs and glands where these biochemical malfunctions have occurred, particularly those affecting the amino acid precursors of glutathione, the master antioxidant in the body. The most important naturally occurring precursors of glutathione that are depleted by mercury are certain amino acids or antioxidants including cysteine, methionine, taurine, ALA, and NAC. When Linda channels that a client needs these substances, so critical to detoxification, it is primarily because *mercury has already depleted them.*

How Mercury Affects Glutathione, the Master Antioxidant in the Body

Glutathione is the body's principal detoxifier and protector against free radical and lipid peroxidation damage. Although it is found in every cell in the body, it is primarily synthesized and concentrated in the liver (detoxifier), spleen (immune system enhancer), and skin. The liver exports glutathione to the blood where it functions as a biochemical washing machine, quenching free radicals and neutralizing heavy metals, pharmaceutical drugs, alcohol, and nicotine. It also protects the mitochondrial energy factory that produces ATP, which is found in every cell in the body.

The reason glutathione is called the master antioxidant is due to the fact that it contains an abundant amount of sulfur-containing thiol. That originates as a tripeptide molecule that must be synthesized from three precursor amino acids—cysteine, glutamic acid, and glycine—before it can work effectively. This reaction occurs, in part, through sulfur oxidation with thiols. When sulfur molecules are attached to mercury, glutathione chelates the mercury and dumps it into the bile for excretion. Paradoxically, however, as methyl mercury *continues* to leach unabated from dental amalgams, the amount of glutathione needed to remove the mercury begins to increase. Now, however, the supply is diminishing.

The reason for this is that mercury has now become a catalyst for the destructive free-radical oxidation of glutathione by virtue of its ability to block sulfur oxidation. Thus, the very process needed to synthesize the production of glutathione is now blocked and remaining amounts are depleted. *This depressed level of glutathione, in turn, reduces the body's ability to detoxify mercury and other toxins out of the liver and reduces overall immunity as well.* Beside heavy metals, one of the worst polluters of the liver is a common over-the-counter drug. In 2009, the FDA tacitly acknowledged that the chronic overuse of Tylenol (acetaminophen) is the leading cause of liver failure in the United States.[3] Tylenol inhibits the body's ability to synthesize sufficient levels of glutathione, making it toxic to the liver.

Cellular Disaster 2: Enzymes. These complex proteins speed up the chemical reaction of every biochemical process. Enzyme deficiency is a devastating cofactor in much chronic disease, affecting our ability to fight off disease or repair injury. Many enzymes are derived from sulfur proteins, which also makes them universally available for binding with mercury throughout the body. The strong bonds that mercury forms with thiols disrupt, deplete, and inactivate many essential enzymatic processes throughout the body. This is very important because a majority of enzymes depend on thiols for their activity. As a consequence, mercury has the destructive power to inhibit the function of critically important antioxidant enzymes. These depleted enzymes result in the malfunction of vital core biochemical processes, which leads to chronic degenerative disease. These include lowered energy production of ATP (mitochondrial/heart disease), decreased production of glutathione and other antioxidants (oxidation of cholesterol that contributes to arteriosclerosis and neurodegeneration), disruption of protein synthesis and DNA/RNA function (gene mutation and birth defects), of cell signaling (immune deficiencies and inflammation), and of membrane structure (leaky gut syndrome, ulcerative colitis, and mercury passing through placenta to the fetus).

The biochemical origins of many diseases are associated with impaired antioxidant protection that eventually manifests as many types of chronic degenerative disease. Just a partial list includes diabetes, renal failure, cancer, digestive disorders (leaky gut and ulcerative colitis), cardiovascular and circulatory disease (atherosclerosis, strokes, hypertension), and such neurodegenerative diseases as amyotrophic lateral sclerosis (ALS, or Lou Gehrig's disease), Alzheimer's, Parkinson's, and autism.

Cellular Disaster 3: Hormones. Methyl mercury vapor from dental amalgam has been found to be a profound endocrine system disrupter. Sulfur is essential in the cellular processes in such hormones as insulin, growth hormone, prolactin, and vasopressin. When mercury binds to these molecules, it reduces their ability to carry out normal metabolic functions.[4] Mercury rapidly crosses the blood-brain barrier and is stored preferentially in the pituitary, hypothalamus, and occipital cortex (the visual processing center of the brain) in direct proportion to the number and extent of dental amalgam surfaces.[5] This is a key reason for mercury's relationship to much neuroendocrine dysfunction and many severe emotional problems. For example, the pituitary gland controls many endocrine system functions and secretes hormones that control many bodily processes, including the immune system and reproductive system. The hypothalamus regulates body temperature and many other metabolic processes. Mercury also commonly lodges in the thyroid, prostate, testes (all discussed in this chapter) as well as adrenals, pancreas, and ovaries, and can be a cofactor in chronic conditions affecting these areas.

Cellular Disaster 4: Vitamins and minerals. Mercury has a tendency to bind with certain vitamins, including the Bs, C, and E, and minerals, including selenium, zinc, calcium, and magnesium. (A discussion of how Linda brilliantly channels these in relation to emotional and neurological issues is covered in Chapter 15.) By binding to and interfering with these nutrients, mercury toxicity mimics the symptoms associated with nutrient deficiencies.[6] This potentially applies to many common conditions. For example, mercury is known as a causal factor in an enlarged prostate, and selenium and zinc deficiencies are common in men with enlarged prostates. The relationship between magnesium deficiency and heart disease, vitamin B_{12} and neurological issues, and calcium deficiency and osteoporosis are clearly established.

Cellular Disaster 5: Inflammatory cytokines. Initially, cytokines are part of the immune system's response against many types of foreign invaders. However, chronic mercury toxicity shifts the immune system into a high state of alert, producing inflammatory cytokines. These destructive proteins take on an autoimmune response, attacking cells and tissues in the body. Inflammatory cytokines are known cofactors in autoimmune diseases ranging from rheumatoid arthritis, asthma, lupus, irritable bowel syndrome, celiac, Crohn's disease to depression, dementia, ADHD, Alzheimer's disease, and autism (see Autoimmune Disease below).

WHERE THE MONSTER STRIKES

Given the power of mercury to disrupt or destroy cell function, it is no wonder that researchers have concluded that dental amalgam is often a cofactor or even the sole factor in so many different types of chronic degenerative conditions. In fact, the evidence against mercury is so overwhelming that Linda remarks, *"Pick a chronic degenerative condition anywhere in the body, and the first clue that needs to be investigated is whether mercury or other toxic metals are somehow involved."* In this chapter we will discuss the organs, organ/glandular systems, and tissues where mercury causes the greatest damage in the body: the immune system, kidneys, gastrointestinal (GI) system, prostate, reproductive organs, endocrine system, cardiovascular system, and liver. The entire next chapter is devoted to the effects of mercury on the brain.

Mercury Suppresses the Immune System

It's long been known in the medical literature that mercury suppresses the immune system. The brilliant Dr. Dietrich Klinghardt has taken this concept further than other researchers and devised what is known as the Klinghardt axiom: "Most—if not all—chronic infectious diseases are not caused by a failure of the immune system, but are a conscious adaptation of the immune system to an otherwise lethal heavy metal environment."[7] Linda concurs with his findings and is convinced that mercury toxicity is a significant cofactor in people with such chronic viral illnesses as herpes zoster; genital herpes; chronic fungal illnesses like candidiasis; and recurrent episodes of such bacterial infections as chronic sinusitis, tonsillitis, bronchitis, and bladder/prostate infections.

Antibiotic resistance: Studies suggest that chronic mercury exposure in amounts released by amalgams provokes an increase in antibiotic-resistant strains of bacteria in oral and intestinal flora in primates.[8] Mercury is the only substance ever shown that induces antibiotic resistance in bacteria, other than an antibiotic.[9] This would seem to contribute to the problem of antibiotic resistance and the need for continual development of new antibiotics.[10]

Autoimmune disease. An autoimmune disease is a condition in which a person's immune system destroys cells in his or her body. It is like a case of mistaken identity where a military force kills its own cellular soldiers through friendly fire. When mercury becomes attached to a cell membrane, it distorts the shape of the cell in such a manner that the immune system recognizes it as abnormal.[11] In the ongoing sophisticated surveillance of your immune system, the mercury-infested cell is now mistakenly slated for immediate destruction by your white blood cells. That is why many autoimmune conditions, including chronic fatigue syndrome, multiple sclerosis, ALS, lupus, fibromyalgia, rheumatoid arthritis, Hashimoto's thyroiditis, adrenal insufficiency, and many allergies, are either caused by or exacerbated by immune reactivity to mercury.[12,13]

According to Dr. Russell Blaylock, at least part of the damage caused by many neurodegenerative diseases is related to autoimmune reactions to cells in the nervous system.[14] Even diabetes or mild elevations in blood sugar levels can result from an autoimmune process initiated by mercury's attack on the pancreas.[15]

Biological terrain alterations. Mercury toxicity is responsible for fundamentally shifting the pH of blood and other body fluids to a state of acidosis. In the ongoing war of the microbial worlds that goes on in the body, this unnatural milieu tilts the microbial balance of power away from beneficial flora in favor of harmful pathogenic forms. The blood and other body fluids are now transformed into a breeding ground for harmful bacteria, viruses, fungi, and parasites that set the body up for much chronic degenerative disease (Chapters 5–7).

Chronic fatigue syndrome. Mercury exposure through dental fillings appears to be a major factor in CFS. Not only does mercury depress levels of energy production of ATP, beneficial intestinal bacteria, and overall immune system function, it promotes growth of *Candida albicans* throughout the body as well as the conversion of inorganic mercury into the more toxic methyl mercury form. CFS is often an amalgam-driven condition that has reached epidemic proportions in America.

Testimonial: Curing Anna's herpes simplex and bladder cystitis

Linda met Anna while working at the Kientalerhof Center for Wellbeing in Switzerland in 2005. After contracting genital herpes approximately nine months earlier, Anna had experienced multiple outbreaks, usually after sexual contact. Severe itching and an overall weakening of her immune system made her feel quite rundown. She noticed that the outbreaks were worse when she was stressed. In addition, for the last two years Anna had had chronic bladder infections, which started after the stress of her mother's death. Her doctor diagnosed the condition as bladder cystitis and gave her an antibiotic, which initially worked. However, the cystitis kept returning, particularly after sexual contact. Anna also had eczema on various parts of her body, which she controlled with cortisone. Almost as an afterthought, she mentioned that she had been on birth control pills for a number of years.

Linda channeled that Anna's most stressed organs were her urological system and liver and that psychological stress exacerbated her condition. Linda also learned from the pre-test that Anna's allergic autoimmune imbalance provoked an inflammatory reaction due to mercury toxicity and toxic emotions. Upon questioning, Linda learned that Anna had a significant number of silver amalgam fillings.

Linda channeled the following information: Both Anna's herpes and chronic bladder cystitis were exacerbated by severe systemic acidosis brought about by mercury toxicity from her silver fillings as well as from nickel and aluminum. The acidic terrain of her blood became the breeding ground for various forms of fungi as well as a parasite infestation. Linda channeled these recommendations for Anna to follow, which she did in short order:

1. Shift to a highly restrictive alkaline diet augmented by a powdered bar-

ley juice drink. As her heavy metal, fungus, and parasite loads decreased, Anna may add back certain foods as she reaches certain detoxification milestones.

2. Have a biological dentist remove all mercury fillings (see Chapter 12). Mercury from leaky amalgam fillings was the main reason for Anna's suppressed immune system. This promoted the proliferation of fungi and parasites that were thriving in an acidic terrain.

3. Immediately get off birth control pills. Linda channeled they were throwing off Anna's endocrine system and contributing to candidiasis, which further weakened her immune system.

4. Treat the miasms homeopathically in preparation for a heavy metal detox.

5. Treat the fungi homeopathically and also take probiotics to restore her intestinal flora balance.

6. Treat the parasites with an herbal remedy.

7. Detoxify kidney/bladder/liver with various herbal and homeopathic detox remedies.

8. Open Anna's lymphatic system with an herbal tincture.

9. Take a mineral/trace mineral supplement. The fungal proliferation made absorption of minerals/trace minerals more difficult, affecting her immune and endocrine systems.

10. Use certain gem essences and Kabbalistic meditations to help transform Anna's negative emotions into their positive counterparts.

11. Treat the herpes with transfer factors, chemical messengers that enhance immune system response. According to Dr. Charles H. Kirkpatrick, M.D., director of the Adult Immunodeficiency Program at University of Colorado Health Sciences Center, "transfer factors have been shown to be an effective means for correction of deficient cellular immunity in patients with opportunistic infections, such as candidiasis or recurrent herpes simplex. . . ."[16]

Linda channeled that Valtrex, prescribed by Anna's doctor to control the herpes outbreaks, was only slightly effective and would not cure the condition. In addition, Linda channeled that Anna did not tolerate Valtrex well, and undesirable side effects would occur over a protracted period of time.

Nonetheless, Anna was reluctant to give up Valtrex, believing that taking it controlled outbreaks better than not taking it. Linda agreed to work around Anna's request and channeled a precise treatment protocol where Anna alternated Valtrex with certain transfer factors to eliminate the herpes virus.

Anna took Linda's recommendations seriously, and after doing the dental work and following the other recommendations, she did a heavy metal detox, which consisted of taking several natural herbal and mineral chelating agents. Over six months, Anna was able to significantly lower her heavy metal load, bring her fungal and parasite burden down to negligent or nonexistent levels, as well as achieve a fundamental shift to a neutral pH level. That, in turn, allowed her immune system to strengthen sufficiently so her alternating transfer factor/Valtrex protocol eliminated the herpes virus once and for all. Anna's story is a wonderful example of angelic multitasking at work.

Approximately nine months later, Anna reported that her bladder cystitis was cured, her eczema had disappeared, and her immune system had regained the vigor of her youth. The last we heard of Anna she was all smiles due to her marriage and the recent birth of her first child.

Kidney Disorders

It is well known that mercury tends to concentrate in the kidneys.[17] A study headed by Professor Murray Vimy, D.M.D., of the University of Calgary in Canada also suggests it can also inhibit kidney function.[18,19] In his study, six sheep received silver amalgam fillings while two sheep, in a control group, received glass ionomer fillings. Renal clearance tests were given just prior to the fillings being inserted and at intervals of 30 and 60 days following the insertion of the fillings. Vimy discovered that after only 30 days of chewing with dental amalgam fillings, the sheep had lost 60 percent of their kidney filtration ability, resulting in a decreased efficiency of kidney function. This was measured by a significant decrease in their insulin clearance, when compared with the control group. They also exhibited a significant increase in urinary sodium in the proximal tubules, proving that urinary sodium excretion increases as mercury inhibits the function of these cells. *Both of these conditions are clear indications of kidney malfunction.*

Digestive Disorders

Mercury leached from amalgam is known to be a common cause of many chronic conditions related to leaky gut and intestinal dysfunction. It causes progressive damage to the stomach and intestinal lining and destroys beneficial flora. This eventually allows disease-causing bacteria, undigested food particles, and toxins to pass directly into the bloodstream, triggering an immune response. These dysfunctions in intestinal permeability result in leaky gut syndrome, which impairs the absorption of food and nutrients.[20] It also causes an accumulation of *Helicobacter pylori* bacteria, a major factor in stomach ulcers.[21] Mercury also creates an acidic milieu that becomes a breeding ground for *Candida albicans*, resulting in gastrointestinal dysbiosis. This confluence of factors is often the core cause of diseases such as ulcers, ulcerative colitis, irritable bowel syndrome (IBS), and Crohn's disease.

Testimonial: Curing Eleanor's ulcerative colitis

As many as one million Americans have inflammatory bowel disorder (IBD), with that number evenly split between Crohn's disease and ulcerative colitis.[22] IBD is characterized as an autoimmune condition that tends to run in families. Ulcerative colitis is a chronic inflammation that results in sores (ulcers) in the large intestine, sigmoid colon, and rectum where waste material is stored.

Eleanor is a fifty-five-year-old woman who suffered for years from diarrhea and the severe pain of ulcerative colitis. After enduring a colonoscopy and barium enema x-ray, her doctor diagnosed her with ulcerative colitis and put her on Asacol, an anti-inflammatory drug for her colon. When she asked him about the cause of ulcerative colitis, he said no one really knew and there was no real cure. He simply surmised that stress made it worse. Rounds of the antacids Zantac and Asacol initially gave Eleanor temporary relief from her symptoms. However, the pain and discomfort returned with a vengeance in short order. The doctor reassured Eleanor that this was the best way to treat ulcerative colitis and that she would just have to learn to live with it. He told her that if she did not improve, she might want to consider a surgical option, which was decidedly not to her liking. She was beginning to lose faith that her doctor could provide the relief she sought from her chronic condition. A friend persuaded Eleanor to see if Linda could provide another viable approach.

Before the first session started, Linda told Eleanor there was a high likelihood that some sort of chronic toxic exposure, intestinal infection, or imbalanced intestinal flora had overwhelmed her immune system's ability to function effectively. This was why the process of chronic inflammation had taken its toll on the lining of her colon. The pre-test and a deeper analysis soon revealed a precise snapshot of her problem. Eleanor's two most stressed organs were her liver (mercury, lead, aluminum at a 50 percent load; fungi and parasites) and gastrointestinal tract (mercury, lead, aluminum at a 50 percent load; GI dysbiosis, parasites, and a low-grade salmonella infection). Eleanor also tested high for acid pH, autoimmune allergy, miasms, enzyme and mineral deficiencies, lymphatic congestion, and emotional stress.

Taken aback by the exceedingly high levels of heavy metals, fungi, and parasites, Linda asked Eleanor if she had any silver amalgam fillings. Eleanor responded that she had eight. Linda insisted that Eleanor see a local biological dentist versed in the Huggins protocol (Chapter 12) who could safely remove the source of her heavy metal toxicity.

In the initial "prepping stage" for the body that always precedes a heavy metal detox, Linda put Eleanor on a highly restrictive alkaline anti-candida diet, gave her homeopathic remedies for fungi, miasms, and lymphatic congestion, and treated the parasite infestation with an herbal blend. Linda also recommended a special herbal blend to help detoxify her highly toxic liver, digestive enzymes to promote the assimilation of nutrients, and probiotics to restore beneficial flora. After getting her eight fillings removed, Eleanor felt a little better. Two months later, Linda had her take a gentle dosage of a heavy metal chelator. Over the next few months all of Eleanor's numbers (heavy metals, fungi, and parasites) began to drop and the episodes of severe abdominal pain and diarrhea began to abate. Soon Linda was able to add a greater variety of food choices to Eleanor's restrictive diet. Eleanor also weaned herself off Asacol without any ill effects. After ten months of treatment, Eleanor's ulcerative colitis had completely disappeared and has never returned. Eleanor is once again enjoying life without the ill effects of a condition her doctor said had no cure.

Prostate Disease

Linda has consistently channeled for affected male clients that there is a significant relationship between prostate disease, ranging from benign prostatic hyperplasia (BPH) to prostate cancer, and mercury derived from dental amalgam. Perhaps the best source of information on that relationship is Larry Clapp, a prostate-survivor-turned-coach who has successfully guided many men through mercury detox as part of a natural approach to treating prostate problems. He is the author of an important book, *Prostate Health in 90 Days Without Drugs or Surgery*.

In a section on his website (www.prostate90.com) entitled "Lessons of 17 Years of Healing through Cleansing," Clapp writes: "The overwhelming lesson since my own cleansing and healing [from prostate cancer] in 1990 and coaching of hundreds of patients over these seventeen years has been the devastating effect on health of heavy metal toxicity, from our dentistry, food chain and environmental sources."[23]

Linda also admires the research of Dr. Rita Ellithorpe, M.D., a urologist at the Tustin Longevity Center in Tustin, California, who has developed effective protocols to significantly shrink the prostate, reduce frequent urination, and improve erectile function by reducing the level of mercury in the prostate. Her work is backed by clinical trials utilizing Detoxamin, a suppository containing EDTA (ethylenediaminetetraacetic acid), a heavy metal chelator, in combination with vitamins, minerals, probiotics, and tetracycline that seems to effectively chelate heavy metals out of the prostate gland.[24,25] When Linda channels that mercury or other metals are a cofactor in BPH, she uses this product in conjunction with an array of natural prostate supplements, including beta-sitosterol, DIM (3,3'-diindolylmethane), Swedish bee pollen, stinging nettles, lycopene, zinc, selenium, pumpkin seed oil, and saw palmetto.

Birth Defects, Damage to Children, and Reproductive Disorders

Studies show methyl mercury passes quite easily through the placenta barrier. A peer-reviewed article published in 2008 analyzed the relationship between maternal dental amalgam fillings and exposure of the developing fetus to mercury. It found a strong correlation between high umbilical cord levels of mercury with the number of amalgam fillings in the mother.[26] Mercury alters activities of five different enzymes in the placenta that may result in fetal kidney damage, mental retardation, defects in the chest wall, cleft palate, and abnormal heart alterations.[27,28]

Birth defects are often the result of genetic aberrations in DNA caused by damage to the genetic code by environmental toxins. Normally, there are two sets of 23 pairs of chromosomes, one set from each parent, for a total of 46 pairs. Mercury, however, has been found to produce "aberrant chromosome numbers." This means that a child with a birth defect might have 45 or 47 chromosomes. Examples of this include Down's syndrome and Klinefelter's syndrome.[29] A deviation of more than one chromosome often results in death of the fetus.[30]

This is why Linda urges any woman planning to get pregnant to first get all her silver fillings safely removed by a biological dentist trained in safe amalgam removal

(Chapter 12) before conception in order to minimize any toxic mercury damage to the fetus.

In 1990, the state of California passed legislation called Proposition 65 that was designed to protect citizens from many forms of environmental toxicity. Mercury and mercury compounds were listed as "known reproductive toxins." The warning states: "Dental amalgam, used in many dental fillings, causes exposure to mercury, a chemical known to the state of California to cause birth defects and other reproductive harm." Since more restrictive legislation was passed in February 2001, the link between birth defects and mercury amalgam fillings must be disclosed to dental patients, who must sign a written consent form acknowledging that they have read and understand this.

Mercury-related damage to infants and developing children is well documented in the medical literature. A study conducted of breast-feeding mothers in Sweden in 1996 found a direct relationship between the number of their amalgam fillings and the level of mercury in their breast milk. The study also concluded that mercury from amalgam fillings posed a greater danger to the health of a developing child than mercury from seafood.[31] Other studies show a link between mercury and infertility,[32] miscarriages,[33] and low levels of progesterone in women.[34]

None of this even takes into account the additional potential damage that Linda channels may be caused by thimerosal, a mercury preservative found in vaccines administered to young children (Chapter 11). That's why Linda advises mothers to insist that their pediatricians give vaccinations that do not contain thimerosal. Linda has channeled that all these sources of mercury are a significant cofactor for epidemic-level increases in childhood neurological conditions and other health problems.

Men are hardly exempt from damage as mercury is known to accumulate in the testes. In addition to having estrogenic effects, mercury has other documented hormonal effects on the male reproductive system, including low sperm counts, defective sperm cells, damaged DNA, aberrant chromosome numbers, chromosome breaks, and low testosterone levels.[35,36]

Testimonial: Curing severe male infertility begets twins!

In the fall of 2005, Linda received a call from a young married couple named Herschel and Naomi who were desperately trying to conceive their first child. Unable to conceive normally, the couple was committed to the expensive process of artificially conceiving a child through in vitro fertilization (IVF). This involves placing collected sperm and eggs together in a petri dish until the sperm penetrates the eggs and fertilization is achieved. Several of the embryos judged to be "best" are transferred to the woman's uterus to improve chances of achieving pregnancy. They had already invested considerable time, money, energy, and emotions in this process without achieving the desired result. Out of desperation they came to see Linda after being referred by multiple sources in their close-knit community who had been successfully treated by her.

Herschel had been diagnosed at the fertility clinic with a type of male factor infertility called isolated *teratozoospermia*. A microscopic staining test, called a Kruger strict morphology test, was used to measure the shape of his sperm cells. This accurately predicts the fertilizing capacity of sperm. Relatively few sperm are rated as normal during this test. A strict morphology score of over 14 percent of normal sperm means there is an excellent capacity to fertilize; between 4 and 14 percent is the normal range (although the lower end of this spectrum represents increasingly impaired fertilizing capacity); and 0 to 3 percent represents a severe impairment or probable inability to fertilize. Herschel took the test three separate times, and each time the result was 0 percent morphology. He was told *there was no known cause for this condition, nor any treatment for it.* Although Herschel produced a sufficient quantity of sperm, its morphology (shape and size of the sperm head, midsection, and tail) was highly abnormal (amorphous), rendering it incapable of penetrating or fertilizing an egg on its own. Another approach was needed.

The fertility doctor, also known as an andrologist, proposed utilizing an alternate procedure called ICSI (intracytoplasmic sperm injection) where the woman is first stimulated with medication to produce an egg that is harvested by an embryologist. A single sperm is then injected into the middle of the egg (cytoplasm) with a needle that carefully pierces its outer cell walls (zona). Initially the IVF/ICSI was deemed successful. But after the embryo was successfully implanted in Naomi's womb, she had a miscarriage eight or nine weeks later. When the fetus was removed, the test showed that it was chromosomally abnormal and therefore deformed.

Herschel and Naomi were despondent with good reason. Since the very shape of the sperm and the fetus were both abnormal, they worried that they would never have normal, healthy children even if they were able to conceive. They had reached the end of the line in terms of what the fertility clinic could do for them. To their credit, they had not yet given up hope and believed that if they continued to be proactive with their prayers and actions, a miracle could still be achieved.

When Naomi and Herschel came to Linda, they had two key questions: (1) If she became pregnant again through another IVF/ICSI procedure, would she have a high likelihood of miscarriage? (2) If she did carry to term, was there a high likelihood that the baby would suffer from severe birth defects?

Step 1: Identifying causal factors and the three hurdles to be overcome. Linda channeled that she must first identify *why* Herschel's sperm tested at 0 percent morphology before determining if it could be sufficiently corrected to test in a normal morphological range (between 4 and 14 percent). Knowing this would help Linda assess the three potential hurdles that Herschel and Naomi faced:

1. The first hurdle was to increase the probability of achieving pregnancy for the next IVF/ICSI attempt. It is statistically known, for example, that although Naomi had gotten pregnant once, the likelihood of achieving fertilization with abnormally shaped sperm was still problematic. Studies have shown that when severely amorphous sperm are used for ICSI, the chance of a live birth ranges from 10 to 20 percent for women under 35 years old.[37] What Herschel and Naomi first needed to know was what could be done to improve those odds?

2. The second hurdle was to determine what biochemical/physiological milestones had to be reached to ensure that Naomi could carry a fetus to full term.

3. The third hurdle was to determine what biochemical/physiological milestones needed to be reached so that the delivered baby would be completely healthy.

Step 2: What the initial interviewing process revealed. When Linda asked, using the pendulum, whether she could correct the underlying health issues so that Naomi could get pregnant and carry a healthy baby to full term, she not only got a resounding "yes," but she started shaking rather violently—a strong sign of angelic confirmation. (It was a moment I will never forget— and a poignant example of the shaking phenomenon described in Chapter 1. I generally do not sit in on Linda's sessions unless both Linda and the client think it's a good idea. Having gained permission, I observed the first session and watched Linda work.)

Linda then channeled that the miscarriage was not due to a problem with

Naomi's eggs or another female-related issue. Clearly, the issue was with Herschel's sperm. Herschel then revealed that he suffered from chronic ear infections, acne, eczema, constipation, and feeling tired and sluggish much of the time. *"Do you have any silver amalgam fillings?"* Linda asked. When he said he had nine silver fillings, that was an "Aha!" moment. In addition, his other health complaints provided a valuable set of clues that all pointed to the primary causal factor—mercury, the thousand-headed monster.

At this point Linda went into a brief trance and asked Archangel Raphael to provide an overview of the situation. She wrote down the following information that she heard: *"[At this time] it is very difficult for Naomi to conceive a normal healthy baby because of how the mercury in Herschel's body affects his sperm."*

The angels also informed Linda that the severity of mercury toxicity affecting Herschel's reproductive organs was such that it would be impossible for Herschel and Naomi to conceive a healthy fetus who would go full term with his current morphology score even with the IVF/ICSI approach. Linda went into trance again and, after hearing the words, wrote, *"The morphology must be at least 4 percent to deliver a healthy baby."* So the goal of Linda's treatment protocol became raising Herschel's morphological score from 0 to at least 4 percent.

The relevant information that Linda channeled from the pre-test was that Hershel's most stressed organ (MSO) was reproductive/endocrine system, his dominant focus (DF) was body chemistry, and the origin of complaint (OC) was "mercury." From the pre-test Linda channeled that he had a hormone deficiency that was 40 percent below normal, a significant number of miasms, a high heavy metal load of 30 percent (principally mercury, but also lead, nickel, cadmium, and aluminum), a chemical toxin (formaldehyde), a 45 percent fungal load involving multiple species of fungi, and lesser bacterial and parasitic conditions. No wonder he was a mess!

The key question that broke the case wide open was when Linda asked for the specific anatomical location of where the heavy metal toxins were located in Herschel's body. Archangel Raphael revealed: "The heavy metals were all over his brain and body, but, more unfortunately, were concentrated in the prostate, seminal vesicles, urinary vesicles, and testicles!" The thousand-headed monster had struck again, and this time in a most odious manner. Heavy metal toxins were inundating Herschel's reproductive organs to such an extent that they were actually responsible for altering the shape of the sperm needed to penetrate the egg! This was the angelic meaning of "body chemistry" as the dominant focus.

Step 3. Treatment protocols. Linda made it clear to Herschel that he had to immediately see a biological dentist. Linda channeled from a list of biological dentists located in the area and recommended one dentist as the best candidate to safely remove his amalgam through the Huggins protocol. Herschel followed Linda's counsel and in a short period of time had all his amalgam fillings safely removed. Concurrent with this, Linda channeled that he begin the following protocols:

1. Start the sequential process of detoxifying with homeopathic remedies the multiple genetically inherited miasms that were binding in mercury and other metals.

2. Detoxify with homeopathy multiple strains of fungi that were weakening Herschel's immune system.

3. Switch to a strong alkaline diet and a daily green drink to alter the pH of the biological terrain.

4. Open Herschel's congested lymphatic system with homeopathy.

5. Take a small dose of the amino acid methionine. Linda channeled that Herschel's liver was highly toxic from heavy metals/fungi and other chemical toxins. He was not "methylating properly," as she described it. She recommended that Herschel take just enough methionine to accomplish this task without chelating mercury from his mouth into his body.

6. Take a specific type of bentonite clay that not only addresses constipation issues but also helps chelate heavy metal toxicity in the gastrointestinal tract and colon without "pulling metals" out of the mouth.

Two and a half months after starting the process, Linda channeled that Herschel's heavy metal load had dropped to 25 percent. Herschel and Naomi eagerly asked if this was enough of a drop to make another attempt at IVF/ICSI a success. After Linda channeled a qualified "yes," she recommended that they wait a while longer as the lower the heavy metal load, the higher the morphology percentage would be. She pointed out that Herschel still had significant health issues that needed to be addressed. No matter, that was good enough for the eager couple and off they galloped to the fertility clinic.

The final results were astonishing and a testimony to the power of God's healing light and his angels. During the next IVF/ICSI cycle, the doctor, in utter amazement, informed them that Herschel's morphology rate had now jumped to 5 percent! This was now at the very low end of the range that Linda channeled was necessary for a high probability of overcoming the three hurdles: achieving fertilization, carrying the baby to full term, and delivering a healthy baby. And that is exactly what happened. Herschel and Naomi went through a second IVF/ICSI process. Several eggs were successfully fertilized and implanted in Naomi's womb. Nine months later she gave birth to beautiful, healthy twins—their miracle babies!

Several lessons may be learned from this case: Clearly, the principal cause of the 0 percent morphology and the abnormal shape of the Herschel's sperm was due to mercury toxicity caused by the release of mercury vapors from dental amalgam. What is particularly amazing to us is that merely by safely removing mercury fillings and taking three mild chelators (methionine, bentonite clay, and a green drink), Herschel's overall heavy metal load dropped 5 percentage points in approximately two and a half months. He did just enough to effectuate a change in morphology from 0 to 5 percent. Since Herschel did not do anything medically during this time other than what Linda channeled for him, there is no other reason why his score suddenly jumped up. Unfortunately, the fertility clinic did not even consider heavy metal toxicity as a likely causal factor of low morphology.

Thyroid Disease

The thyroid, a butterfly shaped gland located in the throat about two inches below the Adam's apple, is responsible for controlling the metabolic rate at which the body burns energy. The thyroid does this by producing several hormones, including thyroxine (T4) and triiodothyronine (T3). These hormones work to control the metabolic rate by stimulating the body to produce specialized proteins and increase cell oxygenation. Approximately 93 percent of the secreted hormone is T4 while only 7 percent is T3. However, in healthy people almost all T4 is converted into T3.

Hypothyroidism develops when the body does not create enough T4. Many different body systems are affected when the thyroid gets out of balance. This is why hypothyroidism is called "the great imitator" due to the many diseases or types of depressive behavior it can mimic. Because of the sheer number of metabolic functions thyroid hormones perform, it is easy to overlook their significance as they relate to other body systems. For example, the thyroid is central to the process of vitamin utilization, digestive processes, hormone secretion, and carbohydrate, protein, and fat metabolism. This is why hypothyroidism is a common causal factor for obesity and the inability to lose weight.

The conventional method of diagnosing hypothyroidism involves a blood test that measures the level of thyroid-related hormones in the blood. However, mounting evidence suggests that a significant percentage of people who test normal still suffer from the symptoms of hypothyroidism, which include tiredness and depression. Many healers suspect that the traditional blood test is often unable to detect subclinical hypothyroidism. A diagnostic problem exists in the world of allopathic medicine as well. Short of a biopsy, there is currently no definitive way to test for the presence of mercury or other toxins in the thyroid.

Studies have documented that mercury is a common cause of hypothyroidism.[38] This is due to mercury impairing the production of T4 as well as its conversion to T3. The thyroid gland, which needs iodine for normal functioning, has iodine-binding sites. For those people with chronic mercury exposure, mercury occupies some of the iodine-binding sites, thereby blocking full utilization of iodine by the thyroid. This can happen even when the measured thyroid level appears to be in the proper range. In fact, normal thyroid tests will not pick up this condition. In addition, mercury does direct damage to the cells and tissues of the thyroid. However, a majority of people who successfully detox from mercury show significantly improved thyroid function.

Cardiovascular Disease

As a consequence of free-radical proliferation, mercury starts a chain reaction that blocks the functioning of hemoglobin, reduces oxygen delivery to tissues, and reduces ATP production—all contributing factors to mitochondrial dysfunction. (These neuromuscular diseases are caused by damage to the mitochondria, small, energy-producing structures that serve as the cells' power plants.) It should therefore come as no surprise that mercury is associated with irregularities in blood hemoglobin, chest pains (angina), rapid heart beat (tachycardia), and much more.[39] However, until recently, the insidious threat that mercury poses to the heart had not been fully acknowledged. In 2007 doctors at Vanderbilt University School of Medicine (hardly a hotbed of alternative medical thinking) published a scathing article indicting mercury. Entitled "The Role of Mercury and Cadmium Heavy Metals in Vascular Disease, Hypertension, Coronary Artery Disease, and Myocardial Infarction," it stated: "The overall vascular effects of mercury include oxidative stress, inflammation, thrombosis, vascular smooth muscle dysfunction, endothelial dysfunction, dyslipidemia, immune dysfunction, and mitochondrial dysfunction. The clinical consequences of mercury toxicity include hypertension, coronary heart disease, myocardial infarction, increased carotid IMT (a thickening of the carotid artery wall) and obstruction, CVA [stroke], generalized atherosclerosis, and renal dysfunction with proteinuria."[40] This certainly covers the waterfront for a whole lot of cardiovascular and vascular diseases!

In their book entitled *Reverse Heart Disease Now*, cardiologists Stephen Sinatra and James Roberts cite additional incriminating studies. "In a recently published Italian study, heart muscle biopsy specimens were taken from healthy individuals and patients with either pump dysfunction due to blocked coronary arteries or idiopathic cardiomyopathy (heart failure without any obvious cause). The blocked artery patients had five times as much mercury in their heart cells as healthy patients. The patients with cardiomyopathy had 22,000 times as much! Researchers speculated that mercury adversely affects mitochondrial activity, which leads to pump dysfunction and heart failure. In another study of the association between mercury and heart attack, researchers used hair analysis to measure mercury levels in 1,833 men. Their experiment showed that men with the highest mercury levels had twice as many heart attacks and almost three times as many cardiac arrests as those with lower mercury content."

Drs. Sinatra and Roberts also noted: "Mercury also inactivates selenium, which is necessary for the regeneration of glutathione, the body's most potent free-radical scavenger. Glutathione helps prevent harmful oxidation and protects against the formation of arterial plaque . . . [New] evidence suggests that mercury inhibits glutathione, and if selenium is deficient, *the combination creates conditions for runaway LDL [cholesterol] oxidation . . .* [This] enters into already inflamed arterial tissue and contributes to arteriosclerosis and plaque . . . Finnish researchers who studied the rate of progression of carotid plaque found smoking to be the foremost accelerator with mercury a close second."[41] A recent study of 30 men going through mercury detoxification showed significant improvement in the reduction in cholesterol and other cardiovascular markers in a majority of participants.[42]

Testimonial: Rabbi Moshe's miracle cure

This story about Rabbi Moshe, an esteemed rabbi and scholar of Kabbalah living in Jerusalem, demonstrates the unique power of Linda's gift. Rabbi Moshe had been experiencing shortness of breath and rapid heart beat for the last several years. In May 2001 a treadmill electrocardiogram showed that he experienced tachycardia and arrhythmia during physical exertion due to a significant oxygen deficiency caused by decreased circulation in the coronary arteries due to a buildup of arterial plaque. The test showed that he was experiencing chest pain accompanied by shortness of breath.

Step 1. The first health reading with Linda. Rabbi Moshe's first channeling session in December 2002 during a trip to Los Angeles revealed an array of health issues affecting his cardiovascular system:

1. Mercury, nickel, and lead toxicity from fillings and bridges (cofactors for tachycardia).

2. Dangerously high electrical current coming from a tooth (a cofactor for tachycardia).

3. Fungal proliferation/gastrointestinal dysbiosis/acid pH.

4. Poor circulation/insufficient oxygen.

5. Excess cholesterol and oxidation of cholesterol due to the proliferation of free radicals.

6. Mineral and trace mineral deficiencies.

7. Emotional stress and exhaustion.

Linda channeled that dental issues were having a profoundly negative effect on the rabbi's heart. When she got out her tooth chart she went over each tooth searching for heavy metals. She channeled that the remnants of both mercury and nickel had not been properly removed in two of his lower right molars (17 and 18), which Rabbi Moshe mentioned were underneath what was part of a five-tooth bridge. Because he was set to return back to Israel the next day, Linda channeled one name from a list of biological dentists in Israel and stressed that upon his return Rabbi Moshe should have the dentist remove two other mercury amalgam fillings as part of the healing process. However, upon further channeling, Linda insisted that the Israeli dentist was *incapable* of safely removing the remaining mercury and nickel in teeth 17 and 18 under the bridge. That would have to wait until the rabbi returned to Los Angeles a few months later when he could see a specific dentist whom she recommended. This was Dr. Vernon Erwin, D.D.S., a talented biological dentist in the Los Angeles area whom Linda channeled was the right dentist not only for his technical brilliance, but also because he works closely with Linda on tough cases. *As we will soon see, this bit of information proved to be critical.*

Step 2. Treatment protocols. Linda recommended a range of different natural cardiovascular remedies, which Rabbi Moshe took for the next six months. These included red yeast extract (to help lower LDL cholesterol), CoQ_{10}, magnesium aspartate, taurine, mild cayenne pepper, and hawthorn berry extract. Other supportive products included an antioxidant, homeopathic fungal remedies, a green drink, probiotics, a liquid trace mineral formula, a lymphatic drainage remedy, a liver detox, a stabilized oxygen product, gem essences (for emotional stress), homeopathics for miasms, and a channeled anti-candida diet.

Step 3. Follow-up tests in Israel. Upon his return to Israel, Rabbi Moshe immediately underwent a blood test prior to beginning the protocols that Linda channeled. The test confirmed exactly what she had detected. Rabbi Moshe was still exhibiting an elevated level of cholesterol as well as a poor ratio of healthy HDL to harmful LDL cholesterol. The results of another treadmill test were reviewed by the chief cardiologist at Hadassah Hospital in Jerusalem. He declared the rabbi's health precarious and relayed that the recent stress test proved he had significant coronary disease. The rabbi was experiencing tachycardia during physical exertion due to a significant oxygen deficiency caused by decreased circulation in the coronary arteries. When the rabbi expressed his interest in exploring alternative methods of treating his heart condition, the cardiologist became quite furious and declared in front of the rabbi's wife, "I guarantee if you take that approach you will be a dead man within two years." He urged the rabbi to immediately undergo an angioplasty procedure and also prescribed Lipitor.

After carefully weighing the risks versus rewards of this course of treatment, the rabbi decided to follow his gut instincts and continue on the path that he had started with Linda. His own research led him to conclude that the doctor's approach to managing his case did not address the root causes of his heart condition that Linda had channeled (heavy metal toxicity, oxidized cholesterol, and dental electroconductivity issues). In addition, he reasoned that he could avoid angioplasty if he addressed these underlying issues and that his cholesterol issues could be effectively managed through a combination of dietary modification and supplements.

Step 4. Confirmation of Linda's evaluation by Dr. Vernon Erwin, D.D.S. When Rabbi Moshe flew back to Los Angeles a few months later with his dental records, I accompanied him to see Dr. Erwin. I explained to Dr. Erwin that Linda was concerned about the correlation between the rabbi's teeth and his heart. After taking a new full-mouth panorex x-ray, Dr. Erwin measured the level of current in the bridge that contained teeth 17 and 18 utilizing an amperage metering device. Dr. Erwin was quite astonished when he tested tooth 18 and the device registered 53 microamps. He told me in the 40 years he had conducted this test, that this was one of the highest readings he had ever seen! A normal level of current coming off a tooth is usually 2 to 3 microamps. He then mentioned that the exact location of the abnormally high current was dangerously close to the vagus nerve, which leads directly to the heart. I will never forget when he said to Rabbi Moshe, "Well, of course you are having heart problems. Your heart is being electrocuted 24/7."

Then Dr. Erwin completely removed the old bridge, including all of the mercury and nickel that Linda had identified. After the procedure was completed, he paused for a moment and said, "Since the rabbi came all the way from Israel to have this done, perhaps we should have Linda come over just to make sure that all the toxic metals were completely removed."

After Linda arrived, she got out a tooth chart and her pendulum. With her left index finger over tooth 17 on the chart, the pendulum, which she was holding in her right hand, spun to the right, indicating that the tooth was clear of all mercury and nickel. She then put her finger over tooth 18. When she asked if this tooth was now free of mercury, the pendulum spun affirmatively to the right. However, when she asked if tooth 18 was free of all nickel, the pendulum spun to the left, indicating nickel was still in the root area of the tooth. Dr. Erwin then checked to see if he could visually confirm what Linda was getting. After taking a close look, he told her he could not see any remaining nickel. She checked again with the pendulum and told him she was still getting the same information.

Dr. Erwin decided do some more exploratory drilling to see if he could uncover the nickel. After drilling a while, he told Linda he still did not see anything. She checked again and reported that she was still getting the same results: toxic nickel was still there. "Keep drilling toward the anterior side of tooth 18 between 2 and 3 o'clock and you will find it," she told Dr. Erwin. He did as she suggested and a minute later announced in an excited voice that he had found it and cleaned it out. Linda then confirmed that the nickel had indeed been completely removed from tooth 18.

Dr. Erwin was completely astonished by what had just happened. He remarked that the nickel had completely ionized very deep in the root area and looked like black soot. Rechecking the x-rays, he told me that what Linda had channeled had been completely undetected by the x-ray because the nickel had ionized into a sootlike substance. He then declared that if Linda had not told him twice to keep drilling, the entire procedure would not have been a success. The whole time the rabbi was sitting in the dental chair, he was aware that he was witnessing an authentic miracle of healing. He remarked in front of us, "Thank you God for allowing this miracle to happen." Upon a follow-up visit with Linda the next day, the rabbi reported that the tachycardia had completely ceased. Linda channeled that as a result of this one procedure the vitality of his heart had improved 35 percent!

Step 5. Follow-up care. After returning to Israel, Rabbi Moshe continued on a regime of supplements that strengthened his heart function and reduced cholesterol and triglycerides before successfully completing a heavy metal detoxification program Linda designed. One year later Rabbi Moshe was feeling much stronger and the shortness of breath had essentially disappeared. Of Linda's healing gift, Rabbi Moshe stated, "I have witnessed a true healing miracle from God through his angels that has had a major impact on my physical health as well as on an emotional and spiritual level."

Dr. Erwin said of the miracle that he witnessed: "We send our thanks and blessings to Linda Freud for her help and cooperation in this fascinating case. Without her mastery in the area of health we could not practice with the precision required to help our patients recover their health. Her observations and revelations were 100 percent accurate and 100 percent helpful in my treatment of the dental condition of Rabbi Moshe."

Liver Diseases

In an article entitled "Mercury Toxicity and Systemic Elimination Agents," authors Dr. Dietrich Klinghardt and Dr. Joseph Mercola describe how mercury finds its way to the liver: From the intestines, mercury is taken into the lymphatic system and then into the veins, where it runs into the gut, the liver, and finally the gallbladder. Mercury and other heavy metals are then excreted via the liver into the bowels and are reabsorbed again in the colon.[43] This process is referred to as *enterohepatic circulation*. The key to eliminating mercury from the body is to break this vicious cycle of excretion and reabsorption. To understand how this can occur, we must examine what mercury does to the liver.

Think of the liver as the Grand Central Station of complex biochemical reactions designed to detoxify and transform internal toxins (like bacteria, fungi, parasites, and certain hormones) and external environmental toxins (like drugs, heavy metals, and pesticides) so they can be excreted. The liver converts environmental toxins from a fat-soluble state, where they would otherwise be stored in fat cells and tissues, into water-soluble chemicals that are excreted out of the body. This process is known as *xenobiotic detoxification* and occurs in the phase I and phase II detoxification pathways. Among the most difficult toxins for the liver to excrete is mercury, which inhibits production of glutathione; blocks many normal metabolic reactions involving enzymes, amino acids, and hormones; and causes significant blockages in phase I and phase II detoxification pathways.

Phase I Detoxification Pathway. This process involves a group of 50 to 100 enzymes found in the membranes of liver cells that are collectively referred to as the cytochrome P450 system. These enzymes play a key role in the detoxification of external and internal toxins as well as in the synthesis of steroid hormones and bile acids. Phase I enzymes directly neutralize some of these toxins, with the remaining toxins processed through phase II detoxification pathways. However, mercury toxicity causes a breakdown between the phase I and phase II pathways by substantially reducing the level of glutathione, causing unprocessed toxins to be converted to intermediate forms that are toxic free radicals. The buildup of these intermediate forms can result in severe toxic reactions that cause cellular damage. What makes alcoholism so toxic begins in phase I when alcohol is converted to acetaldehyde, which is molecularly similar to formaldehyde! A hangover occurs when the liver is overwhelmed by one too many drinks and the acetaldehyde lingers, causing the hangover, until it is finally broken down in phase II into carbon dioxide and water.

Phase II Detoxification Pathways. This second step involves a biochemical process called *conjugation*, where toxins are bound to antioxidants that convert the free radicals into useful or harmless water-soluble substances, which are excreted through bile or urine. There are six different types of hepatic phase II detoxification pathways where different toxic xenobiotics and internal toxic compounds are processed out of the body. To determine which toxins are in which pathways, Linda channels from a comprehensive chart listing the toxins that affect the six pathways (see Appendix B).[44] Once one or more of these have been identified, she then goes to the Remedy database to channel which modalities (herbal, amino acids, antioxidants, homeopathic) are optimal for the detoxification process.

The conversion and elimination of mercury and other toxic metals into water-soluble compounds occurs in phase II detoxification pathways called glutathione conjugation and methylation. This produces water-soluble compounds called *mercaptates*, which are then excreted via the kidneys. The body's ability to excrete mercury out of the liver depends on an adequate level of glutathione, which, in turn, depends on adequate levels of methionine and cysteine. These amino acids prevent glutathione from becoming depleted during the detoxification process. Linda often channels that various amino acids like n-acetyl cysteine (NAC) and methionine or other antioxidants are needed to promote the process of detoxifying mercury out of the liver.

In laypeople's terms, methylation can be thought of as your liver's ability to increase the number of crews needed to repair the damage of oxidation due to oxidative stress and other disruptive metabolic processes. Methylation is significantly impaired by mercury and other heavy metal toxicity, as well as by pharmaceutical drugs, smoking, drinking, and nutrient-deficient diets. Linda consistently channels that birth control pills can negatively affect a woman's ability to methylate toxins out of the liver. Breakdowns in this and the other phase II detoxification pathways are also associated with elevated homocysteine, dementia, birth defects, arthritis, and a buildup of old estrogen. The antidote needed to neutralize corresponding free radicals during the detox process is to take the proper precursor supplements made up of specific amino acids and minerals that are then transformed into the antioxidant glutathione, which is critical to normal metabolic processes of both phase I and phase II detoxification.

The following testimonial is an awesome display of Linda's utter originality in healing a severe case of osteoarthritis through her channeled detective work involving phase I and II detoxification pathways.

Testimonial: Lindsey's curious case of osteoarthritis

Lindsey is a fifty-seven-year-old married woman who has generally been in good health most of her life. She works hard at maintaining both an active exercise schedule as well as eating what Linda refers to as a "clean diet"—a vegetarian diet of organic fruits and vegetables and complex carbohydrates. Lindsey generally avoids sugar, soft drinks, alcohol, coffee, and processed foods. She understands the importance of the proper acid/alkaline diet as well as the need for additional supplements to optimize her anti-aging program. She even had ten silver amalgam fillings removed several years ago and had been progressing on an oral chelation program designed by Linda to remove residual mercury from her body. Lindsey generally tries to avoid pharmaceuticals, preferring natural solutions whenever possible. She has periodically worked with Linda over several years primarily to optimize her wellness program.

However, on one visit Lindsey showed Linda that the middle finger on her left hand had become so terribly swollen beyond its normal size that it was enormous! She initially experienced a small but constant pain around her knuckles, which graduated to the point where she could not even bend the finger without experiencing throbbing, excruciating pain. This had been going on for over two and a half months and was getting progressively worse. In recent weeks her second and fourth fingers on the same hand were now also swollen and sore, and any attempt to bend these fingers sent her into waves of agony. Lindsey assumed her condition came from weekly kick boxing workouts. However, she could not recall any particular incident where she actually injured the finger. She hoped against hope that the swelling and pain would somehow just go away over time. Now the pain had gotten so bad that she knew she had to consult Linda.

Linda channeled her angelic guides and found that Lindsey was suffering from a fairly severe case of osteoarthritis and three cofactors were causing the inflammation. After channeling the phase II detoxification chart, Linda determined that two of the six pathways in Lindsey's liver were blocked, preventing her liver from functioning normally. Here's what Linda discovered:

• The methylation phase II hepatic detoxification pathway was blocked by a residue of mercury. Linda channeled that Lindsey should take NAC to boost glutathione production to assist in detoxing the mercury that remained in her liver.

• The glucuronidation phase II hepatic detoxification pathway was blocked by a buildup of old estrogen, clogging estrogen receptor sites in the liver. Linda recommended that Lindsey take a special herbal/nutraceutical product to assist in clearing out the buildup of old estrogen in the liver.

• Linda channeled that there was additional liver toxicity due to *Candida albicans* and *Aspergillus niger* strains of fungi. Linda recommended that these be treated with various Sanum or San Pharma homeopathics designed to eliminate these fungal forms (see Chapter 6). She also added a probiotic product designed to assist in fungal detox and restoration of intestinal flora.

• Linda also channeled a special herbal joint formula to reduce inflammation.

After only one week of being on the protocol the swelling and pain in Lindsey's finger had gone down considerably. In only three weeks, it completely disappeared and her other fingers returned to normal as well. In a fairly short period, Lindsey was able to phase out of the daily protocol. The condition was completely healed and has never returned.

There are several interesting aspects of this case. If Lindsey had gone to an allopathic doctor, the standard protocol would probably have consisted of giving her a COX-2 inhibitor drug like Celebrex, which is a nonsteroidal anti-inflammatory drug (NSAID). While this product is effective, it would not address the real reasons she had the condition, but only work to mask the inflammatory symptoms. This would mean she would probably have to stay on the pharmaceutical for an extended period of time. Given the long-term side effects of this drug, that was not a very appealing option (read the mandatory "black box" warning on Celebrex). The angels guided Linda to find the real underlying causes and address them through natural methods. This resulted in Lindsey's condition being healed with no side effects.

What is also unusual about Lindsey's case is that the osteoarthritis did not happen as a result of poor lifestyle changes—smoking, drinking, diet, and drugs, which are often considered major cofactors in osteoarthritis. It happened for a series of reasons that are either overlooked or simply not acknowledged by the traditional allopathic approach. After relaying this story to me, Lindsey remarked that she considered Linda to be her healer and "a real miracle worker." She also mentioned that although she might see other practitioners on occasion, "I never make a serious move regarding my health without consulting Linda."

CHAPTER 11

Neurotoxicity and Mercury: The Brain Polluter of Wasting Diseases

Mercury is a potent neurotoxin and should be suspected as the underlying cause of every chronic neurological illness unless proven otherwise.[1]

—DR. DIETRICH KLINGHARDT

FROM A MEDICAL PERSPECTIVE, the single most important thing that Linda does is identify, rank, and prioritize physical, energetic, and genetic toxins anywhere in the body. She can do this more effectively than any other health care practitioner I am aware of. Because it is so difficult for doctors to identify neurotoxins in the brain, perhaps nothing is more important than her ability to do this. Neurotoxins, which disrupt vital functions of the nerve cell, are often the root cause of a host of neurological disorders that include autism, ADD/ADHD (attention deficit/ hyperactivity disorder), Asperger's disorder, Alzheimer's disease, MS (multiple sclerosis), ALS (amyotrophic lateral sclerosis), and Parkinson's disease. They are also often associated with a whole range of serious mental illnesses, ranging from dementia to schizophrenia, as well as less serious but very troubling personality disorders.

Because of the severe levels of neurological and emotional damage inflicted on the unsuspecting recipient of multiple mercury fillings, mercury poisoning is often referred to as "Mad Hatter's disease." The origins of the expression "mad as a hatter" come from England where in the 1800s hat manufacturers used quicksilver (mercury nitrate) to turn fur into felt. A significant number of millinery workers were afflicted with a spate of severe emotional and neurological problems when they breathed in the highly toxic fumes. These included suicidal tendencies, emotional outbursts, depression, anxiety, cognitive memory decline, and slurred speech, as well as body tremors.

In fact, mercury has long been known in the scientific literature as a potent neurotoxin when inhaled from vapors emitted from mercury amalgam fillings, ingested from seafood, or injected as a preservative component in a vaccine. Mercury amalgam dental fillings have been found to be the largest source of both inorganic and methyl mercury in most people who have several amalgam fillings.[2] Studies have shown that mercury is a neurotoxin that either kills or damages brain cells and nerve cells.[3] Programmed cell death (apoptosis) is documented to be a major factor in degenerative neurological conditions like ALS, Alzheimer's, MS, and Parkinson's. Some of the main reasons this occurs are because mercury depletes glutathione, generates dangerous reactive oxygen species (ROS), kills brain tubulin cells, induces cytokine inflammation, and inhibits enzymes, nerve growth, and production of neurotransmitters.

Over the last twenty-five years several medical research laboratories have conducted peer-reviewed studies that clearly establish methyl mercury vapors from amalgam fillings and other environmental sources as major contributors to a whole range of neurological conditions shown in Table 11-1.

TABLE 11-1. PSYCHOLOGICAL, BEHAVIORAL, AND NEUROLOGICAL EFFECTS FROM MERCURY TOXICITY

CENTRAL NERVOUS SYSTEM AND NEUROLOGICAL SYMPTOMS

Chronic headaches	Loss of ability to perform hand movements	Ringing in ears
Convulsions		Speech disorders
Difficulty walking	Mental disability	Tremors of hands, feet, lips, eyelids
Dim vision	Muscle coordination problems	
Dizziness	Muscle paralysis	Tingling of fingers, toes, lips, nose
Epilepsy	Muscle twitches	
Facial twitches	Narrowing of field of vision	Unexplained leg jerks
Hearing difficulty	Noises or sounds in head	Vertigo
Insomnia	Numbness of arms and legs	Voices in head

PSYCHOLOGICAL AND BEHAVIORAL SYMPTOMS

Anxiety	Emotional instability	Insomnia/sleep disorders
Apathy	Fatigue	Irrational behavior
Chronic fatigue	Fits of anger	Irritability
Confusion	Forgetfulness	Lack of energy/lethargy
Depression	Hallucinations	Lack of self-control
Drowsiness	Inability to concentrate	Loss of appetite

Lowered intelligence	Nightmares	Suicidal tendencies
Manic depression	Restlessness	Tiredness
Moodiness	Short attention span	Your doctor says, "It's your nerves"
Nervous excitability	Short-term memory loss	

NEUROLOGICAL CONDITIONS

ADD	Asperger's disorder	Myoneural transmission resembling myasthenia gravis
ADHD	Autism	
ALS (Lou Gehrig's disease)	Multiple sclerosis	Parkinson's disease
Alzheimer's disease		

There has been a huge increase in the incidence of degenerative neurological conditions in virtually all Western countries over the last two decades.[4] The increase in Alzheimer's has been over 300 percent, while the increase in Parkinson's and other motor neuron diseases has been over 50 percent. The primary cause appears to be a significant increase in the exposure to toxic pollutants.[5]

Linda concurs with Dr. Dietrich Klinghardt about the relationship between mercury and neurological diseases and has consistently channeled that the core causal factors behind the majority of such wasting neurological diseases as ALS, Alzheimer's, MS, and Parkinson's, as well as the new childhood epidemics of autism, Asperger's, and ADHD are conceptually similar. By this she means that in many of these conditions some form of "undiagnosed toxicity" affects different parts of the brain, promoting a specific disease etiology. Such are the nefarious ways of the thousand-headed monster. Although there are many different types of neurotoxins that may play a part, the most dangerous of these are heavy metal toxins and, of these, clearly the most dangerous is mercury.

The Effect of Galvanic Current from Mercury Fillings on Neurological Disorders

Any engineer will tell you that when you place two or more dissimilar metals in a salt solution, it creates a battery much like the one in your car. The electrical current produced is referred to as a *galvanic current.* Mercury amalgam fillings typically contain 50 percent mercury and 50 percent of up to four dissimilar metals including silver, copper, tin, and zinc. Our saliva, much like a salt solution, is an excellent conductor of electrical current. The roots of upper molars are located only two inches from the brain. One does not have to be an engineer to understand that electrical currents created this close to the brain may be a significant causal factor in various neurological and emotional conditions.

In his book *Whole-Body Dentistry*, Dr. Mark Breiner, D.D.S., a biological dentist in Connecticut, states that the five metals in amalgam, when placed in saliva, can generate enough current to interfere with brain or heart function.[6] For a toxic individual, this phenomenon may initially manifest as an unpleasant electrical sensation or metallic taste in the mouth. A biological dentist is trained to measure current coming off teeth with amalgam fillings (through voltage, amperage, and milliwatt) against a baseline of low levels of current in teeth with no fillings. The higher the negative galvanic readings of a filling, the faster vapors from these metals move through the blood-brain barrier into the brain.

The brain normally operates with a galvanic current of 6 to 9 nanoamperes. The current released from amalgam fillings may bombard the brain at a rate of up to 100 or more microamperes.[7] There is a correlation between neurological autoimmune conditions such as MS and epilepsy and emotional conditions such as depression and high levels of current coming from teeth with amalgam fillings.[8] Amazingly enough, some of this information was reported in an article published in 1936 by the *Journal of the American Dental Association.*[9]

PROVING THE CAUSAL RELATIONSHIP BETWEEN AMALGAM FILLINGS AND NEUROLOGICAL CONDITONS

What was first needed to prove a causal relationship between mercury amalgam fillings and the neurological conditions mentioned above was to show that mercury leaching from dental amalgams could penetrate through the blood-brain barrier. It would then be in a position to migrate to the various sites in the brain known to be responsible for these terrible wasting neurological conditions. That first level of proof was clearly established in a joint international study of cadavers entitled "Correlation of Dental Amalgam with Mercury in Brain Tissue" conducted by Dr. Daniel Eggleston, D.D.S., of the University of Southern California School of Dentistry and Dr. Magnus Nylander, D.D.S., of the Karolinska Institute of Sweden. The results of this study were published in the prestigious *Journal of Prosthetic Dentistry* in 1987 and showed a direct correlation between the levels of mercury found in the brain and the number of amalgam fillings.[10]

In 1989 the International Academy of Oral Medicine and Toxicology funded studies by researchers headed by Drs. Murray Vimy, Fritz Lorscheider, and Leszek Hahn at the University of Calgary showing that mercury vapors released from 12 mercury amalgam fillings placed in the mouths of sheep and monkeys for 28 days showed pathological damage in many parts of the body and brains.[11,12,13] Then in 1997, studies conducted by a team headed by Dr. Boyd Haley, Ph.D., a protein biochemist and former chairman of the Chemistry Department at the University of Kentucky, demonstrated that the inhalation of mercury vapors produced molecular lesions in the brains of rats that were very similar to lesions seen in 80 percent of Alzheimer's-diseased brains.[14] However, the precise mechanisms underlying degeneration remained elusive—until a revolutionary study appeared in 2001.

The conclusive level of proof was provided by direct visual evidence in real time showing how mercury damages brain cells (neurons). This was detailed in a study at the University of Calgary by researchers headed by Dr. Naweed Syed, Ph.D. The study, entitled "Retrograde Degeneration of Neurite Membrane Structural Integrity of Nerve Growth Cones Following In Vitro Exposure to Mercury," was published in the March 2001 issue of NeuroReport, a British medical peer review journal. It revealed direct, visual evidence of how even low levels of mercury cause neuron degeneration.[15]

Dr. Syed, head of the Cell Biology and Anatomy Department at the University of Calgary and research director of the Hotchkiss Brain Institute, is a highly respected researcher who has received numerous awards for his contributions to neuroscience. His research has been published in such prestigious journals as *Nature, Science, Neuron,* and *Journal of Neuroscience,* as well as *Time* magazine, and he has appeared on the Discovery Channel. His laboratory researches how brain cells reach out, recognize, and connect with each other through an intricate matrix of synapses that form the basis of all brain functions. The scientists also investigated how the morphology and physiology of neurons are altered by environmental toxicity, injury, and stress.[16] Snail neurons are perfectly suited for this research, because well over 97 percent of the amino acid sequence that uses microtubules (the main protein building blocks in the structure of a neuron) are exactly the same across species.[17] Because Dr. Syed's laboratory is one of the very few in the world which has the capacity to grow neural tissue cultured from snails, it offers a unique opportunity to observe exactly how mercury affects healthy brain cells in humans in real time.

Dr. Syed's lab devised an experiment to simulate how amalgam fillings affect the brain and central nervous system. The researchers isolated and cultured neurons from snails and then exposed the neurons to a concentration of mercury far lower than would appear in the urine of anyone with seven to eight mercury fillings. Utilizing state-of-the-art neurobiological techniques coupled with time-lapse photography to monitor growth cone behavior in neurons, they showed precisely how mercury ions actually alter and destroy cell membrane structure in developing neurons that result in molecular lesions in the brain.

As a result of the worldwide interest in the work of Dr. Syed and his associates, the University of Calgary produced a jaw-dropping video entitled "How Mercury Causes Brain Neuron Degeneration" that demonstrates exactly what happens to neurons when exposed to very low levels of mercury. This five-minute video is on Linda's website (www.thehealinggift.com). For those readers interested in a technical explanation of the neurological anatomy described in the video, read "A Brief Primer on Neuronal Function That Explains the Significance of the Video." Otherwise, feel free to skip over the next section.

A Brief Primer on Neuronal Function That Explains the Significance of the Video

Neurons are the most significant cells of the brain as well as the most fundamental component of the nervous system. There are over 100 billion neurons in the brain that are grouped into networks and control and coordinate many functions in the body and behaviors in the brain. In both children and adults, the ongoing development of the brain and central nervous system requires that neurons continue to be generated and undergo migration to specific areas of the brain. Developing neurons contain extensions called neurites, which branch out and become an intricate wiring system composed of axons and dendrites in the adult neuron. Using an analogy of a tree to describe a neuron, an axon is the trunk of a neuron "tree" that sends electrochemical messages to other neurons. A dendrite is a branch attached to the trunk that receives messages from other nerve cells. At the tip of each neurite is a structure called a growth cone, which contains the sensory, motor, integrative, and adaptive functions of growing axons and dendrites. Its function is to seek out and connect with other neurons as well as other cellular structures in order to form structural circuits with a space between them called a synapse. These, in turn, allow for the flow of electrical impulses and neurotransmitters.

The growth cone establishes various connections by sampling the extracellular environment, which allows it to make decisions about the direction of the neurite extension. Growth cones contain an enzyme, a structural protein called tubulin, which forms the neurite membrane. During normal cell growth, which involves a process called tubulin synthesis, tubulin molecules link together end to end to form a skeletal structure called a microtubule, which supports the neurite structure. These, in turn, surround neurofibrils, a protein filament that is a component of the neuronal axon.

The video shows that after a very low-level mercury solution was applied by micropipette (syringe), it took only 17 minutes for the rapid degeneration of the growth cone in the nerve cell, with the neuron disintegrating and shrinking to half its original size! After the devastation wrought by mercury, the protein tubulin is stripped away, leaving a bare, unsupported nerve fiber. The bare fibers of the neuron eventually form aggregates or tangles. The video shows that *mercury damages the brain by disrupting the binding sites that connect the tubulin during the process of tubulin synthesis. This destroys the ability of tubulin to bind together and form the membrane sheath that both holds and supports the growth cone in a nerve.* Dr. Syed explained in conversation that these structural proteins, like bricks held together by cement, provide the framework for connecting brain cells. Enzymes activated by mercury chew up the cement and the building blocks fall apart.[18]

Figure 11-1 shows a neuron before exposure to mercury and after exposure. The twisted filament remains of mercury devastation on the right are called "denuded neurofibrillary tangles," and they are the result of the brain's failed attempts to make microtubules, essential for cellular communication and the transmission of neurotransmitters.

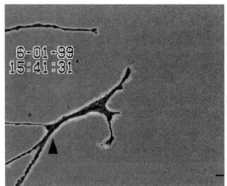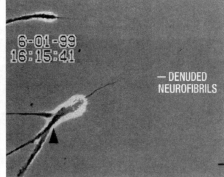

Figure 11-1. Neurons before (left) and after (right) mercury exposure.
Used with permission of Dr. Naweed Syed, Ph.D., University of Calgary.

Interestingly enough, when other metals and minerals, including aluminum, lead, cadmium, and manganese, suspected of having a role in Alzheimer's, were tested in the same manner as mercury, there was no observed degeneration of the growth cone, and tangles were not produced.[19]

I spoke with Dr. Syed about his research and he told me an interesting story. Following the release of the article in *NeuroReport* in 2001, he received telephone calls from members of the royal families of Denmark and Sweden. They thanked him for his work and informed him that use of amalgam had been banned for all members of the royal families and that they would press to get it banned in their respective countries. Dr. Syed was pleased to report that had happened.[20]

Dr. Syed was gracious enough to share the results of his current research with me. He has strong evidence demonstrating that snail neurons grown in the presence of low levels of mercury also fail to establish synaptic connections between neurons that are fundamental for all brain function![21] These studies, completed in 2008, will remain unpublished until such time that the results can be reproduced in rat brain cells.[22] Dr. Syed said that this is even more significant than his original research, as learning and memory rely on the formation of new synaptic connections. Failure to establish these synapses in the presence of mercury renders the nervous system dysfunctional. He believes his newest research reinforces the link between mercury and autism spectrum disorders—either from mercury crossing through the placenta to the fetus or from thimerosal found in vaccines. The implications of this groundbreaking research are profound for all the wasting neurological conditions discussed below.

MERCURY'S RELATIONSHIP TO MAJOR NEUROLOGICAL DISEASES

What do the studies supported by the video mean for the sufferers of various neurological diseases? Let us take Alzheimer's, Parkinson's, multiple sclerosis, and autism as examples.

Alzheimer's Disease

According to the Alzheimer's Association, 5.1 million Americans age sixty-five and older have Alzheimer's disease, which has a devastating impact on its victims and loved ones. By 2050, that number is projected to rise to between eleven and sixteen million. It is the sixth leading cause of death, and currently over $148 billion are spent annually on care and treatment.[23] Despite the billions of research dollars, the official position of the Alzheimer's Association is that "the cause of Alzheimer's disease is unknown, and there is no real cure on the horizon." Unfortunately, the focus of existing pharmaceutical research is based primarily around efforts to mask Alzheimer symptoms rather than to discover what causes the disease.

As we have seen, in recent years the link between mercury released from silver fillings and Alzheimer's disease has gone from hypothetical conjecture to strong scientific suspicion. In light of the scientific studies presented here, *it would be difficult not to conclude that mercury toxicity, particularly from dental amalgams, is a significant cofactor behind this debilitating condition.*

Dr. Boyd Haley's autopsy research proved that elevated blood levels of mercury were a significant cofactor in people with Alzheimer's disease. The two most important diagnostic markers that came out of his research are: (1) Denuded neurofibrillary tangles were linked to low levels of mercury that disrupted tubulin synthesis in rats. These same diagnostic markers appear in 80 percent of people with Alzheimer's. (2) Elevated levels of beta-amyloid plaque, the main component of neuritic plaque, are correlated with even low levels of mercury. This is now universally accepted as a marker for Alzheimer's. Haley states that "neurofibillary tangles . . . and amyloid plaques are the result of Alzheimer's disease, not the cause of it. The cause is exposure to environmental toxicants including mercury that attack enzymes with the most reactive thiol groups."[24]

Commenting on the results of the 2001 study from University of Calgary, Dr. Haley stated, "[Many] of the characteristic markers that we look for to distinguish Alzheimer's disease can be produced in normal brain tissues or cultures of [snail] neurons by the addition of extremely low levels of mercury. In addition, [our] research [in 1997] has shown that Alzheimer's-diseased patients have at least three times higher blood levels of mercury than controls. *How much more research is necessary before the appropriate regulatory bodies respond with restrictions on the use of mercury-leaking dental amalgam fillings?*"[25] (Emphasis added by DF.)

Parkinson's Disease

The primary cause of Parkinson's disease appears to be substantial exposure to such pollutants as toxic metals and pesticides. This results in brain inflammation and oxidative damage due to free-radicals that affect a small part of the brain called the *substantia nigra* and its connections.[26] A recent study suggests that Parkinson's patients have a genetic defect that alters their ability to form conjugating enzymes, a vital method of cellular detoxification.[27] This condition makes them more susceptible to oxidative stress in that part of the brain, and mercury radically increases oxidative stress. Interestingly, another study found that patients with Parkinson's disease have a higher number of amalgam fillings than did controls.[28]

Multiple Sclerosis

Multiple sclerosis is caused by the erosion of myelin, a substance that helps the brain send messages to the body. Heavy metals such as mercury can bind to myelin, causing an autoimmune response. In such cases, the progression of MS can be halted by removing the source of the metal.[29] Not surprisingly, MS patients have been found to have much higher levels of mercury in cerebrospinal fluid compared to controls.[30] In fact, German studies have found that MS patients usually have high levels of mercury in their bodies, with one study finding levels as much as 300 percent higher than controls.[31] Most recovered after mercury detox, with some requiring additional treatment for viruses and intestinal dysbiosis. Very high levels of mercury have also been found in brain memory areas such as the cerebral cortex and hippocampus in patients with diseases such as MS, who often have memory-related symptoms.[32] The bottom line: *Studies have found that the neurological effects of mercury toxicity are indistinguishable from those of MS.*[33] (Emphasis added by DF.)

Autism

Autism is a complex neurobiological disorder that cuts across all racial, ethnic, and social groups and is four times more likely to strike boys than girls. It is actually a variety of different disorders that include classic autism, Asperger's disorder, Rett's syndrome, childhood disintegrative disorder (CDD), and pervasive developmental disorder (PDD). It impairs a child's ability to communicate and relate to others. Unfortunately, it lasts to varying degrees throughout that person's life. Only twenty years ago the statistics were 1 in 10,000. *In 2009, 1 in 150 individuals is diagnosed with autism, making it more common than pediatric cancer, diabetes, and AIDS combined.*[34] What happened?

An expose by Robert Kennedy Jr. reported on a 2005 study revealing that autism is virtually unknown among Pennsylvania's large Amish populations—a strong indication that vaccines are indeed a principal culprit of the epidemic.[35] Naysayers could say, "Well, this resistance is a racial component much like Tay-Sachs in Jewish people or sickle cell anemia in African Americans." But this argument hinges on the Amish being a racial group. However, the Amish are not a racial group; they are a religious group—a group that does not vaccinate their children.

Although autism is not linked to mercury amalgam fillings, this video should be of great interest to parents of autistic children, as it strongly suggests that mercury, in the form of thimerosal, a preservative found in childhood vaccinations, is largely responsible for their children's condition. Brain inflammation due to oxidative stress, caused by thimerosal is believed to be a major factor in autism.[36]

Only 30 micrograms (mcg) of mercury were used in Dr. Syed's snail neuron study, far less than most children are given in vaccines. In fact, it has been reported that some children have received up to 237 mcg of mercury from multiple vaccines containing thimerosal, an amount far greater than needed to completely destroy over half the neuron shown in Figure 11-1.[37] In reality, mercury toxicity causes a child to suffer a breakdown of all sensory input integration, processing, and relaying of information between the central nervous system and peripheral nervous systems, resulting in autism. Amazingly, this confirms what Linda has channeled about autism: that the autistic brain is basically devoid of communication among its various parts!

The great tragedy, Linda channels, is that a substantial percentage of these neurologically based degenerative diseases could be completely eradicated if the FDA just banned mercury fillings and purged mercury from our vaccines and environment.

CHAPTER 12

Chelating Out of the Darkness: Linda's Rules for Mercury Detoxification

*The key to everything is patience. You get the chicken
by hatching the egg, not smashing it.*
—ARNOLD H. GLASOW

*No physician can ever say that any disease is incurable.
To say so blasphemes God, blasphemes Nature, and depreciates
the great architect of Creation. The disease does not exist,
regardless of how terrible it may be, for which God
has not provided the corresponding cure.*
—PARACELSUS

AFTER YEARS OF RESEARCH AND REFINEMENT, Linda has taken the art of heavy metal detoxification to unprecedented levels. In broad strokes, she adheres to the Klinghardt detoxification axiom: To successfully detoxify the body, three issues have to be addressed simultaneously—the detoxification of the physical body, the treatment of latent microorganisms and parasites, and the treatment of unresolved psychoemotional issues.[1] Her uniquely sophisticated and thorough process is one of the reasons why she has such a high success rate. The science involved in peeling what Linda calls this "toxic onion" is quite complex. Miasms are treated with remedies in a sequential manner, while all other aspects of the detox are concurrently treated in a multitasking approach. *Our angelic guides have revealed that a proper heavy metal detox should never commence until several preparatory steps have been taken to prepare the body for the detox. If a heavy metal detox is attempted out of sequence, the results can be potentially harmful.*

172

LINDA'S RULES FOR MERCURY DETOXIFICATION

Aided by these channeled precautionary steps, Linda is able to guide the client through the process to minimize or even completely eliminate major detox reactions. Here is an overview of the preparatory steps that Linda follows to treat a client suffering from mercury poisoning due to dental amalgams.

DETOX PREP RULE 1.
Never Attempt Any Heavy Metal Detoxification Protocols Unless All Your Dental Amalgams Have First Been Removed

Contrary to what some health care practitioners or dentists might believe, years of experience and angelic guidance have shown us that it is *absolutely detrimental* for a client to begin a mercury detoxification program prior to having all mercury amalgams removed. The reason is that if any mercury remains within the tooth structure when a chelating (excreting) agent is taken, it is almost certain that the mercury vapors in the amalgams will leach in an accelerated manner either into the body to be deposited in organs or tissues and/or through the blood-brain barrier into the brain, eyes, and ears. This, in turn, can lead to severe emotional outbursts of depression and anger as well as a range of degenerative health conditions.

Since she started doing this work, Linda has had a significant number of clients come to her after a botched detox. If, for example, a person with a number of amalgam fillings takes megadoses of vitamin C, a known heavy metal chelator, he or she has a good chance of getting even sicker from mercury poisoning! The reason is that vitamin C chelates mercury out of the fillings and redeposits the toxic vapors all over the body and brain at a greatly accelerated rate. Although we recognize that vitamin C is essential for good health, the same substance that is very beneficial can also be very harmful *if taken out of sequence.* By this we mean taking it prior to the removal of all mercury amalgam fillings. After that, the possibility exists that vitamin C may turn out to be the chelator of choice.

DETOX PREP RULE 2. Get Thee to a Biological Dentist

Never have just any dentist remove your mercury amalgams. Use only a biological dentist who has received specialized training in the safe removal of such fillings and other toxic dental materials. There are several key differences between the typical dentist and a biological dentist. The typical dentist merely blasts out amalgam fillings with a drill without taking the necessary safety precautions for the patient (let alone for him- or herself and the dental assistant!). A biological dentist is a *holistic practitioner* who has studied the complex relationship between the teeth and the rest of the body and who only uses nontoxic dental materials. In addition, he or she uses many precautionary techniques, including the use of a custom-fitted rubber dam that creates an effective barrier between drilled-out mercury sludge and any body tissues.

If you have your regular dentist drill out amalgam fillings without taking specific precautions, you run a significant risk of getting far sicker than you already are! Without proper protection, the drilled-out toxic mercury vapors can easily go up your nose or down your throat, redepositing in your brain or organs. So serious an issue is this that Linda channels it is better *not* to have your amalgam fillings removed rather than to have them removed incorrectly. Unfortunately, no dental school in America teaches these precautionary techniques!

Specific methods and techniques have been pioneered by different biological dentists and taught by the International Association of Oral Medicine and Toxicology (IAOMT). Another comprehensive system called the Huggins protocol is taught by Dr. Hal Huggins, D.D.S., of Colorado Springs, Colorado. For a list of dentists in your area who have been trained in these methods, visit the website of DAMS (Dental Amalgam Mercury Solutions) at www.dams.cc.

DETOX PREP RULE 3.
Have Your Health Care Practitioner Do a Blood Test for Genetically Inherited Miasms and Then Clear Them Out of Your Body

The removal of genetically inherited miasms is one of Linda's most important original contributions to the art of mercury detoxification and is, in part, responsible for her incredible track record in this area. Genetically inherited miasms, in particular tuberculosis and syphilis, bind in mercury in body tissues, making it incredibly difficult to chelate them out of the body. Think of them as magnets that bind in heavy metals. Once the underlying miasmatic burden is removed, the whole detoxification process is dramatically easier. According to Linda, "The poison can now slide out instead of being violently ripped out as if it were bound in by magnets, glue, or Velcro." This process using Polysan colloids (www.biomedicine.com) must be done in a sequential manner, detoxing one miasm at a time (see Chapter 8).

DETOX PREP RULE 4. Do Not Start a Mercury Detox Program until All Pathways of Elimination Are Opened Up

Linda feels it is essential that all pathways of elimination (the sewer systems of the body) be open and flowing before mercury is dumped into them. That requires flushing out toxins in the lymphatic ducts, kidneys, and colon as well as cleansing the liver and skin. Here is a brief overview of what's involved.

• **Lymphatic system:** Perhaps no system in the body is more neglected by mainstream medicine than the lymphatic system. Since its healthy maintenance requires detoxification protocols that are generally not understood, it is often overlooked as a core cause of inflammatory processes and immune system dysfunction. Heavy metal toxicity and the pathogens that accompany it play a key role in contributing to lymphatic congestion, which Linda consistently channels in almost everyone with silver amalgam fillings. Sadly, there is even a lack of awareness of this among a majority of American holistic practitioners, whereas in Europe the value of lymphatic massage and drainage remedies is more appreciated.

The lymphatic system is a one-way drainage network of vessels, ducts, nodes, lacteals (capillaries in the small intestine that absorb digested fats), and lymphoid organs (spleen, thymus, and tonsils) that pervades the entire tissue structure of the body. It returns filtered plasma (blood without red blood cells) back to the blood and is responsible for waste disposal and immune response. Lymph nodes produce two components that help bolster immunity: (1) macrophages, specialized waste disposal cells called antibodies that collect pathogens and toxins and deposit them in various sites of elimination; and (2) lymphocytes, which assist in producing antibodies. Transported by lymphatic fluid, both of these perform a lymphatic patrol function, with macrophages capturing invaders in the drainage system and lymphocytes destroying invaders in the lymph nodes. Impaired lymphatic flow results in the buildup of toxic waste materials, which reduce production of macrophages and lymphocytes. The breakdown of these processes clogs the lymph nodes and directly contributes to inflammatory conditions and a depressed immune system, which lasts indefinitely unless treated.

Cleansing the lymphatic fluid of mercury, along with the bacteria, fungi, and parasites that often accompany it, is critical in promoting and maintaining the integrity of the immune system. This helps prevent infectious diseases and inflammatory conditions such as arthritis from forming. Linda utilizes three different approaches based on the severity of lymphatic congestion. Light congestion requires taking various homeopathic, herbal, or enzymatic products that she channels. Moderate congestion requires taking the same products along with daily use of a lymphatic rebounder and self-massage techniques in the affected areas. Heavy congestion requires lymphatic massage by a therapist specially trained in the science of lymphatic circulation. This provides manual stimulation to get the stuck fluid moving in the right direction.

• **Kidneys:** Mercury from amalgam exerts real stress on kidney function and can exacerbate chronic degenerative kidney disease. Linda consistently channels the importance of detoxifying the kidneys prior to and during the mercury detoxification process. It is therefore of utmost importance to Linda to preserve kidney function during the entire process. Before detox this may involve tonifying and strengthening the kidneys with certain herbal or homeopathic remedies to prepare them for the onslaught caused by this horrific poison. The ability to safely excrete mercury through the kidneys during the detoxification process represents a big challenge for Linda. This must be a carefully measured and slow process as detoxing mercury too rapidly can cause lasting damage to the kidneys. In addition to insisting on proper hydration, Linda channels from a list of kidney drainage remedies. These include herbal tinctures, enzyme formulas, and homeopathics, which support proper kidney function. In challenging cases, she also recommends acupuncture and Chinese herbal blends for the kidneys to correct kidney yin deficiency, a chronic weakness that often happens during the detox process.

Linda has found that people who have heavy metal toxicity in the kidneys frequently exhibit intense fear and other irrational behavior in their daily lives. This conforms with a medical axiom from both TCM and Kabbalah that the kidneys are "the seat of fear" in the body. Once mercury toxicity has been identified as a causal factor behind this fearfulness, Linda channels either a flower or gem essence that gently but effectively takes the edge off the fear or other negative emotions that have been exacerbated by mercury toxicity.

• **Colon:** Linda recommends cleansing the colon and intestines prior to and during a mercury detox through colonics provided by a qualified colon hydrotherapist, along with a high fiber diet. There are also colon cleanse products, including various herbal blends and medicinal clay products, that are highly beneficial.

• **Liver:** Herbal, amino acid, and homeopathic remedies are used for liver detoxification. Acupuncture may also be recommended to reduce such TCM syndromes as stagnant liver Qi, which often accompanies mercury toxicity.

As discussed in Chapter 10, Linda places great emphasis on rebuilding levels of glutathione, the master antioxidant and detoxifying agent in the body. She channels from a list of glutathione precursors including n-acetylcysteine, methionine, taurine, and alpha lipoic acid.

• **Other organs, glands, or systems:** The bladder, gastrointestinal tract, lungs, or prostate may need to undergo various forms of detoxification. As mentioned in Chapter 10, the prostate is like a sponge for heavy metals and other toxins.

• **Skin:** Sweating out heavy metal toxins lodged in fat tissues through the skin, the body's largest organ, is best handled by infrared sauna and steam. However, in Linda's experience, this level of detox does not appear to reach toxins stored in organs.

DETOX PREP RULE 5. Alkalize the Diet

Years of research and channeling have led us to an integration of three different dietary paradigms: (1) Metabolic Typing, a brilliant customized nutritional approach based on one's biochemical individuality as determined by lab analysis of the Krebs cycle and the autonomic nervous system (see *The Nutrition Solution* by Harold Kristal and James Haig). (2) Glycemic Index, a method of measuring the quality and quantity of carbohydrates of a particular food in relationship to its ability to raise blood glucose levels. (3) Anti-candida diet, a highly alkaline, vegetarian approach to diet that largely trumps the other two approaches for an individual suffering from mercury toxicity or a compromised immune system until such time that mercury detoxification is completed. So complicated is the interrelationship of food, lifestyle, and healing that one of our next books will be largely devoted to that subject. We also recommend reading *Conscious Eating* by Dr. Gabriel Cousens, M.D., for valuable insights into this process.

What we can say in broad strokes here is that people who suffer from mercury toxicity are *always* overly acidic. "Acid pH diet" and "acid pH toxins" are the most common variables that show up in the pre-test for these clients. An acidic diet is the equivalent of pouring gas on a fire. In fact, an acidic diet will exacerbate the severity of many of the conditions related to mercury toxicity listed in Table 9-1 and/or block or stall any detoxification program.

Diet, by itself, rarely cures a disease caused by toxicity. It is wishful thinking that diet alone will be able to rid the body of mercury or other heavy metals. However, the correct individualized healing diet is an important piece of a bigger puzzle and an integral part of a holistic healing strategy. It enhances the detoxification process by providing more energy and vitality in the healing environment. An anti-candida diet is expressly designed for people who have chronic degenerative disease brought on by heavy metals or other environmental toxins.

To help clients become co-creators in their healing, Linda discusses the purpose of the alkaline anti-candida diet with them. She notes that the diet must not "feed" the fungus and parasites by increasing acidity in the body. Quite the contrary, the diet is designed to alter the biological terrain to starve out unhealthy pathogens. This is analogous to draining the swamp, as discussed in Chapter 2. People who are quite sick are sometimes initially taken aback by the restrictive nature of the diet that Linda channels. The severity of the alkaline anti-candida diet is commensurate with the severity of the client's toxicity and fungal, parasite, acidosis, and suppressed immune system issues. In general, the key attributes of a more severe anti-candida diet are:

• Reduction or elimination of animal protein in the diet (meat, poultry, dairy products, eggs).

• No raw or refined sugar, products with these sugars, or artificial sweeteners. Stevia and (in milder cases) agave are acceptable sweeteners.

• No processed foods or products with white flour or yeast.

• No alcoholic beverages, coffee, mushrooms, vinegar, or fermented foods made with vinegar.

• Elimination or reduction of acid-forming fruits (oranges, grapefruits, bananas, and others), vegetables with high sugar/starch content (beets, potatoes, carrots), and fish.

• Eat organic food whenever possible.

Linda channels from a comprehensive list of foods broken down by category, including vegetables, fruits, meats, poultry, fish, grains, dairy, nuts and seeds, and spices. She points out that the diet is temporary and fluid, and will change over time. It becomes less restrictive, with a greater variety of food choices added, as heavy metals, other toxins, fungi, and parasites are reduced during the detoxification process. The upside for reluctant participants, she explains, is that they will fundamentally begin to feel better. She reminds clients that the angels have precisely guided this information, but it is up to them to follow it.

Linda is a big believer in what are called "functional foods"—foods that accomplish a particular medicinal goal. For example, raw cultured vegetables, which may be purchased in most natural food stores or made at home, help to reestablish our inner bacterial ecology. Rich in lactobacilli (beneficial bacteria) and enzymes, raw cultured vegetables are highly alkaline, cleansing, predigested, and unpasteurized. According to Donna Gates, author of the *The Body Ecology Diet*, these delicious sauerkraut-style salads may initially produce gas and bloating as they stir up toxins in the intestinal tract.[2] That's why Linda recommends using probiotics at the beginning of the detox process before introducing raw cultured vegetables. There are recipes for raw cultured vegetables and other dietary suggestions on www.thehealinggift.com. In addition, Linda strongly endorses devices like juicers, sprouters, dehydraters, and nut-milk makers as useful components of the detoxification process.

If the client has a busy lifestyle and his or her case is not too severe, Linda has the client agree to adhere to what she calls the "80/20 diet." This diet is designed for a person who typically eats out often and who cannot easily control his or her diet. In such cases, Linda counsels that these people should establish a realistic goal of achieving 80 percent compliance, with 100 percent compliance at home and less when eating in restaurants. Linda makes it quite clear, however, that the greater the compliance the faster and more dramatic the healing results will be.

DETOX PREP RULE 6. Eliminate Harmful Pathogens

These include fungi, parasites, bacteria (see Chapters 5–7), and viruses. At the same time, it's necessary to restore beneficial intestinal flora with probiotics.

DETOX PREP RULE 7. Stabilize the Endocrine System Function

This is often done with herbal, nutraceutical, and homeopathic formulas. For more challenging cases, Linda may refer the client to an integrative physician experienced in bioidentical hormone therapy (Chapter 16).

DETOX PREP RULE 8. Address Neurological and Emotional Issues

This involves remedies ranging from flower/gem essences to orthomolecular nutrients as well as meditation techniques to treat conditions as diverse as brain fog and depression (Chapter 15).

LINDA'S HEAVY METAL DETOXIFICATION PROCESS

After completing the prep part of the process, the client is fundamentally stronger and prepared to begin the main event: the challenging process of mercury detoxification. Linda is often asked how long this will take. That is difficult to answer; it may range from as little as a few months to well over a year or longer. It depends on the degree of mercury toxicity (the total mercury load) as well as the client's ability to cope with what occurs during the process. What has changed by this time is that all the barriers to a successful detox have been removed: miasms have been eliminated, while the lymphatic, kidney, and liver excretionary pathways have been sufficiently opened. The client can more easily handle the toxic onslaught of mercury moving out of the body with a minimum of resistance or complications.

Chelating mercury out of the body and brain is not an exact science. It's closer to an art form because the degree of toxicity and the precise location of toxicity and biochemical individuality are different in every person. Nonetheless, it is possible to make some broad generalizations about how to proceed, including a list of basic dos and don'ts.

The origin of the word "chelation" comes from the Greek word for "claw." Chelation literally claws mercury out of tissues where it has burrowed. Without supervision from someone with real expertise in this area, chelating mercury can be a difficult and painful experience fraught with discouraging pitfalls. Even when dealing with an integrative physician or other health care professional experienced in such matters, it is something that, at least in the critical first phase of the process, must be closely monitored, with adjustments for lowering the dose or temporarily stopping the process entirely at the first sign of a negative reaction.

Close communication is necessary because, as Linda puts it, "With chelation you may take two steps forward and then one step backward on more than one occasion before you cross the goal line." Again, what Linda uniquely brings to the table is direct angelic guidance, which is the best support we know of to minimize discomfort during detoxification. Here are the basic rules of Linda's mercury detoxification process.

DETOX RULE 1. Do Not Make Stressful or Important Life Decisions While You Are Detoxifying

You must be in the proper head space to undergo mercury detoxification. The prospects of marriage, divorce, pregnancy, or career change should all be put on hold at least until the detox process is well underway. This is because negative, irrational emotions and outbursts sometimes surface during the detox process. These negative emotions are biochemically triggered and magnified as the poison is redeposited and eventually moves out of the brain and body. Linda frequently counsels people starting detox to have minimal contact with people whose behavior is toxic to them. Preferably, they should have their own support group of friends and like-minded individuals who understand the physical and emotional ups-and-downs of this process.

For more information on the trials and tribulations of someone who has gone through this process, we recommend the informative weblog www. mercurylife.com written anonymously by a self-described "thirty-something attorney and engineer who has spent the past seven years battling fallout from mercury toxicity." He issues this caveat: "When you chelate, you stir up, or 'mobilize,' mercury and other toxic metals from the various places it is stored in your body. Because the chemical chelators have a stronger affinity for the mercury than do the proteins in your body, the chelators can bind to the mercury and pull it away from its tight bonds with your organs and other tissues. But, unfortunately, only a portion of the mobilized mercury will then actually be excreted by your body, through [various] routes. This probably reflects, in part, the extreme toxicity of these substances to your excretory organs."[3]

In an article entitled "Mercury Detoxification Perpetuating Factors, Problems and Obstacles," Dr. Klinghardt describes some of the challenges: "There is a difference between mobilizing and detoxing. Mobilization means stirring [mercury] up in its hiding place. Mobilization may lead to excretion. [However,] it also may lead to redistribution. The body had done the best it could by storing [mercury] wherever it stored it. By mobilizing, we are telling the body that we know better where to put it. [The truth is] we don't. Detoxifying or detoxing means mobilizing and moving it out of the body. There are no true detoxifying agents. All we have is mobilizing agents. The body has to do the excreting with the help of the proper agents. The body is not always able to do this! Often perpetuating factors are present that disable the body's mechanisms to detox."[4] Linda describes the mobilization process with this visual: Imagine shaking one of those crystal ball Christmas ornaments containing a snowman where the snow flies up in the air and resettles. Moving mercury around is only the first step.

DETOX RULE 2. Have Your Health Care Practitioner Pick the Proper Chelating Agent

Picking the proper agent is tricky because one size rarely fits all. This is why it is important for Linda to channel from her list of natural chelators. There are two types of heavy metal chelators: natural and pharmaceutical. Nutritional remedies include cilantro, chlorella, vitamin C, selenium, zeolite, garlic, methionine, EDTA suppositories, apple pectin, germanium, seaweed, spirulina, blue-green algae, MSM (methylsulfonylmethane), and homeopathic remedies. For more information on these, see www.thehealinggift.com.

Sometimes, there are special considerations. If one is dealing with a child, for example, it is advisable to use a homeopathic form, as anything stronger would be too intense for the child. Because Linda does not work with pharmaceutical chelators, in cases where one is needed, she works in conjunction with a physician trained in using them. The two principal pharmaceutical products are DMSA and DMPS, which are much stronger than natural remedies. As noted earlier, both can be damaging to the kidneys and liver and must be used carefully.

DETOX RULE 3. Think of Mercury Detoxification as the Tortoise and the Hare Running a Race—the Hare Never Wins This Race

The proper dosage of the chelator is more critical than in any other process Linda uses. If mercury detox proceeds too rapidly, there can be disastrous results emotionally, neurologically, and physically. Without proper management, the process can leave a person feeling highly depressed, accompanied by irrational outbursts of anger or fear. This is the dreaded Mad Hatter's disease described above. The Freuds—both Linda and Sigmund—assure you that no amount of psychological counseling can eliminate these biochemically triggered, temporary psychotic episodes. Dr. Vaughn Harada, D.D.S., a retired biological dentist in Santa Monica, California, whom I saw many years ago, gave me a unique, visual insight when he described the neurological and emotional damage people experienced if they detox too rapidly: "Imagine being in a small room with the windows and doors closed shut and violently shaking a dusty rug with the dust flying all around the room. That is the feeling that you experience in your head when you detoxify from mercury too quickly."

Moving mercury out too fast can also result in serious physical problems, including kidney or liver damage, disruption in endocrine function, increased fungus and parasite disease, chronic fatigue syndrome with weakened immune response, and a potential spate of other unforeseen problems. *It's particularly important that the kidneys and liver have plenty of time to recover and repair during the detox process.*

DETOX RULE 4. Know That Mercury Detoxification Is a Push-Pull, Stop-Start Proposition

The key is to start very slowly on a low dose of natural chelator and watch to see how you physically and emotionally react to it. It's best to stay at a very low dosage level that you can comfortably handle without any or minimal adverse physical or emotional reactions. This period may last from a few days to a couple of weeks or even longer in severe cases. You must literally check in with yourself, both physically and mentally, on a daily basis to see if you are able to handle detoxifying on any given day. *After you have successfully handled a very small dose of the chelating agent, you may be ready to push the envelope very slightly and increase the dosage by a very small, incremental amount. But be sure to check with your practitioner first.*

Linda and her angelic guides recognize the importance of being able to function in one's occupation without being negatively impacted by a mercury detox. This is another reason why a detox must proceed slowly, for to move too rapidly might leave one bedridden and unable to function. The trick is to carefully pick your spots when you detox. For example, if you have an important business meeting or other function for which you must perform, you certainly do not want to be chelating that day. Completely stopping the process the day before usually allows enough time to reestablish a clear head needed to control and focus emotions. On the other hand, you should push the detox process when you have time to relax over the weekend.

Linda highly recommends using the Eng3 ActiveAir device during any heavy metal detoxification. This sophisticated computer-controlled inhalation device biophysically alters the air to fight oxidative-stress-related disease. It is also useful for a wide range of chronic diseases as it strengthens the immune system, speeds recovery, and optimizes energy. It is especially beneficial for optimizing cardiac health. We both use this device quite often as part of our own anti-aging program. For details, see www.thehealinggift.com.

DETOX RULE 5. Replenish Beneficial Minerals That Are Lost During Chelation

In addition to mercury, heavy-metal chelating agents pull many beneficial minerals and trace minerals out of the body that must be replenished with mineral supplements. Failure to compensate for the loss of minerals will lead to or exacerbate different forms of chronic degenerative disease.

DETOX RULE 6. Plan for the Worst, Be Prepared to Put Out Fires, and Anticipate Potential Flare-Ups Ahead of Time

To guide you through the detox process, your practitioner must develop a master plan to deal with strengthening the organs, glands, and systems that are at risk for damage due to the resettlement of mercury that invariably occurs before it is fully excreted out of the body. In addition to acupuncture, that arsenal should include alkalizers, minerals, antioxidants, amino acids, probiotics, and homeopathic fungal remedies. It should also include flower/gem essences; essential fatty acids (salmon or cod liver oils or flax, evening primrose, or borage oils); B vitamins and other nutraceuticals (natural pharmaceuticals) for neurological and emotional issues; herbal, amino acid, and glandular support to control endocrine disruption; and kidney, liver, and lymphatic drainage remedies.

What the angels provide is a delicate strategy for not only picking the right chelator, but also providing absolutely precise levels of dosages so that clients can push the envelope without suffering physical or emotional effects. This is one of the miracles of Linda's work.

CHAPTER 13

A World of Natural Supplements

Effective health care depends on self-care; this fact is currently heralded as if it were a discovery.
—IVAN ILLICH

Everyone has a doctor in him.
We just need to help him in his work.
—HIPPOCRATES

IN PRESENTING LINDA'S GIFT, I realized there was so much information about how Linda uses a vast array of natural supplements and remedies that it was impossible to adequately describe all of them in this book. Therefore, an entire book is in the planning stages that will detail Linda's experiences with supplements, diet, and other lifestyle issues.

I have chosen instead to discuss some of the medical reasons why Linda uses various categories of supplements and remedies. These include vitamins, minerals, antioxidants, essential fatty acids, probiotics, enzymes, amino acids, herbal remedies, homeopathics, green drinks, medicinal clay, and certain devices. A discussion of the most popular of these is found on www.thehealinggift.com. Table 13-1 provides an overview of the categories of natural healing modalities that Linda works with.

At the dawn of a new era of socialized medicine, we are at the crossroads where we must finally make some hard lifestyle choices: Either embrace the principles of anti-aging medicine to significantly slow down the aging process through detoxification, nutritional supplements, bioidentical/homeopathic hormone therapies, healthy diet, exercise, and other lifestyle adjustments or succumb far more quickly to degenerative disease through a mechanized-factory medical system, where medical decisions are often driven by economic

TABLE 13-1. CATEGORIES OF NATURAL HEALING MODALITIES THAT LINDA WORKS WITH

Adaptogens

Alkalizing products

Allergy remedies

Amino acids

Antibiotics
  Herbal, homeopathic,
  enzyme and
  orthomolecular

Anti-inflammatory/pain
  remedies

Antioxidants

Blood pressure remedies

Blood sugar/insulin regulators

Cardiovascular remedies

Chemical detox remedies

Colds/flu remedies

Colon/intestinal remedies

Digestive remedies

Endocrine system remedies
  Herbal, homeopathic,
  glandulars, plant extracts,
  bioidentical hormones
  from a doctor

Enzyme formulas

Essential fatty acids
  Fish oils/plant oils

Eye remedies/nutrients

Flower/gem essences

Fungus/yeast remedies

Green drinks

Homeopathic remedies

Immune system support

Kidney detox remedies

Liver detox remedies

Lyme disease protocols

Lymphatic drainage

Mercury/heavy metal chelators

Miasm remedies

Mineral/trace mineral formulas

Neurological remedies

Osteoporosis formulas

Oxygen supplements/devices

Parasite remedies

Pesticides/insecticides

Phenolics/chemicals detox

Probiotics

Protein supplements

Radiation detoxification

Respiratory remedies

Sexual tonics

Sleep remedies

Vitamins

Water devices

Weight management

Women's formulas

---

considerations. Your options are to either seize the bull by the horns and take personal responsibility for promoting *your own good health* or risk being a premature statistic on a government chart. On a personal note, while not statistically significant, we have significant anecdotal proof that the healthiest people we know in their eighties and nineties are people who have been actively taking nutraceuticals for the last forty years. They are our role models.

To take control of your own health demands that you become an educated consumer—a student of health. Our mantra is *"Make health your passion."* This requires putting an end to all destructive lifestyle and dietary habits. There is little sympathy here for such preventable conditions as alcoholism, drug addiction, or smoking. You are on your own now, and a government system of rationed health care will not save you. You must approach wellness with the same degree of passion that you approach any other project. Don't rely on your overworked, stressed-out doctor who has only a few minutes to spend on your complicated health issues. It's not really about money either. It's about acquiring the knowledge and mindfulness needed to take good care of your body. Even if you don't possess these now, you can acquire them—if you choose to do so. We hope you will.

Over eighty million Americans have some form of cardiovascular disease. While the pharmaceutical approach can certainly be beneficial, its potential side effects are no joy ride. Just as any mechanic will tell you, your engine will last longer if you just change the oil every 3,000 miles. *With careful planning, drug therapy does not have to be the inevitable consequence of aging.* Yet, how many consumers take the time to research the merits of CoQ_{10}, magnesium, niacin, essential fatty acids from fish oil, plant sterols, D-ribose, carnitine, pomegranate extract, and beta-glucan for their heart?

We are not preaching that you should ignore your doctor's advice. Far from it. What we are saying is that to achieve optimal wellness you need to make sure your doctor has a working knowledge of natural solutions in addition to the pharmaceutical approach he or she learned in medical school. Do your homework prior to visiting your doctor so that you can intelligently discuss which natural supplements should become part of your healing regime.

Nutritional supplements and detoxification protocols helped to save both of our lives when we were very ill. They empowered us to heal as they addressed the real causes behind our illnesses—real toxins and pathogens, real deficiencies and excesses requiring real solutions. As we became enthralled with their potential as vehicles for optimum wellness, they became an integral part of our lives. This empowerment, in turn, was our bridge to the spirit world. Make no mistake about it: Supplements and alternative medicine are *not* the spirit world. They are, however, a bridge to it. Therefore, we feel blessed, due to Linda's gift, to be on the cutting edge of an industry that has done so much to improve the quality of life for so many.

SOME OF THE MANY REASONS WE TAKE SUPPLEMENTS

Taking supplements is no longer optional or merely desirable. Here are several reasons why supplementation is essential for either obtaining or maintaining good health.

• **Nutritional value is missing in our mass-market food supply.** As a result of the dumbing down of the quality of our food supply by agribusiness, many nutrients can no longer be obtained purely from food to the same extent that was possible years ago. In the rush to get as much produce to the supermarket shelves as quickly and as cheaply as possible, nutritional quality has become the sacrificial lamb in this equation—pun intended! This is a consequence of small family farms being largely replaced by agribusiness concerns driven by short-term, high-yield economic interests. They have no financial incentive to be good stewards of the land or to provide high-quality nutritious organic food for their customers. Constant overuse of land for crop production has left the topsoil largely depleted of minerals and trace minerals. Therefore, the fruits and vegetables one buys from the typical supermarket are actually low in nutritional value compared with produce from a bygone era, from an organic farmer, or from one's own garden.

• **Depletion of nutrients from heavy metal toxicity.** In his book *New Optimum Nutrition for the Mind*, author Patrick Holford speaks at length about the depletion of nutrients due to heavy metal toxicity. He characterizes metal and heavy metal toxins as "antinutrients" that are associated with mood swings, aggressive behavior, attention deficit, depression, disturbed sleep patterns, and problems with cognitive memory. The toxins he refers to include mercury, lead, cadmium, aluminum, and copper. He states that these toxins "interfere either with our ability to absorb or use essential nutrients, or in some cases, promote the loss of essential nutrients from the body."[1] Just a few examples of depleted nutrients that need to be replenished due to the deleterious effects of these antinutrients include vitamins (B vitamins and folic acid), minerals (zinc, calcium, selenium), essential fatty acids, amino acids (methionine, taurine, n-acetyl cysteine), and antioxidants (alpha lipoic acid, CoQ_{10}).

• **Depletion of nutrients from pharmaceutical drugs.** Dr. Hyla Cass, M.D., has written a much needed book entitled *Supplement Your Prescription* that describes the side effects drugs cause by depleting nutrients and then provides solutions to compensate for that. For example, statin drugs like Lipitor, Zocor, and Pravachol deplete CoQ_{10}, which is associated with mitochondrial dysfunction affecting certain forms of heart disease.[2,3] Acid-blocking drugs such as Prilosec, Prevacid, and Nexium prevent absorption of vitamin B_{12} and magnesium, leading to depression and other mood disorders.[4] They can also block protein digestion, affecting amino acid and neurotransmitter production. Tylenol (acetaminophen) quickly depletes glutathione levels, which leads to liver disease. Alternative health practitioners have found creative solutions with supplements and diet that can provide benefits similar to these medications without side effects.

• **Psychotropic drugs may be a "wrong-headed" solution.** The use of psychotropic drugs to treat depression and anxiety is soaring. However, with them comes a price tag that includes undesirable physical and emotional side effects. However, if a psychiatrist or other mental health care professional is not addressing certain nutritional issues like omega-3 or B vitamin deficiencies or certain physical conditions and syndromes like hypothyroidism or chronic mercury toxicity, then no amount of psychotropic drugs or psychotherapy can really correct the situation. In Chapter 15, I offer a fascinating look at how Linda successfully uses vitamins, minerals, amino acids, essential fatty acids, other brain nutraceuticals, and flower and gem essences to successfully treat many forms of depression—all without the side effects that often accompany psychotropic drugs.

- **Safety issues.** There are several areas of treatment where a natural approach is safer than the pharmaceutical approach because very few side effects, if any, are ever encountered. An example is controlling inflammation caused by arthritis. While Vioxx was effective at counteracting arthritic pain, it was also shown to cause or exacerbate cardiovascular disease; so it was removed from the market in 2004. Its main replacement, Celebrex, has fared better but still has real problems. It is unnecessarily strong for many people, placing them at extra risk of such major side effects as gastrointestinal hemorrhage, kidney injury, and death.[5] Linda achieves effective control over arthritic pain through a combination of various natural remedies without any side effects. These may include homeopathic creams, hydrolyzed beef collagen, hyaluronic acid, glucosamine, fish oil, and specific enzyme, herbal, and mineral blends. She is also a big believer in acupuncture, chiropractic treatment, prolotherapy (also called sclerotherapy), magnet therapy, and photonic light stimulation for pain management.

- **Strengths and limitations of homeopathy.** Homeopathy, which is enormously popular in Europe and India, is one of the safest forms of medicine in the world. Linda finds homeopathy quite useful in treating many types of disorders (see "Hybrid Homeopathy"). In certain areas of treatment, such as the removal of miasms, no other approach works. Homeopathy is one of Linda's favorite ways to treat fungal disease, as it more effectively targets specific forms of fungi instead of a broad-spectrum pharmaceutical drug that may be toxic to the liver. It is also effective in treating certain viruses as well as detoxifying and draining many environmental toxins out of the lymphatic system and organs. Homeopathy is clearly the safest choice in many other situations. For example, certain sensitive adults and young children who have very delicate constitutions or are extremely toxic cannot handle anything stronger than homeopathy. They require its subtle energetic approach that, although quite thorough, may take a somewhat longer time to achieve the desired effect than other natural methods.

Contrary to what many homeopaths will tell you, however, there are other areas of treatment where homeopathy is of limited or no value because it does not address the underlying cause of the problem. For example, if a person is deficient in alpha lipoic acid, a precursor to glutathione, a homeopathic will not correct this. Only alpha lipoic acid can. Because the biochemical individuality of each person is different, certain people simply resonate better with an herbal or orthomolecular nutrient approach than with homeopathy. Sometimes a stronger approach than homeopathy is needed. For example, if a person is doing a liver or gallbladder cleanse, an herbal approach to detoxification may be more effective than a homeopathic approach.

Hybrid Homeopathy

Linda and I have developed a formulation and manufacturing process called Hybrid Homeopathy(tm) that we believe is more advanced and efficacious than any other homeopathic process we are aware of. This complex process is a blend of channeled homeopathic ingredients and dilutions combined with gem essences, proprietary structured water, and full-spectrum light. The homeopathically diluted ingredients include amino acids, herbs, enzymes, glandulars, vitamins, minerals, and other nutrients.

Gem essences are known to address specific negative emotional states associated with certain conditions. In addition, our research has shown that gem essence resonances help "amplify" the potency of the homeopathic resonances they are combined with. Hybrid Homeopathy can be thought of as homeopathic "rocket fuel" that works rapidly like other treatment modalities, but with the safety of homeopathy. Our first product is called Power for Women, which is specifically formulated for women's physiology to enhance stamina, strength, and metabolism as it improves the quality of exercise or aerobic routines. It contains no ephedra or caffeine. A similar product called Power for Men is planned as well as additional products for reducing stress, and improving sleep and weight loss. For details, see www.thehealinggift.com or www.alwaysyoung.com.

• **Universal need for antioxidants.** Linda consistently channels that the vast majority of her clients require some type of antioxidant. Any long-term exposure to drugs or heavy metal toxicity, ranging from amalgams to spinal cord or hip replacement surgeries where different types of metals are now in the body, means that a client has to be on some form of antioxidant as long as that metal is in the body. However, this need is not limited to people with heavy metal toxicity. Many other environmental toxins also promote free radical proliferation and require an antioxidant in response.

Countering Side Effects of Pharmaceutical Drugs

As pharmaceutical drugs have become the predominant method of treating chronic degenerative diseases, holistic healers have found that the unique and unfortunate medical side effects of the drugs are often best remedied by natural supplements. Here are a few examples that Linda constantly encounters.

• **Countering imbalances with probiotics.** Bacteria are an underappreciated concept in promoting wellness. Some bacteria are essential for life, while other bacteria can cause death. There is a constant "war of the worlds" going on in the body between beneficial bacteria and other destructive forces that can overwhelm them if left unchecked. These forces include heavy metals, broad-spectrum antibiotics, birth control pills, steroids, smoking, alcohol, electromagnetic pollution, stress, and an overly acidic diet.

Probiotics refer to various strains of beneficial bacteria that collectively colonize in the intestinal tract. *Lactobacillus* strains are most active in the small intestine, while *Bifidobacterium* strains work best in the large intestine and colon. A healthy intestinal wall encourages optimum absorption of nutrients, including vitamins and minerals, and supports healthy digestion and elimination.

The most common causal factors of probiotic deficiencies that Linda sees in clients are due to heavy metal toxicity and overuse of antibiotics. As discussed earlier, mercury causes severe acidosis, promoting a milieu that accelerates the fermenting process and turns the body into a "mini-brewery." This breeds fungi and promotes harmful bacteria. Broad-spectrum antibiotics, which are often derived from fungi, are equal-opportunity destroyers of bacteria. They can kill beneficial bacteria as easily as they can kill infectious bacteria. If antibiotics are taken without alkalizing the diet, the resulting acidic terrain soon becomes a breeding ground for fungi, parasites, and eventually more harmful bacterial forms that overwhelm beneficial bacterial flora in the digestive and intestinal tracts. Linda has channeled that if one has no recourse but to take a pharmaceutical antibiotic, probiotics should be "standard issue" to support and replenish a healthy balance of flora. Taking probiotics, in conjunction with an alkalizing diet, are the best way to remedy bacterial imbalances created by antibiotics.

• **Detoxifying steroids and other drugs from the liver.** Linda has seen wonderful improvement in liver health and function in clients when she channels amino acids such as n-acetyl cysteine and methionine, certain herbal blends and tinctures, or homeopathics, which are particularly good at removing drug toxins from the body.

• **Weaning off antidepressants.** Working under the auspices of Dr. Thom E. Lobe, Linda channels a slow, methodical, phased program to ease clients off antidepressants using a combination of supplements that may include B vitamins, amino acids, herbs, homeopathics, and flower/gem essences (see Chapter 15). This transition to natural mood-regulating methods promotes a positive outlook without any side effects.

Caveat

The information and products we have discussed here are solely to support health and not intended to diagnose, treat, prevent, or cure any disease, and they should not be used as a substitute for diagnosis and treatment by your personal physician.

PART TWO

Emotional Healing

CHAPTER 14

Our Work with Sigmund Freud: A Preamble to the Emotional Database

There is no light without shadow
and no psychic wholeness without imperfection.
—C. G. JUNG

ALTHOUGH THIS BOOK IS PRINCIPALLY about Linda's extraordinary healing gift, we could not have created the Emotional Database without Sigmund Freud's guiding influence from the spirit world —a force that has aided our medical, emotional, and spiritual development for the past sixteen years. Therefore, in addition to introducing Linda to the world, a secondary purpose of this book is a *coming-out party* to introduce Sigmund Freud's new insights on a broad array of topics to an entirely new audience in the 21st century (see Figure 14-1). At the same time, being able to update Freud's theories by communicating with him from his lofty perch in the spirit world where he currently resides—a state which most traditional scientists dismiss as a ridiculous impossibility—gives a much needed stamp of validity to metaphysical reality.

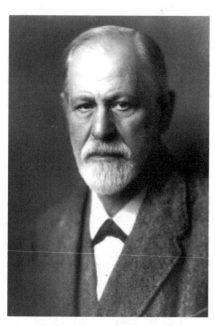

Figure 14-1. Sigmund Freud.
Used with permission of the Freud Museum, London.
Photograph: Max Halberstam.

We are making an audacious claim: Linda is in active communication from the beyond with a dead person, specifi-

194

cally Sigmund Freud who died in 1939. Assuming you can temporarily suspend disbelief, the logical question (as much as any of this is logical!) is: Why Sigmund Freud? If you were to pick a famous historical figure who could prove beyond a reasonable doubt that Linda Freud is capable of communicating with a dead person, that person would need to exhibit certain unique qualifications to validate him for this new role.

That person would need to have a scientific background and be capable of understanding the inner workings of the mind from a psychological and spiritual perspective. He would need to be unafraid of taking a leadership role in promoting ideas that were controversial, not just in his time, but even more so today. He would need to be unafraid to acknowledge from the spirit world those theories he still stands by as well as those he now admits were wrong. He would need to regard his previous time on earth as part of an evolutionary process of his soul's journey from lifetime to lifetime. Above all, he would need to be a communicator, who is interested in sharing what he has learned in the spirit world to help those now on earth evolve their personal and collective consciousness.

Who better than Sigmund Freud could transcend boundaries between the material and the metaphysical worlds! These qualifications contain a certain transcendent logic about why Sigmund Freud (1856–1939) is the most important spirit guide who communicates with us on a regular basis. We have had a close relationship with him since the early 1990s, and pay rapt attention to his incredible, newfound wisdom acquired in the spirit world. Our relationship with Sigmund is quite complicated, but certainly one reason is genetic. I am a distant relative of his several generations removed.

We are happy to report that Sigmund has made enormous progress in the spirit world over the last seventy years since he transitioned out of his physical body. He is a powerful and pioneering soul, who has also been other famous individuals in previous incarnations (see Chapter 17). Over the years Sigmund has given us a clear and honest assessment of certain aspects of his life's work, which he now believes is a mixed bag of brilliant insights and erroneous conclusions. His ego does not gloat over his successes, and he is humbled and even distressed by his blunders.

It is important to realize that when Freud started psychoanalysis, his "science of the psyche," the field of psychiatry was generally held in low esteem by the scientific community as late as 1906.[1] His goal for psychoanalysis was to transform the field of psychiatry by developing and refining new methods of understanding the unconscious mind. Clearly, a Magellan of the mind, Freud chose to explore psychic territory in new ways even though he was often unaware of where it would ultimately lead. Therefore, since he, along with his associates in the Psychoanalytical Society of Vienna, were the primary explorers and architects of this new science, he had to, *by necessity,* achieve significant successes as well as make significant mistakes. If viewed within the context of his time, he was a complete and original genius, who dared to break new ground where others feared to tread. If viewed within the context of *our* time in the early part of the 21st century, some of his theories have clearly stood the test of time, while others have been replaced or declared passé.

However, try as we might, none of us can escape his shadow. Sigmund Freud started a train of thought whose influence is still strongly felt individually and culturally. His contributions to psychoanalysis are so extensive that they require twenty-four volumes to completely cover the gamut of human experience—from mining the unconscious through the interpretation of dreams to providing a profound understanding of human sexuality. Linda has channeled that from an angelic perspective his archetypal persona is viewed as "a guardian of conscious and unconscious mind."

However, unlike certain angels, who view much of humanity with some disdain, Sigmund Freud understands all too well the inherent shortcomings and limitations of human beings. Although there are other historical figures who could conceivably fit this bill, no one is better equipped or more prepared to make this historical qualitative leap in human understanding than Sigmund Freud. His life, his accomplishments, his own psychoanalysis, and his written correspondence with colleagues are, in large part, an open book. As noted Freud biographer Peter Gay said in an article he wrote in 1999 about Freud for *Time* magazine:

> There are no neutrals in the Freud wars. Admiration, even downright adulation, on one side; skepticism, even downright disdain, on the other. This is not hyperbole. A psychoanalyst who is currently trying to enshrine Freud in the pantheon of cultural heroes must contend with a relentless critic who devotes his days to exposing Freud as a charlatan. But on one thing the contending parties agree: for good or ill, Sigmund Freud, more than any other explorer of the psyche, has shaped the mind of the 20th century. The very fierceness and persistence of his detractors are a wry tribute to the staying power of Freud's ideas.[2]

The controversy surrounding Freud's theories about such things as the unconscious, the origin of neuroses, the Oedipal complex, and the primacy of the sex drive continues to this day. In 2006, *Newsweek* featured Freud smoking his trademark cigar on its cover with a title that screamed: "Freud Is *Not*

Dead!" The issue contained multiple articles that showed the utterly pervasive influence his thought processes still have on our culture as well as the newfound respect that neurologists and other scientists now hold for certain aspects of his work. *If only they knew just how alive he really is!*

Sigmund is using Linda, in this and in future books, as his vehicle to help retool the field of psychology in the 21st century from above. He wishes to communicate a dazzling amount of information about alternative healing modalities, new consciousness technologies, and profound discoveries about spirituality that reveal humanity's true relationship to God. Therefore, we ask the reader to understand that the ideas presented in this section are truly a collaboration among Sigmund Freud, Linda, and me.

It is interesting to note that Freud's first abiding passion, while still a student at the University of Vienna, was neurology, and he has repeatedly told us that he relishes his role as a scientist above all else. It is therefore no wonder that he is the guiding force behind the research in the Emotional Database. He was a powerful soul for change in his lifetime, and he remains the same powerful force for change from the spirit world. From this clear vantage point, he is now quite aware of those discoveries he made in his lifetime that were correct as well as those that were incorrect. To complete his own personal tikkun (karmic or past-life correction process), he embraces the opportunity we are offering him in this book and feels duty-bound to make amends and rectify those concepts he erroneously propagated in his lifetime.

SIGMUND WELCOMES US TO HIS WORLD

So pervasive is his influence on Linda's work that a rather curious phenomenon has occurred at various times since the early 1990s. Like chess pieces moved around on a metaphysical chessboard, we have, in one fashion or another, been introduced to several people who are the reincarnation of individuals who worked directly with Sigmund Freud as psychoanalytical or medical associates. Although we are sworn to protect their confidentiality and cannot reveal their current names, we can say with certainty that Linda has identified the following associates who worked with Sigmund Freud in some professional capacity: Dr. Ernest Jones, his biographer, close associate, best friend, and confidant; Sándor Ferenczi, close associate and friend; Dr. Otto Rank, an associate who later turned on him; Dr. Ernst Wilhelm von Brücke, his professor of neurology from the University of Vienna; and Professor Jean-Martin Charcot, his teacher from the University of Paris who taught him hypnotherapy. The following two stories involve clients who were, metaphorically speaking, "brought" by Sigmund to Linda for both physical healing and a metaphysical awakening.

The Reincarnation of Oskar Pfister

A very positive article about Linda's gift entitled "Channeling Help from Afar" appeared in the July–August 2004 issue of *Alternative Medicine* magazine written by researcher Burton Goldberg, author of the landmark *Alternative Medicine: The Definitive Guide* (see www.thehealinggift.com). Linda received an overwhelming response from this article, and many people achieved remarkable improvement in their health as a result. Among the e-mails she received was one from a thirty-seven-year-old Asian-American named Joseph, who sought help from a mysterious, debilitating type of chronic fatigue syndrome that had severely compromised his immune system and caused his weight to drop to 112 pounds. Since 2000 he had spent tens of thousands of dollars with numerous mainstream doctors, alternative practitioners, and medical laboratories, with very little to show for it.

In working with Joseph, Linda discovered that he had severe liver toxicity (from heavy metals, chemicals, fungi, parasites), multiple miasms, multiple bacterial and viral infections, food allergies, gastrointestinal dysbiosis, chronic fatigue, and adrenal exhaustion and other hormonal imbalances. Linda set about systematically identifying and eliminating these toxins and pathogens, and over time the healing program she channeled restored his health. The story of what Joseph had to do to achieve this is certainly worthy of being a testimonial in this book.

However, what was far more astonishing is the revealment of a past-life relationship between Joseph in his last past life and Sigmund Freud, which stayed concealed until Joseph was basically healed. Fortunately, Joseph, who has a passion for metaphysical knowledge, was highly motivated to have a deep understanding of past-life associations related to his prolonged illness and assorted idiosyncratic behaviors he had experienced in his life. It soon became obvious why he had a strong drive for spiritual understanding as well as a highly developed analytical mind. Linda revealed that he was none other than the reincarnation of Oskar Pfister (1873–1956), a card-carrying member of Sigmund Freud's inner circle of psychoanalysts! In fact, Linda channeled that Sigmund maintained such a strong personal interest in Joseph/Oskar that he guided him to pick up a copy of the magazine and e-mail Linda for an appointment. Linda notes she always felt the presence of Sigmund during Joseph's readings but did not think to ask why until Joseph finished his healing.

Joseph is one of Linda's clients who early on grasped the spiritual significance of her extraordinary gift and desired to understand, once the "fire had been put out," why he had to endure such physical suffering in this lifetime. When Joseph came for a fateful reading in June 2006, Linda started the session by receiving channeled instructions to get a book on Sigmund Freud by Professor Peter Gay entitled *Freud: A Life for Our Time*. With her pendulum, she scanned the entire index that listed every important psychoanalytical/medical collaborator whom Freud had worked with in his career. When she came to Oskar Pfister's name, the pendulum swung wildly to the right and she simultaneously received several profound shakes that both Joseph and I witnessed— a startling confirmation of metaphysical reality. Sigmund then revealed to Linda his deep desire not only to help cure his close friend, but also to help guide him to discover the same types of spiritual/scientific discoveries that Sigmund has made in the spirit world. Linda channeled that in addition to certain past-life corrections for Oskar, it was Joseph's destiny to experience disease as a gateway to new spiritual understandings in this lifetime.

Between 1909 and his death in 1939, Sigmund Freud maintained a close personal and professional relationship with Reverend Oskar Pfister, a Swiss Calvinist minister, teacher, and psychoanalyst practicing in Zurich (see Figure 14-2). Pfister had the unique distinction of practicing psychoanalysis on his parishioners in addition to his ministerial duties. As a "healer of the soul," Pfister became a psychoanalyst because he felt that traditional church dogma was inadequate for achieving transformational cures. In psychoanalysis, he

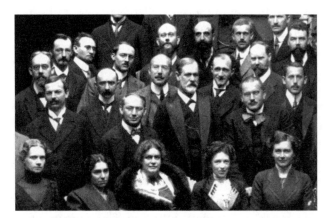

Figure 14-2. Center portion of the photograph of the Weimar Conference of the International Psychoanalytic Association, 1911. Sigmund Freud is in the center, Carl Jung is second to his left, and Oskar Pfister is the first on the left in the second row. *Used with permission of the Freud Museum, London.*

found an effective method for relieving the spiritual and emotional suffering of his parishioners. Pfister embraced psychoanalysis and became one of Freud's most loyal supporters. For over thirty-seven years, Pfister practiced his "psychoanalytic pastoral ministry," occasionally running afoul of the conservative Lutheran Church.[3]

According to *Psychoanalysis and Faith: Dialogues with Reverand Oskar Pfister,* "Between 1909 and his death in 1956 he also published numerous books and papers in which he described his work and observations, in particular on psychoanalytic technique, on the . . . importance of sexuality in the formation of neuroses, on religion and hysteria, the psychology of art, philosophy and psycho-analysis, analysis in pastoral work, Christianity and anxiety, and related themes."[4] In 1919, Pfister helped to establish the Swiss Society for Psychoanalysis, which still retains its affiliation with the International Psychoanalytic Association (IPA).

The relationship between Freud and Pfister spanned three decades of unbroken and mutual respect and friendship.[5] They shared their scientific findings about the application of psychoanalysis in personal meetings and correspondence. "Their temperaments, and the honesty and integrity which characterized both, often brought them into sharp conflict, but they also always showed true tolerance and mutual understanding."[6] Pfister's unshakable devotion to psychoanalysis and their deep, abiding friendship allowed him to escape Freud's negative views on religion, which makes their relationship all the more remarkable. In 1983, the American Psychiatric Association, in collaboration with the Association of Mental Health Clergy, established the Oskar Pfister Award to "honor those who have made significant contributions to the field of religion and psychiatry."[7]

The Reincarnation of Marie Bonaparte

In 2007, Sigmund arranged for a seemingly chance encounter with a woman whom I met at Starbucks in Pacific Palisades, California. While I was quietly enjoying a flavored latte as I read the newspaper, a woman sitting at the next table with a male friend suddenly asked me what time it was. After telling her the time, the three of us struck up a conversation that eventually led to the inevitable "What do you do for a living?" I replied that I was writing a book about my wife's work as a medical intuitive. The woman, whose name was Diane and who appeared to be in her late thirties, asked what her name was. When I said Linda Freud, she gasped in astonishment and said a friend had told her all about Linda. She had been meaning to call her but hadn't because she was currently working with another local healer, albeit with very limited success. Diane then briefly mentioned her medical problems, which included a severe case of chronic fatigue syndrome from which she had suffered for the last seven years. It had physically and neurologically affected her to such an extent that she was frequently bedridden for days at a time, which kept her from leading a normal life.

Diane subsequently saw Linda, who channeled a very complex set of causal factors that her other healers had totally missed. After initially being overwhelmed by the sheer volume of information that flowed forth from the angels in her first session, Diane quickly recovered, exhibiting the steely will of a fighter and survivor—attributes that were necessary to overcome her level of adversity. Still, Diane complained of her frustration with feeling so sick much of the time. She could not understand why she had been "singled out" to experience such a debilitating health condition in the prime of life. Her lack of progress with a bevy of high-priced doctors and alternative practitioners had made her the "problem child" of her family, most of whom considered her a hypochondriac with deep-seated emotional problems. This is an all-too-common pattern that Linda sees in people who have been misdiagnosed by doctors and then relegated to the category of life's losers by their families who believed in the infallibility of doctors.

However, Diane clearly did not fit that mold. Linda and I observed that she was a truly bright, engaging woman. Something was clearly wrong with this picture, as her life made absolutely no sense whatsoever. I told Diane that in a case as befuddling as hers there must be a metaphysical/spiritual reason why on some level she had been "ordained" to suffer so much in this lifetime. Since both Diane and her family had exhausted all conventional logic, she had to look outside the box to find real answers to her horrible physical problems. The idea that there could be either spiritual lessons or past-life information to be learned from her illness was an utterly new concept for her.

In her third session with Linda, a tantalizing tidbit of information burst forth. After Linda was in a trance state for a few minutes, Sigmund came to her and revealed: *Diane was the reincarnation of one of his patients, students, and closest friends, Princess Marie Bonaparte.* Martin Freud, Sigmund's son, called her "the best and dearest friend of father's last years."[8] Marie Bonaparte (1882–1962) was a direct descendant of Napoleon's brother Lucien on one side and the developers of Monte Carlo on the other. She married into one of the most respected royal families in Europe. Her husband, Prince George, was a brother of the late king of Greece and a member of the royal family of Denmark.

Freud first met Marie in 1925 when he was sixty-nine years old. Marie saw him for psychoanalysis and subsequently became his student. Marie was not only a completely devoted disciple of Freud's, but also an important psychoanalyist in her own right. In 1926 she founded the Psychoanalytical Society of Paris (Société Psychoanalytique de Paris) and translated Freud's work into French. From this professional relationship, a mutual and dear personal friendship developed. Marie tried for years to persuade the Nobel Prize Committee in Stockholm to give Freud the Nobel Prize and also utilized her fortune to assist in publishing and republishing his works.

Upon further research I discovered that Marie Bonaparte was the woman who in 1938 bribed the Nazis so Sigmund and his immediate family could escape the clutches of the coming holocaust (see Figure 14-3). From Austria, he and his immediate family went to Switzerland, France, and finally to England. During this extremely stressful period, Sigmund entrusted Marie to smuggle a sizable amount of gold out of Vienna for him. She arranged for the Greek Embassy in Vienna to dispatch it by courier to the King of Greece, who shortly

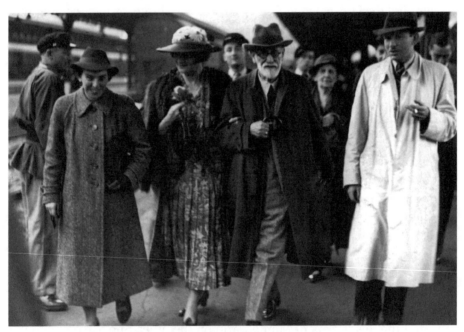

Figure 14-3. From left to right: Anna Freud, Marie Bonaparte,
Sigmund Freud, and William Bullitt.
Used with permission of Getty Images. Photographer: Pictorial Parade.
Collection: Hulton Archive.

thereafter transferred it to the Greek Embassy in London.[9] Sigmund had the burning desire to reciprocate the favor and help his dear friend Diane/Marie by directing her to Linda and assisting in her healing.

In researching Marie Bonaparte's life in a book entitled *Marie Bonaparte: A Life* by Celia Bertin, Linda discovered that Marie had a difficult childhood. Her mother had died when she was an infant and her father was emotionally distant and rarely at home. As a result, the young heiress was raised largely by nurses and governesses. Depite the monetary advantage, her childhood was emotionally barren—marred by a lack of warmth and parental concern. As a result, she developed night terrors, morbid fears of illness, and various obsessional anxieties.[10] In addition, as psychiatrist Robert M. Chalfin observed in a review of the book for *The Psychoanalytic Quarterly*, "Marie Bonaparte came to analysis from a life that reads to a degree like a popular novel with its 'poor little rich girl' and unfulfilled womanhood motifs."[11] This is eerily familiar, as Diane has told Linda that this is the same karmic pattern that she has endured in her life. Furthermore, when Linda channeled Sigmund, he revealed that Marie's obsession with illness had manifested in Diane's life, though admittedly Diane's health problems were far more severe.

Sigmund told Linda that he had overly focused on repressed sexuality and other related issues during Marie's psychoanalysis. He also revealed that "when someone does something very special to help you in a lifetime, it is incumbent to reciprocate the favor from the spirit world if one is able to." Sigmund expressed a strong desire to work through Linda to facilitate a cure for Diane/Marie.

When we got together for the interview for this book, Diane related that when she saw me sitting in Starbucks reading the newspaper, she felt compelled to speak to me after hearing a male voice in her head say clearly, "You must speak to that man." That voice was Sigmund's.

CHAPTER 15

The Emotional Database

There can be no transforming of darkness into light
and of apathy into movement without emotion.
—C. G. JUNG

THE EMOTIONAL DATABASE IS A COMPILATION of information showing all the ways that emotions affect health or that toxins affect emotions. It includes lists of all negative and positive emotions, potential neuroendocrine and endocrine issues, allergies, neurotoxins, and such remedies as nutraceuticals, herbs, and flower and gem essences. Negative emotions may be a direct causal factor behind a physical condition or an indirect cause—meaning they bind in a neurotoxin, much like a miasm. Negativity arising from unresolved past-life issues and a lack of connection to God are all part of Sigmund Freud's new way of thinking through the complexities of the body/mind/spirit connection, discussed in Chapter 17.

Sigmund acknowledges that depression and anxiety are far more complex than he had originally envisioned in his lifetime. He is now convinced that they should both be thought of as "whole body diseases" which, if unchecked, can have disastrous consequences for physical and emotional health. In addition to unresolved childhood or adult traumas, a whole range of potential new causal factors must be added to the mix. For instance, a significant degree of depression and anxiety can arise from biochemical imbalances involving four different types of brain chemicals—neurotransmitters, neuropeptides, cytokines, and hormones. This refers to the controversial field of *psychoneuroimmunology*, which focuses on the incredibly complex biochemical relationship between psychological states and the nervous, endocrine, and immune systems (see Chapter 16). The old way of thinking viewed the brain and the body as quite separate and distinct. Today's more scientifically accurate approach reveals that a vast interconnectedness of brain chemicals profoundly influences the control the brain has over the body and vice versa.

This approach to understanding hidden physiological cofactors behind emotional problems demands an awareness of biochemistry, toxicological issues, nutritional deficiencies, brain injury, and exercise physiology. (The relationship between neurotransmitter imbalances and depression is reviewed later in this chapter.) Hormonal imbalances also deeply affect emotions. Chronic levels of stress due to unresolved issues of environmental and/or emotional toxicity contribute to estrogen dominance in women, low testosterone levels in men, and an underactive thyroid and adrenal exhaustion in both. These underappreciated syndromes can either cause or exacerbate depression and anxiety. The effects of these complicated issues on women are discussed in Chapter 16.

Sigmund Freud now offers a new paradigm on the body/mind/spirit connection that represents a more integrated approach to treating emotional problems. His new way of thinking about depression necessitates that new tools and modalities be introduced into the psychotherapeutic process. For instance, he has requested that such topics as neurotoxins, neurotransmitters, cytokines, and hormones be included within the context of the Emotional Database, even though they are also part of the Physical Databases. The inclusion of such topics gives Linda the ability to channel information that reestablishes and optimizes brain chemistry and function. Sigmund believes in the need to integrate psychotherapy with various natural supplement modalities such as vitamins, minerals, amino acids, antioxidants, essential fatty acids, flower and gem essences, homeopathics, glandulars, and herbals. He also acknowledges the emotional benefits of exercise, yoga, meditation, and acupuncture, and is fascinated by the relatively new field of neurofeedback.

In his book, *The UltraMind Solution,* Dr. Mark Hyman, M.D., echoes Sigmund's sentiment: "Years of psychoanalysis or therapy will not reverse the depression that comes from profound omega-3 fatty acid deficiencies, a lack of vitamin B_{12}, a low-functioning thyroid, or chronic mercury toxicity." "Depression," he declares, is not a "Prozac deficiency."[1]

EMOTIONS AND PHYSICAL TOXINS

In addition to emotional, physiological, and socioeconomic causal factors traditionally accepted in the field of psychology, Freud now believes biochemical imbalance exists that causes certain cases of depression, anxiety, and anger that may be derived from various types of environmental toxins. Toxins that affect emotions manifest either in the brain or in other organs. The most common categories include heavy metals, inorganic compounds and solvents, organic substances, pesticides, and drugs. A list of these harmful neurotoxins is in Appendix C. After scanning this list to determine the presence of a particular neurotoxin in the brain or toxin in an organ, Linda then asks if this substance is a cofactor for depression or other identified emotional issues. Toxins can be viewed from two perspectives: those that directly or indirectly cause negative emotions or those that are bound in by negative emotions.

1. **Toxin-generated emotions.** This category covers emotional imbalances that are directly or indirectly caused by a neurotoxin in the brain or toxins in the body. Common toxic sources include specific heavy metals such as mercury and aluminum, chemicals such as MSG (monosodium glutamate), and toxins in various classifications of drugs that contribute to toxicity in the brain or an organ. This toxicity produces negative emotional side effects that can be significant cofactors for depression. That means one of the following scenarios:

• Although depression may have existed to a certain extent beforehand, it is now greatly exacerbated by these specific neurotoxins. These may cause certain brain imbalances by worsening brain wave, neurotransmitter, and hormonal function as well as helping to create inflammatory conditions like elevated homocysteine levels and elevated cytokines levels, all of which may cause depression.

• It is known in both TCM and Kabbalah that people who display great levels of anger often exhibit some form of liver disease. People who are very fearful often exhibit some form of kidney disease. However, Sigmund takes it one step further: Toxicity in the liver or kidney can trigger anger or fear.

2. **Emotions binding in toxins.** This is the flip side of toxin-generated emotions. The relationship between emotions and toxins cuts two ways. While certain toxins, such as mercury, aluminum, or MSG can generate or exacerbate negative emotions, other toxins, such as lead, are bound in by negative emotions. Sigmund asserts that it is quite problematic to achieve any meaningful results in the detoxification of lead until the negative emotion(s) that bind in this poison have been identified and resolved. In essence, he explains, the negative emotions are functioning in much the same way as a miasm. That is why he has developed a highly effective protocol for Linda to eliminate lead toxicity that first involves identifying the specific negative emotion(s) from a master list in the Emotional Database (see Appendix D). After

he has identified the particular negative emotion(s), he then guides Linda to channel from a list of flower or gem essences (discussed later in this chapter). The flower or gem essence literally loosens up the stuck negative emotion(s) so that a chelating agent can then come in and do its job. By altering the vibrational energy in the auric fields that surround the body, these essences take the edge off various negative emotions. This process represents a real breakthrough in safely treating such emotions without side effects.

3. **Pathogen-generated emotions.** Pathogens including bacteria, viruses, parasites, and fungi can also have a profound effect on emotions. A 2008 article in *Scientific American* points out that certain forms of mental illness, formerly believed to originate from neurological or psychological problems, may be caused or exacerbated by viral or microbial infections.[2] Linda has channeled that more often than not where there is neurological smoke (toxins), there is a greater likelihood for fire (pathogenic activity in the brain). This may manifest as a fungal, parasitic, bacterial, or viral infection. So pervasive and misunderstood are their effects on mental health problems today that early on I realized the necessity of compiling a master list of these possibilities to help Linda channel pathogenic cofactors behind emotional problems.

DEPRESSION RESULTS FROM LOW LEVELS OF NEUROTRANSMITTERS

Neurotransmitters are responsible for mediating the sensory and emotional responses to every pleasurable and painful mood and sensation we feel. They help regulate how well we sleep and the degree of our sexual drive. They help control our energy level, our appetite, and even the particular foods that we crave. There are two types of neurotransmitters: excitatory neurotransmitters, which stimulate or activate neurons, enabling mental functioning to occur at warp speed, and inhibitory neurotransmitters, which slow down or stop excitement in the receiving neurons.[3]

The electrical functioning of the brain as it processes neurotransmitters between its various lobes and the central nervous system is vital to a healthy brain. This processing occurs optimally when each neuron is correctly programmed to produce, transmit, or receive a specific neurotransmitter. However, certain neurologic and psychiatric conditions result when excesses or deficiencies in these biochemicals cause the brain or the body to either overwork or shut down.

A deficiency of any of the principal neurotransmitters can not only affect neurological functioning, but also lead to functional disruptions in the endocrine system, which, in turn, is critical for all metabolic functioning in the body. It is not overstating the case to say that optimizing levels of the four major neurotransmitters—serotonin, dopamine, GABA, and acetylcholine—is a core component of the body/mind/spirit connection.

Serotonin

Serotonin originates from the amino acid tryptophan, which can be found in a variety of high protein foods. This feel-good neurotransmitter plays an important role in regulating many aspects of body function and the emotions associated with them. These include appetite, sexuality, sleep, dream states, body temperature, blood pressure, and digestion. Low levels of serotonin are often associated with mood disorders, including clinical depression, anxiety disorders, anger, aggression, bipolar disorder, and obsessive-compulsive disorder. They also exacerbate such physical disorders as migraines, fibromyalgia, irritable bowel syndrome, vomiting, and tinnitus. A byproduct of serotonin is the hormone melatonin that is most commonly associated with sleep patterns and keeping our circadian rhythms in sync.

Women have greater difficulty maintaining serotonin levels than men due to the complex relationship between a woman's serotonin levels and her monthly menstrual cycle. The shifting emotional sands that a woman may experience during her periods can include increased moodiness, irritability, and sensitivity to pain. Women with low levels of serotonin are likelier to experience feelings of depression and anger. Men with low levels of serotonin are more prone to violent rages. One of the many downsides of alcohol and drug addiction is that they often produce low serotonin levels.

Dopamine

Dopamine originates from the amino acid phenylalanine, which is found in high protein foods. It is then transformed in the liver into tyrosine and phenylethylamine (PEA). PEA is the natural mood elevator of sexuality, which, in one of God's wry biological ironies, is also found in chocolate. Tyrosine goes through additional transformations until it evolves into dopamine. Along with two additional byproducts of dopamine—noradrenaline and adrenaline—these neurotransmitters and stress hormones are collectively members of the biochemical family called catecholamines. Both participate in what is referred to as the fight-or-flight response, a physiological coping mechanism that prepares the body to deal with imminent danger or excitement (see Chapter 16).

Dopamine is the primary neurotransmitter of reward, working through receptors located in the limbic region of the brain, which controls the flow of emotions. Reward comes in many natural forms such as food, positive social interactions, and laughter (hence the biochemical meaning of "laughter is the best medicine"). A temporary elevation in dopamine levels can lead to an improvement in alertness, mood, euphoric feelings, and libido. A disruption of dopamine levels occurs in neurological disorders such as Parkinson's disease. It also occurs in neuropsychiatric disorders like ADHD, depression/apathy, and schizophrenia as well as in pharmaceutical/recreational drug and alcohol addictions.

When people have healthy levels of dopamine, they exhibit higher levels of energy, are motivated to set and achieve long-term goals, and experience pleasure more intensely. This occurs during what is aptly called an adrenaline rush. Adrenaline, which is also called epinephrine, is a hormone and neurotransmitter produced and triggered by the adrenal glands during dangerous high stress or physically exhilarating situations.

Noradrenaline, which is also referred to as norepinephrine, functions as both a neurotransmitter and a hormone. As a neurotransmitter, it assists in the regulation of various states of "positive" stress, including sexual arousal, dreaming, and moods. It also stimulates the release of a sex hormone called oxytocin, which promotes sexual arousal, feelings of emotional attachment, and lactation in nursing mothers. Low levels of dopamine/noradrenaline may therefore be at the root of intimacy problems. Noradrenaline can also influence the rate of metabolism and the secretion of insulin. When one is under stress, noradrenaline doubles as a stress hormone by increasing blood pressure, constricting blood vessels, and quickening heart rate.

Deficiencies in serotonin and dopamine are both responsible for depression. However, pharmaceutical research has advanced the idea that a low level of serotonin is directly responsible for depression, while a low level of noradrenaline/adrenaline, precursors of dopamine, is responsible for lack of motivation due to depression.[4] The stressful demands of life cause the brain to require higher levels of serotonin and noradrenaline/adrenaline to cope with the emotional and physiological needs of a person under stress. Depression and apathy are exacerbated when there is a lack of the proper building-block nutrients, principally derived from food and/or supplementation. These are needed to facilitate the conversion of essential amino acids and other brain chemicals into neurotransmitters.

GABA

GABA (gamma-aminobutyric acid) originates from glutamic acid, an amino acid produced in the temporal lobe of the brain. GABA, the major inhibitory neurotransmitter of the central nervous system and the retina, has a calming, relaxing effect on the brain. It is also associated with calming, rhythmic theta brain waves found in various lobes of the brain. Its dampening effect on the nervous system is brought about because GABA counteracts and balances out the stimulating neurotransmitters. For example, GABA controls the release of dopamine in the reward center of the brain, which helps to regulate the brain's internal rhythm.

At normal levels, GABA positively affects the personality in a manner that allows one to handle the stresses of everyday life and stay organized. When GABA is deficient in the brain, its flowing internal rhythm goes out of kilter, resulting in anxiety, nervousness, and irritability, coupled with bouts of insomnia. The tranquilizer Valium is an example of a GABA-enhancing drug.

Acetylcholine

Acetylcholine is derived from the synthesis of choline, a B-complex vitamin, and acetyl-CoA, an important molecule in metabolism, which occurs in the parietal lobes of the brain. It is associated with the ability to process sensory stimuli (touch, taste, smell, vision, and sound) as well as access stored information. These thinking functions include those qualities associated with basic intelligence—innate learning ability, powers of concentration and alertness, and memory.

Persistent forgetfulness is an example of a brain malfunction brought on by a deficiency in acetylcholine. This results in the brain's inability to connect new sensory stimuli to previously stored memories. Low levels of acetylcholine affect brain speed, which determines the rate at which electrical signals are processed throughout the body and brain. A deficiency in acetylcholine can result in memory lapse, depression, mood disorders, and learning disabilities and is a contributing factor in Alzheimer's disease.

A CLASH OF PHILOSOPHICAL APPROACHES IN TREATING DEPRESSION

Given that the lack of sufficient serotonin, dopamine, and noradrenaline are the core causes of much depression, it is important to differentiate between a pharmaceutical antidepressant approach and natural supplements.

The Pharmaceutical Approach

As an example of one pharmaceutical approach, antidepressant drugs called selective serotonin reuptake inhibitors (SSRIs) artificially maintain high levels of serotonin in the brain. It is known that depression can be caused if a lack of stimulation occurs in the receiving neuron when neurotransmitters and other electrochemical messages are passed from one neuron to another through the synapse. Normally, serotonin passes through the synapse where it is picked up (the reuptake process) by the receiving neuron and broken down. However, by inhibiting reuptake, drugs like Prozac, Paxil, and Zoloft cause serotonin to stay in the synapse for a longer period of time than it normally would. This gives serotonin the opportunity to be recycled and recognized over and over again by the receptors of the receiving neuron so it can be stimulated. In this way it tricks the brain into thinking there are more serotonin molecules than there really are. However, this process cannot go on indefinitely, and eventually those serotonin molecules break down, leaving the brain with serotonin depletion—and more depression.

Unfortunately, these medications also poison metabolic pathways in the body, causing multiple side effects in a statistically significant number of people, including insomnia, nausea, weakness, sexual dysfunction, and weight gain. In addition, they are not the universal panacea for depression they are touted to be; some studies suggest they are completely ineffective in approximately one-third of cases of depression.[5] Further, more serious issues exist in a small number of cases. The warning label that consumers receive when they buy Paxil, for example, is depressing all by itself! It states: "Pooled analyses of short-term placebo-controlled trials of antidepressant drugs (SSRIs and others) showed that these drugs increase the risk of suicidal thinking and behavior (suicidality) in children, adolescents, and young adults (18–24) with major depression disorder (MDD) and other psychiatric disorders."

SSRIs are hardly the only example. Stimulant drugs like Ritalin, prescribed for ADHD in children or teenagers, are designed to mimic dopamine effects. Over time, however, Ritalin depletes users' ability to make their own dopamine, noradrenaline, and adrenaline. This disruption of dopamine neuronal systems may, in turn, also contribute to the eventual abuse of cocaine, amphetamines, alcohol, nicotine, and other dangerous drugs.[6] In addition, drugs such as Ritalin, Adderall, or Dexedrine are known to raise blood pressure and heart rate. A recent study showed that children using these type of stimulant drugs were 20 percent more likely to visit an emergency clinic or doctor's office with cardiac-related symptoms, such as a racing heartbeat, than children who had never used or discontinued treatment.[7] It is no wonder that in 2006 the FDA added a "black box" warning to these ADHD medications about possible serious heart risks. These problems are readily acknowledged by the medical profession, which would seemingly have enough incentive to explore other options.

Alas, as noted elsewhere in this book, the Hippocratic oath ("Above all else, do no harm") too often takes a backseat to the economic and political realities of contemporary medicine. As a result, physicians have been slow to recognize and adopt an approach that is both far safer and extremely effective. Suffice it to say, vast pharmaceutical fortunes have been made by creating convoluted work-arounds, *patentable* solutions that initially seem effective for controlling depression. However, in the long term a statistically significant number of people develop unpleasant side effects or find that the drug no longer works.

Linda is not channeling that SSRIs and other types of pharmaceutical approaches for the treatment of depression or anxiety do not have merit. However, in all but very severe cases of depression, the nature of the field itself is changing. *A doctor or other health care professional now has a plethora of viable, safer options available that should first be explored before immediately jumping to a pharmaceutical solution.* Some of the important ones are discussed later in this chapter and in Chapter 16. Conversely, if a health care practitioner who is familiar with these natural supplement approaches does not achieve success in quelling a patient's depression or anxiety, then a pharmaceutical approach should be taken.

The Nutraceutical Approach

Treating depression with nutritional supplements works from the supposition that it is both safer and more effective to raise the level of neurotransmitters in the brain by providing the basic, natural building blocks. These consist of certain amino acid precursors and other nutrient cofactors needed to make them. The deficiency in precursors is often a central component in depression, and may be due to such issues as poor diet, neurotoxins, hormonal imbalances, or negative emotions. Dr. Hyla Cass, M.D., a pioneering holistic psychiatrist who treats neurological/emotional issues with nutraceuticals, amplifies this idea: "If [the origins] of your mood problems are due to a deficiency in the materials that make up the neurotransmitters, then simply inhibiting their reuptake won't solve your problems in the long run. This is one reason why the drugs stop working after a while."[8] Since neurological construction materials can generally not be patented, pharmaceutical companies have no financial interest in an approach that delivers them naturally to the brain.

Picking up on the theme of deficiencies in "neurological construction materials" as a core causal factor behind depression, Sigmund Freud has guided Linda to pursue a diagnostic evaluation of the biochemistry of these deficiencies from a nutritional, endocrinological, and lifestyle perspective. He cautions that *this approach is not meant to replace psychotherapy, but rather to augment and fine-tune it.* He now believes that psychotherapists would achieve fundamentally better overall results if they integrated these concepts into their practice. Nutritional imbalances affecting neurotransmitters that deal directly with depression (serotonin and dopamine) may be caused by deficiencies in one or more of the following cofactors: (1) precursor amino acids (tryptophan and tyrosine) and various types of nutrients (B vitamins, especially B_3, B_6, B_{12}, folic acid, zinc, magnesium, iron, manganese, calcium, SAMe, TMG, 5-HTP, essential fatty acids, among others) affecting the metabolic pathways; and (2) blood sugar imbalances due to excessive sugar (see Chapter 16) and stimulant drug intake. (See "A Word of Caution: Don't Take Matters into Your Own Hands.")

A Word of Caution: Don't Take Matters into Your Own Hands

If you are currently on a pharmaceutical(s) for the treatment of depression and anxiety and are experiencing negative side effects or a lack of effectiveness, you may want to switch to a natural approach. The information in this chapter will provide guidance about the possible natural remedies that may be of help. In all cases you should only take natural remedies under your doctor's supervision. You must take care not to abruptly stop taking pharmaceutical medication as this may cause intense withdrawal symptoms. The process of weaning off pharmaceuticals should only be done under the supervision of your doctor. Do not substitute the facts in this book (or any book) for your doctor's medical opinion.

NUTRIENTS FROM DIET OR SUPPLEMENTS PROVIDE BUILDING BLOCKS FOR NEUROTRANSMITTERS

Figure 15-1 shows the "family tree" of the two biochemical pathways for serotonin and dopamine neurotransmitters that are primarily responsible for positive mental functioning or negative emotions like depression and anxiety. These pathways start with essential amino acids obtained from food and are followed by a delicate symphony of nutritional cofactors, including vitamins, minerals, nonessential amino acids, and other brain chemicals. Various biochemical reactions occur along the pathways. Like dominoes falling in a certain order and manner, these reactions produce adequate levels of 5-HTP, serotonin, and melatonin in the indoleamine pathway, and dopamine, noradrenaline, and adrenaline in the catecholamine pathway. Deficiencies in these nutritional cofactors also work like dominoes; if one is deficient, the next substance in the pathway is produced at an inadequate level and so on down the line. Toxicity, inflammation, and stress may cause such disruptions in these pathways as well.

As she works under the auspices of Dr. Thom E. Lobe, it is fascinating to watch Linda use Figure 15-1 to channel where deficiencies exist in the two neurotransmitter pathways that are often associated with depression. When

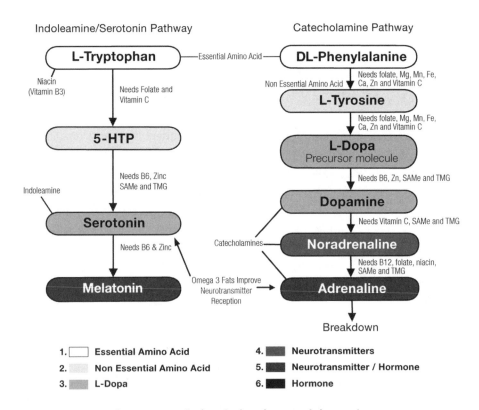

Figure 15-1. Biochemical pathways of depression.

she channels Figure 15-1, her angelic guides or Sigmund Freud direct her to deficiencies or imbalances that have a cascading effect on everything that comes below them. As noted in Figure 15-1, the most common deficiencies are in amino acids, B vitamins, SAMe and TMG, essential fatty acids (omega-3 fatty acids), melatonin, and various minerals. Herbs, flower and gem essences, and bioidentical hormones (see Chapter 16) can also be useful in addressing imbalances.

Because of the significance that potential nutritional deficiencies may have on depression and anxiety, Linda recommends that people suffering from these or other serious emotional conditions have their doctor or health care professional use clinical laboratory testing services that specialize in identifying nutritional imbalances and toxins that may be cofactors in their condition.[9]

Amino Acids

Tryptophan is found in fish, turkey, chicken, eggs, and cheese as well as beans, oats, and tofu. Increasing your levels of these foods or taking a tryptophan or 5-HTP supplement can improve one's mood and help lift depression. It is preferable to take tryptophan before going to sleep as it induces drowsiness. More often then not, Linda channels that 5-HTP (derived from an African plant named *Griffonia simplicifolia*) is even more effective in assisting in the relief of depression. The three catecholamines—dopamine, noradrenaline, and adrenaline—originate from phenylalanine, which is then transformed into tyrosine.

Both of these amino acids are found in high-quality protein foods such as fish, chicken, and eggs as well as beans, nuts, and seeds. Increasing your levels of these foods or taking supplemental forms of these amino acids may improve energy, mood, and attentiveness. The conversion process of tryptophan to 5-HTP, as well as phenylalanine to tyrosine, occurs in enzymes in adrenal, intestinal, brain, and peripheral nervous tissue.

B Vitamins

The collective B family of vitamins is vitally important for brain function and mental health. Since these water-soluble vitamins pass rapidly out of the body, they must be replenished on a daily basis by either diet and/or supplementation. Acting as catalysts called coenzymes, B vitamins perform many vital neurological functions, including the conversion of nutrients into glucose, the primary fuel in the brain. In fact, it is surprising to learn that the brain consumes more glucose than any other organ! This is why low levels of glucose are often a major contributory factor in depression, fatigue, apathy, and brain fog.

When Linda channels that a client's depression is affected by low glucose levels, she immediately channels a diet that adheres closely to the tenets of the Glycemic Index in addition to ample B vitamins. This approach takes into account a particular food's carbohydrate quality, which determines its ability to raise the speed with which it raises blood glucose levels. The dietary goal is to avoid sudden insulin spikes and sugar lows that contribute to depression. Complex carbohydrates that do not break down quickly are in; other complex and refined carbohydrates that break down quickly are out. Linda's dietary mantra for treating depression is "Not high carbs versus low carbs, but slow carbs versus fast carbs."

What also makes B vitamins critical for brain health is their ability to control homocysteine, an amino acid naturally produced by the body, through the process of methylation. As described in Chapter 10, defects in methylation are a natural consequence of inflammation from heavy metal toxicity and drug toxins; now we add a lack of B vitamins to the mix. Methylation refers to biochemical processes that keep thousands of neurotransmitters, hormones, and other essential biochemicals in balance by donating methyl groups which help the body adapt to changing circumstances.[10] Methylation also assists in the creation of brain-friendly fats called phospholipids, a major component in cell membranes.

Recent discoveries confirm that there is also a genetic predisposition that determines how well a person "methylates."[11] There is growing evidence that people who are prone to severe depression or schizophrenia don't methylate properly.[12] The goal then is to overcome bad genetics by supplementing specific methylating nutrients (B vitamins, SAMe or TMG, and zinc) to correct these imbalances. This is yet another area where Linda's gift of customizing precise dosage levels of nutrients is invaluable for her clients.

Heavy metals and drug toxins block or alter the methylation process, resulting in elevated levels of homocysteine and depressed levels of SAMe, the mood-enhancing neurotransmitter serotonin, and the sleep-inducing neurotransmitter melatonin—a biochemical recipe for depression, insomnia, and dementia. A 2000 study showed that depressed people with the highest elevations in homocysteine have significantly less SAMe needed to create mood-enhancing neurotransmitters.[13] High levels of homocysteine also promote inflammation by damaging blood vessels delivering blood to the brain. At more dangerous levels, homocysteine can contribute to heart attack, stroke, and liver damage.

B vitamins break homocysteine down into methionine, a sulfur-containing amino acid. This combines with ATP (adenosine triphosphate), the cellular energy molecule in the body, to produce SAMe (S-adenosyl-methionine), an amino acid-like substance that is necessary for the production of mood-enhancing neurotransmitters like serotonin as well as other transmitters. SAMe levels are closely associated with mood.

Vitamins B_3 (niacin), B_6 (pyridoxine), B_{12} (cobalamin), and folic acid—the "four horsemen" of the B vitamins—help restore and control the critical process of methylation. Supplementation with B vitamins can revive production of neurotransmitters as well as have a significant bearing on alleviating depression caused by abnormalities in methylation. Here is an overview of these most essential B vitamins. (See "Caution: Certain Over-the-Counter and Prescription Drugs Deplete B Vitamins.")

Caution: Certain Over-the-Counter and Prescription Drugs Deplete B Vitamins

Most consumers are unaware that many common pharmaceuticals, including aspirin, diuretics, stomach-acid suppressors (such as Nexium and Prilosec), estrogen, and the anti-diabetic drug metformin (Glucophage), can interfere with the metabolism of one or more B vitamins, which can result in elevated levels of homocysteine.[14,15] You should also know that because many B vitamins are produced by beneficial bacteria in the intestinal tract, various antibiotics, including sulfa drugs and tetracyclines, kill these intestinal flora, which, in turn, reduce the body's ability to produce B vitamins.[16]

- **Vitamin B_3:** Niacin affects brain function by removing toxic chemicals and assisting in the production of sex- and stress-related steroid hormones made by the adrenal gland. It helps in the amino acid conversion of tryptophan to 5-HTP, which leads to serotonin. Niacin is also involved in the production of acetylcholine, which improves cognitive memory. Dr. Abram Hoffer, M.D., Ph.D., the founder of orthomolecular psychiatry, discovered that high doses of niacin were often effective in treating even severe cases of schizophrenia.

• **Vitamin B$_6$:** In its active form, pyridoxine is called pyridoxal-5'-phosphate (P5P). It is a cofactor in approximately 100 different enzymatic reactions and is vital to methylation processes that produce neurotransmitters and reduce high homocysteine levels. It is a catalyst for the enzyme that converts 5-HTP into serotonin and is also involved in the production of dopamine, noradrenaline, and GABA. P5P is also crucial in a wide range of biochemical reactions, including the metabolism of amino acids and glycogen as well as hormone modulation. It is also associated with sulfur metabolism and heavy metal detoxification.

A 2008 study of men and women at Tufts University found four groups particularly deficient in vitamin B$_6$: those over 65, women of reproductive age, African-American males, and male smokers.[17] In women, B$_6$ deficiency most commonly affected current and former users of oral contraceptives. Common symptoms included depression, hormonal imbalances, and water retention. Replenishing B$_6$ eases depression and anxiety associated with premenstrual syndrome and menopausal symptoms. In either sex, this deficiency can also be due to other drugs, stress, or alcohol.

• **Vitamin B$_{12}$:** Cobalamin is vital to the methylation process and works with folic acid to convert tryptophan into 5-HTP as well as tyrosine into dopamine. It is also critical to the production of acetylcholine. B$_{12}$ helps to control inflammation by reducing homocysteine levels and fights depression by inhibiting monoamine oxidase (MAO), an enzyme that reduces serotonin and the three catecholamines. It is also essential for the formation and maintenance of myelin, the protective covering around nerve cells in the brain and elsewhere. Studies also show that deficiencies in B$_{12}$ in the elderly are associated with depression and a decrease in cognitive memory. However, when given B$_{12}$ by injection or sublingually, they often recover a good deal of their mental capacity.

• **Folic acid:** This is needed to make catecholamines (dopamine, noradrenaline, and adrenaline) and 5-HTP, a precursor to serotonin. Folic acid is beneficial in treating depression, bipolar disorder, dementia, anemia, insomnia, irritability, forgetfulness, peripheral neuropathy, and restless leg syndrome. It helps to make red blood cells, which are important in preventing anemia, and also lowers levels of homocysteine. People who have a poor response to antidepressant drugs may have low levels of folic acid.

SAMe (S-adenosyl-methionine) and TMG (trimethylglycine)

SAMe and TMG, both amino acid-like substances produced in the body, are critical in the conversion process of amino acids to neurotransmitters. Figure 15-1 shows that in the indoleamine/serotonin pathway, SAMe and TMG normally donate their methyl groups to facilitate the transformation of 5-HTP into serotonin. The same process occurs in the catecholamine pathway for the production of dopamine and the subsequent transformation of noradrenaline into adrenaline.

Both SAMe and TMG are available as nutritional supplements. A SAMe supplement reduces homocysteine levels and restores SAMe to healthy levels. Researched extensively, SAMe is effective in treating depression as well as arthritis. However, it is not recommended for people with bipolar disease. In addition, it is expensive and rather unstable. A less costly and more stable product that may be of benefit for treating depression is TMG, which converts homocysteine back to methionine and then into SAMe.

Essential Fatty Acids (Omega-3)

Up to 60 percent of brain tissue is made up of essential fatty acids (EFAs). Therefore, it should come as no surprise that brain health is adversely affected by EFA deficiencies. Since EFAs are not made or synthesized by the body, however, they must be obtained through diet. The unique role that healthy essential fatty acids play in improving neurotransmitter reception of both serotonin and the catecholamines is of real significance in the treatment of depression. A panel headed by renowned psychiatric researcher Dr. Joseph Hibbeln, M.D., of the National Institute on Alcohol Abuse and Alcoholism was appointed in 2007 by the American Psychiatric Association to review multiple population and clinical studies on the effects of omega-3 from fish and fish oil on a range of depression disorders. Their report concluded that people who consume high levels of omega-3s from fish and fish oil (EPA and DHA) are substantially less likely to suffer from depression, bipolar disorder (manic-depression), anxiety, and related mood disorders.[18]

Melatonin

Perhaps no single daily health factor can affect a person's quality of life more than chronic insomnia. Sleep is absolutely essential for the repair and rejuvenation of both the body and the soul. One of the primary biochemical markers for clinical depression is a deficiency in serotonin, which often creates a direct biochemical link among melatonin deficiency, insomnia, and depression. Without enough serotonin, the brain is challenged to manufacture enough melatonin needed for restful sleep. That is why the old home remedy of having a glass of milk, with its high levels of tryptophan, before you go to sleep is actually grounded in science.

The pineal gland, located at the back of the midbrain just above the cerebellum, produces the highest quantities of serotonin and melatonin in the brain. It is the brain's internal clock that is responsible for regulating our cycles of wakefulness and sleep. When darkness predominates for a period of time, the pineal gland is prompted to transmute serotonin into melatonin. Serotonin can therefore be thought of as a daytime neurotransmitter that prepares the brain to be awake during the day. Melatonin is the nighttime neurotransmitter that shortens the time needed to fall asleep. It induces a profound relaxation of muscles and nerves necessary for restorative sleep and a healthy dream state.

Mild cases of chronic insomnia can result in personality aberrations such as anger, irritability, fatigue, and an inability to concentrate. In more serious cases, insomnia and sleep deprivation can significantly raise levels of cortisol and ACTH (discussed in Chapter 16), two hormones associated with an inflammatory cytokine known as interleukin-6 (IL-6). This destructive protein has been linked with numerous autoimmune diseases (see Chapter 10). Linda consistently channels that age-related decline in melatonin levels is often due to a progressive buildup of several potential cofactors—neurotoxins and/or calcification of pineal gland tissue, and unresolved negative emotions.

In addition to being highly beneficial for treating insomnia, Linda channels that in certain cases taking a melatonin supplement can be a useful adjunct in treating depression as it helps to increase the conversion rate of thyroid hormone T4 into T3 as well as calm down excessive cortisol activity due to stress (see Chapter 16).

Minerals

A veritable symphony of biochemical interactions exists among minerals, neurological processes, and emotions. In addition to the most important minerals discussed here—zinc, magnesium, and iron–Linda regularly channels for deficiencies or excesses in such minerals as manganese, copper, chromium, calcium, potassium, and selenium.

- **Zinc.** The most commonly deficient mineral and the most critical nutrient for mental health,[19,20] zinc is involved in methylation and is important in controlling inflammation, a critical factor in brain dysfunction.[21] Zinc deficiency is associated with many emotional and neurological disorders, ranging from depression, anxiety, and apathy to schizophrenia, autism, and MS. It is also a cofactor in over 200 different enzymes, some of whose functions involve the synthesis of serotonin, noradrenaline, and GABA. Adequate levels of zinc are essential for the development of brain cells as well as optimum regulation of such important hormones as thyroid-stimulating hormone (TSH), progesterone, estrogen, and testosterone. In addition to deficiencies in iodine, iron, and selenium, Linda finds that a deficiency in zinc can be a contributing factor in hypothyroidism, which itself often triggers severe emotional problems (see Chapter 16).

  Zinc has an antagonistic relationship with such other metals as copper and mercury that can negatively affect emotions when deficient. For instance, a zinc deficiency can cause copper in the body to increase to toxic levels, which can trigger paranoia and anxiety. This may be remedied by taking a zinc supplement.

  A zinc deficiency caused by mercury toxicity results in depressed levels of metallothionein, a protein that promotes normal excretion by binding in and metabolizing proper levels of various metals in the brain. Deficiencies in metallothionein have been linked to ADHD and autism. Zinc helps rid the body of mercury by boosting metallothionein.[22] It is interesting to note that *Linda consistently channels zinc (and selenium) deficiencies in people suffering from emotional issues due to heavy metal toxicity from mercury, lead, or cadmium.*

- **Magnesium.** This relaxation mineral relieves different kinds of stress ranging from irritability to muscle cramps. A deficiency in magnesium can be a significant contributor to anxiety and mood disorders. It is involved in over 300 enzymatic reactions in the body and is a cofactor in the synthesis of serotonin, dopamine, and GABA. In addition to stress, excesses in caffeine, sugar, alcohol, phosphoric acid (from colas), acid-blocking drugs (Prilosec, Prevacid, Nexium), antibiotics, oral contraceptives, and diuretics are capable of blocking the absorption of magnesium. This, in turn, can contribute to reduced levels of serotonin, dopamine, and GABA.

- **Iron.** Levels of iron can be an important cofactor in optimal neurological functioning as iron is involved in the synthesis of serotonin, noradrenaline, and GABA. Iron plays an important role in the conversion of phenylalanine to tyrosine, which is a precursor to thyroid hormones. An iron deficiency can therefore contribute to hypothyroidism. Iron deficiencies can also reduce the body's capacity to transport oxygen in the blood and increase the absorption of lead. They can also upset the delicate mental health applecart that exists between zinc and copper. Depression, apathy, and exhaustion may be symptoms of chronic iron deficiency. However, excess levels of iron may also cause or worsen psychiatric problems, promote oxidation and free radicals, and be a cofactor in Parkinson's disease.[23]

Herbs

Nature's amazing pharmacy of herbal remedies can be a safe and effective way of controlling depression. Determining the main causal factor(s) as to *why* depression exists is the key variable in determining which herbs will be effective. Common physiological and emotional causes of depression that can be addressed by herbal remedies include neurotoxicity, neurotransmitter and endocrine imbalances, vasodilation, and stress. If you are on prescription drugs, be sure to consult your health care professional regarding possible drug interactions before taking herbal remedies.

Herbs that address neurotransmitter imbalances include:

• **St. John's wort.** This herbal extract has become increasingly popular, particularly in Europe, as a natural and safer alternative to antipsychotic medications in treating mild to moderate depression. It works not only by inhibiting reuptake of several neurotransmitters, including serotonin, noradrenaline, and dopamine, but also by enhancing GABA activity. Studies have shown that it is just as effective as SSRIs and produces far fewer side effects.[24] *However, Linda consistently channels that it is of limited value in treating depression that is primarily due to neurotoxicity.* Do not combine St. John's wort with any pharmaceutical antidepressants, and consult with your doctor before taking it with any other types of drugs.

• **Kava.** Used as an oral spray or tincture, kava appears to enhance GABA activity. It promotes relaxation by acting on the limbic system, the emotional center of the brain, as well as by being a muscle relaxant. Avoid alcohol consumption while taking kava, and consult with your doctor regarding other possible drug interactions.

• **Ginkgo biloba.** An extract from the leaf of the ginkgo tree, ginkgo biloba may be effective in treating elderly people with depression. Studies show that it increases levels of serotonin as well as improves blood circulation and works as an antioxidant.[25] Other antistress herbs include valarian, hops, and passion flower. Consult with your doctor about possible drug interactions.

• **Adaptogens.** These natural herbal products increase the body's resistance to stress, trauma, anxiety, and fatigue. Linda has had success incorporating them into her treatment of depression. They include rhodiola, Siberian ginseng, ashwagandha, schisandra, and maca root.

Herbs that address various endocrine imbalances (see Chapter 16) include:

• For perimenopausal and menopausal imbalances in women: black cohosh, genistein, maca root, chasteberry, dong quai, and licorice.

• For reduced libido in either sex: damiana, muira puama, deer antler, and maca root.

• For blood sugar issues: extracts of cinnamon, gymnema sylvestre, fenugreek, bitter lemon, ginseng, hops, and acacia bark.

Flower and Gem Essences

Linda is a firm believer in using flower and gem essences in the treatment of depression and anxiety. Her experience with her more sensitive clients confirms that negative thoughts and feelings that operate in the subtle fields just below the radar of consciousness (see discussion of energy fields in Chapter 18) can be transformed into their positive counterparts. In fact, she views flower and gem essences not only as a method of treating emotional disorders, but also as a proactive means of promoting spiritual growth.

Bach Flower Remedies are a gentle, safe method of managing various negative emotional states or personality characteristics. In the 1920s and 1930s, Dr. Edward Bach (1886–1936), a brilliant British medical doctor and homeopath, developed a complete system of thirty-eight flower remedies, each prepared from the flowers of wild plants, trees, and bushes. The remedies contain a small amount of flower material in a 50/50 solution of water and brandy. The best known of these is Rescue Remedy, also known as Five Flower Combination (rock rose, impatiens, clematis, star of Bethlehem, and cherry plum). It is effective for treating stress, anxiety, and panic attacks in emergency situations and is available in better natural food stores (www.bachcentre.com).

Bach believed that certain plants possess particular vibratory wavelengths that embody the energetic frequency of a specific emotional or spiritual quality of the soul. He believed that the root cause of much physical illness was due to spiritual and emotional blockages. According to Bach, every human being has an immortal soul (his or her spiritual self) and a mortal personality (that he or she represents here on earth). The higher self functions as a mediator between the soul and the personality, containing that which is noble in the human spirit. While the soul is aware of its mission, destiny, and karma, the personality is not. When the personality is out of spiritual alignment with the soul, it is because it is choosing to persist in the illusion that it is separate from it.[26] By acting against the intentions of the higher self and soul, there is an energetic disharmony or distortion that manifests as negative emotions that, if not corrected, progress into physical illness (dis-ease).

Bach described how his remedies work to correct these imbalances and reestablish an inner communication: "The action of these remedies is to raise our vibrations and open up our channels for the reception of the spiritual self; to flood our natures with the particular virtue we need, and wash out from us the fault that is causing the harm. They are able, like beautiful music or any glorious uplifting thing that gives us inspiration, to raise our very natures, and bring us nearer to our souls and by that very act to bring us peace and relieve our suffering. They cure, not by attacking the disease, but by flooding our bodies with the beautiful vibrations of our higher nature, in the presence of which disease melts away as snow in the sunshine. There is no true healing unless there is a change of outlook, peace of mind, and inner happiness."[27]

Although Linda still likes flower essences, in recent years she has come to favor gem essences as they seem to be more powerful in targeting deep-seated emotions. Gem essences are made using a dilution process that is somewhat similar to that used in homeopathy. Like flower essences, their higher vibrational frequencies help to balance and align chakras and auras—the subtle energy systems of the body (see Chapter 18).

Caveat

The information and products we have discussed here are solely to support health and not intended to diagnose, treat, prevent, or cure any disease, and they should not be used as a substitute for diagnosis and treatment by your personal physician.

CHAPTER 16

The Connection Between Emotions and Women's Hormones

The great question which I have not yet been able to answer,
despite my thirty years of research into the feminine soul,
is "What does a woman want?"

—SIGMUND FREUD

PERHAPS NO PHYSIOLOGICAL FACTOR IN WOMEN is as misunderstood in terms of its effect on negative emotional states as hormones. Linda finds that the four most common hormonal issues that affect the emotional well-being and psyche of her female clients are estrogen/progesterone ratio imbalances, a low or hypothyroid condition, adrenal exhaustion, and blood sugar disorders.

Many women endure emotional turmoil throughout their lives due to hormonal imbalances. For example, problems related to imbalances in estrogen/progesterone ratios can include depression, anxiety, irritability, mental fog, low libido, and fatigue. Physical problems may include sudden weight gain, migraines, hot flashes, heart palpitations, insomnia, night sweats, painful intercourse, and low bone density. These conditions can have profound emotional repercussions that blur the lines of distinction between what is a physical causal factor and what is an emotional causal factor. For example, not only is the estrogen/progesterone ratio imbalance responsible for many significant physiological changes that occur throughout the course of a woman's lifetime, but it is frequently a mysterious player in the emotional upheavals of daily life. Its nuances, shadings, and colorations can leave men and even women baffled.

Sigmund Freud is now the first to admit that a more enlightened understanding of the female endocrine system that was lacking in his time will bring science and psychology significantly closer to unraveling the mysteries of the female psyche. Linda is convinced that no other area of anti-aging

225

management is as individualistic and complicated for women as effectively balancing their hormones. (See "What Are Hormones?")

What Are Hormones?

Every gland in the endocrine system produces its own unique molecular messengers called hormones. They exert an influence on many aspects of cellular function, ranging from repair to replication. They are similar to neurotransmitters in the sense that they are chemicals of communication: both issue instructions telling brain cells, various organs, and components within the endocrine system how to behave. A key difference is that neurotransmitters are manufactured from precursor compounds such as amino acids, glucose, and a dietary amine called choline. In contrast, hormones, with the exception of thyroxine, melatonin, and human growth hormone, are created from cholesterol and are called steroid hormones.

This cascade of steroid hormones begins with pregnenolone, which is then converted into other hormones, including DHEA (dehydroepiandrosterone), progesterone, cortisol, androstenedione, testosterone, and various forms of estrogen. While the first part of our discussion focuses on the relationship between estrogen and progesterone, a holistic therapeutic approach recognizes that all the steroid hormones in the chain are interrelated, each performing a unique biochemical function that must be in balance. The lofty goal of treatment is to restore, to the greatest extent possible, hormone levels of middle-aged/menopausal women to those of women in their twenties and early thirties. This is an important quality of life issue—a meaningful component of anti-aging that allows women to retain a youthful physical and emotional state well into their sixties and beyond. Slower aging for middle-aged women leads to a more graceful, softer landing in women's advanced years, instead of the jarring, premature health collisions so many women endure.

REPRODUCTIVE HORMONES

Estrogen and progesterone are essential for the healthy functioning of a woman's physical and emotional states of well-being in addition to her reproductive system. Sudden and dramatic fluctuations in the level of these hormones may occur either in monthly cycles or in cycles that run over a course of years. What makes understanding female reproductive hormonal issues such a complex phenomenon is that each woman has a unique pattern and severity of estrogen/progesterone fluctuations. Therefore, in order to understand how conditions like PMS and menopause can wreak physical and emotional havoc on a woman, no matter how well adjusted she may otherwise be, first requires a brief crash course on estrogen and progesterone as well as an understanding of the breakdown that occurs in perimenopause and the onset of menopause.

Estrogen

Estrogen refers to a powerful group of three hormones called estradiol, estrone, and estriol. Estradiol, which is converted into estrone and then estriol, is by far the most potent form of estrogen, followed by estrone. Estriol is considered a weaker but safer form of estrogen. Collectively, estrogen expresses the essence of feminine energy and sensuality throughout the course of a woman's life. It is the same essence that triggers puberty when a girl makes the physical and emotional transition into fertility. It is the same essence that initiates perimenopause when fertility begins its gradual decline for many women starting around age thirty-five. This is followed by the more precipitous decline called menopause, the cessation of menstruation, which begins for most women around the age of fifty.

The importance of estrogen cannot be underestimated. Produced in the ovaries, adrenal glands, fat cells, and placenta during pregnancy, estrogen, or the lack thereof, can have a significant impact on over 300 tissues and systems in a woman's body. Estrogen is essential in promoting the toning and suppleness of the breasts, uterus, urinary tract, and blood vessels as well as the distribution of body fat and body hair. Each component of estrogen plays a very important role during a woman's lifetime.

• Estradiol starts to be actively produced during puberty and remains the main form of estrogen until menopause. It is most responsible for "feminizing" the body and for initiating ovulation, vaginal lubrication, enlarging the breasts and pelvis, and preventing bone loss. Emotionally, it affects a woman's psyche by promoting a healthy libido.

• Estrone is produced in fat tissue as well as the ovaries. However, with the onset of menopause, the ovaries tend to make less estradiol, while fat cells continue to pump out estrone. This form of estrogen now makes up a greater portion of the total amount and is why estrogen levels during menopause tend to be higher in heavier women.[1]

• Estriol is normally produced in large amounts during pregnancy and acts in a protective, benign manner to counterbalance the effects of the other two forms of estrogen. It is responsible for preventing hot flashes and night sweats, promoting more youthful, supple appearance of skin, and lubricating the vagina. For women with mental fog due to a deficiency in estriol, Linda often recommends that clients see a holistic gynecologist who can prescribe a bioidentical form of estriol. Bioidentical hormones are described later in this chapter.

Progesterone

Progesterone has a profound counterbalancing effect on estrogen that can have a significant bearing on a woman's emotions, neurological functioning, and her physical well-being. While estrogen has an excitatory effect on the body and the brain, progesterone has an opposite, calming effect. The primary role of progesterone is to prepare the uterus for the implantation of the fertilized egg at the time of conception. Progesterone then closes the uterine cervix so that the fertilized egg and subsequent fetus remain inside the uterus during pregnancy. Acting as a natural birth control agent, high levels of progesterone shut down ovulation for the duration of the pregnancy.

During the final trimester, women typically secrete up to 20 times more progesterone than during the last two weeks of their normal menstrual cycle. Despite the additional discomfort of excess weight and apprehension concerning the birthing process, many of Linda's pregnant clients have told her that they never felt better in their lives. Linda has channeled this is primarily due to the high levels of progesterone that promote a state of well-being and increased energy. The corollary is also true for women who experience postpartum depression, which is due to a precipitous drop in progesterone levels following the birthing process.

The many positive attributes of progesterone explain why bioidentical progesterone replacement therapy is so important to a woman's anti-aging program. Just a few of its physical benefits include increasing metabolism and promoting weight loss, balancing blood sugar levels, enhancing the action of thyroid hormones, normalizing sleep patterns, reducing cyclical migraines, stimulating new bone production, and enhancing cell oxygen levels. Emotional benefits include reducing depression and anxiety, and enhancing libido.

However, as essential as estrogen and progesterone are for the healthy functioning of a woman's body, her physical and emotional states of well-being can be tied to sudden and dramatic up-and-down fluctuations in the level of either or both of these hormones. These can occur in monthly cycles or in cycles over a number of years.

ESTROGEN DOMINANCE 101

What makes female hormonal issues so complex is the unique pattern of each woman's estrogen/progesterone fluctuations. Premenstrual syndrome (PMS), perimenopause, and menopause involve an imbalance in the normal ratio of estrogen to progesterone due to the complicated phenomenon of estrogen dominance. Without enough counterbalancing progesterone, estrogen levels stay unnaturally high toward the end of the menstrual cycle, causing PMS. A deficiency in estrogen is the most common clinical indicator of perimenopause and menopause. However, much of the emotional and physical discomfort that many women experience from these issues can clearly be attributed to an out-of-control ratio of progesterone to estrogen.

It is estimated that 75 percent of PMS sufferers have high estrogen levels in relation to progesterone.[2] Linda channels that this is a significant reason why perimenopausal women who suffer from PMS are more greatly affected by stress, mood swings, and depression. An overload of estrogen stops the body from breaking down cortisol. This causes higher levels of cortisol, often associated with depression and anxiety, to remain in the body for a longer period of time. It also increases copper levels, which, in turn, can deplete the body of zinc, a biochemical combination discussed in Chapter 15 that is associated with depression.

A common misconception that some mainstream gynecologists have labored under for years is that estrogen dominance in perimenopause and menopause only results from extremely high levels of estrogen. However, the pioneering work of Dr. John Lee, M.D., Dr. Jonathan Wright, M.D., and others have proven otherwise. These conditions are primarily caused by the ratio of *normal* levels of estrogen to relatively low levels of progesterone or by the ratio of *low* levels of estrogen to extremely low levels of progesterone.

Linda observes that most of her middle-aged female clients, including herself, who are nearing or experiencing menopause, have suffered to one degree or another from estrogen dominance. While their level of estrogen can drop between 40 and 60 percent at the onset of menopause, their level of progesterone can drop even more dramatically. Although the adrenal glands may continue to produce progesterone for a while, the level of progesterone dries up to nearly zero following menopause. The body now lacks sufficient progesterone to counterbalance elevated levels of estradiol and estrone.

The key emotional consequences of estrogen dominance experienced by menopausal women explain why many women suffer from depression, fatigue, anxiety, and brain fog. In an even more disturbing trend, Linda sees a

growing number of young, fertile women with similar symptoms. Corresponding physical conditions include hypothyroidism, painful breasts, fibrocystic
breast disease, abnormal clotting, and increased risk of breast and uterine cancer. However, something is very wrong with this scenario. With rare exceptions *these are not the type of problems that afflicted our grandmothers' generation!*
What on earth has happened to women's health over the last quarter of a century?

In his book *Natural Hormone Balance for Women,* gynecologist Dr. Uzzi
Reiss, M.D., offers a fascinating take on this hormonal aberration. He draws
from years of clinical experience to contrast the nature of the typical problems
that financially challenged religious Jewish and Arab women experienced in
his practice in Israel in the 1970s to what a significant number of affluent
women in Beverly Hills are experiencing in his practice today. "From 1972 to
1976, I practiced in Israel in an area where most women follow a traditional
pattern of multiple pregnancies. My patients included Palestinian as well as
North African and religious Jewish women. *I rarely saw any of the conditions
that we commonly see today in gynecological practice.* They didn't have cancer,
menstrual cramps, abnormal bleeding, PMS, migraines, fibroids, adeno-
myosis, or endometriosis. Their main complaint was that after so many pregnancies, they had varicose veins and a prolapse of the uterus."[3]

However, Dr. Reiss does not believe that lower birthrates in the United
States alone are the main reason why women in Beverly Hills have higher levels of "aggressive" estrogen that are commensurate with a rise in breast cancer, autoimmune disease, infertility, and other health issues. *Instead, he believes
that environmental toxins and pharmaceutical drugs are the main forces that have led
to an accumulation of aggressive estrogens.*[4]

Linda has channeled that such drugs as birth control pills, hormone
replacement therapy (HRT), anti-inflammatory drugs, antibiotics, high blood
pressure and thyroid-regulating drugs, and insulin along with estrogen-
mimicking chemicals found in detergents, plastics, and pesticides can increase
levels of aggressive estrogen. Other cofactors may include dietary issues
(excess sugar and processed foods), obesity, neurotransmitter imbalances,
exposure to electromagnetic fields (EMFs), and emotional stress.

Linda has channeled that the worst culprits include:

• **Birth control pills.** These pills contain strong, synthetic estrogens that
along with synthetic progestins do not resemble natural progesterone. Thus,
the pill supplies aggressive estrogen *without* estriol or progesterone protection. Birth control pills also aggravate inflammation in women with polycys-

tic ovaries. This is a common and debilitating condition in up to 20 percent of women who suffer from acne, increased hair growth, weight gain, tendency toward diabetes, and irregular periods.[5]

• **Hormone replacement therapy (HRT).** Perhaps the most damning piece of evidence against such synthetic hormone replacement drugs as Premarin, Provera, and Prempro, which are meant to regulate decreasing estrogen levels, comes directly from a *government-sponsored study*, the Women's Health Initiative, in 2002. The study backfired on the pharmaceutical interests and was stopped after 5.2 years instead of a projected 8.5 years. Since the risks of synthetic hormones outweighed the benefits, it was determined that there was no reason to continue the study.[6] In addition to the admission that these products protect neither the bones nor the heart, the results were truly shocking. In particular, one study found that Prempro, an estrogen/progestin combination drug, resulted in a 26 percent increase in breast cancer, a 29 percent increase in coronary artery disease, a 41 percent increase in strokes, and a 100 percent increase in blood clots in leg and lungs (pulmonary embolisms)! Given these drugs are derived from the urine of a pregnant horse, it was astonishing for us to learn that of the twelve different estrogen compounds found in mare urine, only one is an exact replica of human estrogen!

• **Xenoestrogens.** These are endocrine-disrupting chemicals (EDCs) that often exacerbate problems of excess estrogen. More than at any other time in history, these toxic chemical compounds are commonly found in our food, water, air, and soil. Xenoestrogens include growth hormones used in dairy and meat production, and organochloride pesticides such as polychlorinated biphenyls (PCBs) found in freshwater and saltwater fish, and other organochlorides, and pesticides. They are also found in plastics, cosmetics, shampoos, hair dyes, detergents, and other household products. They contain a molecular structure so similar to estrogen that they mimic the effects of estrogen as they disrupt hormonal balances throughout the body. Linda is very concerned about the potential effects of EDCs on young girls who experience sexual transformation well before the age of 13, the age that in earlier eras was considered the norm for reaching puberty. Linda has channeled that xenoestrogen "parading" as estrogen is a likely cofactor in cases where estrogen is implicated in breast, ovarian, and uterine cancers.

• **Inadequate water filtration system.** Pharmaceutical toxins are polluting our drinking water. According to a 2007 article in *E/The Environmental Magazine* written by Greg Peterson, "The EPA suspects that part of the problem is consumers flushing old or unwanted drugs down toilets or drains . . . [and the EPA acknowledges that] many of America's wastewater treatment plants are not designed to remove pharmaceuticals and personal care products. Meanwhile, federal officials continue to study the human health effects of the pharmaceutical compounds found in waters known as endocrine disrupters, including possible links to neurological problems in children and increased incidence of some cancers . . . Several [research] studies of the Potomac and Shenandoah rivers have revealed inter-sex fish, a wide range of abnormalities in which both male and female characteristics are present in the same fish."[7]

LOW THYROID AND DEPRESSION

In the fall of 2008 Oprah Winfrey, one of the most influential women in America (and a major queen from a past life, according to Linda), announced on her talk show that after suffering for an extended period of time from exhaustion, sleeplessness, and depression, a battery of medical tests confirmed that she had been suffering from thyroid disease. She is hardly alone. In fact, it is estimated that as many as fifty-nine million Americans have thyroid conditions. Most cases are women whose symptoms have been ignored or simply misdiagnosed. The reason is that the ambiguity of the symptoms frequently causes both patient and healer to mistake the symptoms for emotional problems, stress, perimenopause, or menopause. Far too many of Linda's female clients report that their doctors had relied on a vague euphemism called "normal aging" or, worse, had pronounced the problem as being entirely "psychosomatic."

As mentioned in Chapter 10, hypothyroidism is also called "the great imitator" because it can mimic many forms of depression. Linda consistently channels that a biochemical chain reaction—a combination of undiagnosed heavy metal toxicity and estrogen dominance that suppresses thyroid function—leads to hypothyroidism. Research proves that hypothyroidism reduces the function of serotonin receptors, a core cause of depression.[8] Mood disorders such as bipolar disorder have been linked to people with altered thyroid function.[9] In fact, hypothyroidism can also be caused by lithium-based mood stabilizers that are often used to treat bipolar disorder.[10] Fatigue, confusion, and a decline in cognitive memory function are common repercussions of hypothyroidism.

Linda often channels that heavy metal toxins, chemicals (PCBs, chlorine, and fluoride), or radiation lodged in the thyroid are core causal factors for hypothyroidism and the emotional issues that plague many women with this condition. The ability to diagnose the presence of such toxins in tissues is a perfect example of how Linda's gift outshines conventional testing protocols. With the exception of energetic protocols such as EAV (Dr. Voll's electro-acupuncture) and ART (Dr. Klinghardt's autonomic response testing) or Linda, we are unaware of any conventional method short of a biopsy for accurately testing for the presence of these types of toxins in the thyroid gland. Linda has had great success in improving the physical and emotional well-being of clients by detoxing these poisons out of the thyroid. She also channels a customized diet that accentuates specific nutrients to optimize thyroid function. These include iodine, found in seafood and sea vegetables, which is necessary to make T4 in the thyroid gland. Vitamins A, B complex, C, and E, as well as selenium, zinc, magnesium, iron, manganese, and the amino acid tyrosine are also needed in the conversion of T4 to T3. A note on tyrosine supplementation: Linda consistently channels that tyrosine should only be considered if the woman is a vegetarian. Although it is important for thyroid metabolism, tyrosine can, in many cases, actually suppress thyroid function.

Linda frequently channels that there is a symbiotic relationship between a hypothyroid condition and adrenal exhaustion in her female clients. In such a situation, both glandular imbalances affect each other and need to be treated concurrently. This linkage is an interesting confirmation of the Five Element Theory of TCM whereby the thyroid gland and the adrenal gland are controlled by the element of fire. Linda channels that chronic stress from either emotions and/or environmental toxicity can produce elevated cortisol levels in the adrenals. This, in turn, inhibits T4/T3 conversion that controls the production of the hormone thyroxine, which depletes thyroid function.

In regard to adrenal exhaustion, the field of psychoneuroimmunology (mentioned in Chapter 15) uses a biochemical perspective to determine what TCM and homeopathy have long known: the body/mind connection is inextricably linked to the disease process itself.

STRESS AND THE HYPOTHALAMIC-PITUITARY-ADRENAL AXIS

Adrenal exhaustion is usually due to a combination of emotional and/or physical stress and environmental toxicity. It is a common cofactor in many physical and emotional problems stemming from hormonal imbalance that Linda sees in her practice. Although adrenal exhaustion occurs in men and women, Linda finds it slightly more common in women.

Adrenal exhaustion is caused by an imbalance in the hypothalamus-pituitary-adrenal (HPA) axis. The HPA axis, discovered in the 1930s by the brilliant Canadian endocrinologist Dr. Hans Selye, is a neuroendocrine feedback loop mechanism the body uses to cope with stress, which can include psychological, physical, and biological factors as well as environmental toxins. These forces take the body out of a state of homeostasis—the body's self-regulating thermostat that maintains the synergistic functioning of the organ systems. A stress response is how the brain responds biochemically to reestablish normal homeostatic balance.

Dr. Selye demonstrated the existence of stress disease he called the "general adaptation syndrome" (GAS). His and subsequent research shows that the body adapts to maintain a state of homeostasis through the integration of a matrix of biological systems (cells, glands, and organs) acting in concert with various chemicals (neurotransmitters, peptides, hormones, cytokines) through the central, peripheral, and autonomic nervous systems. Chronic levels of stress involving the HPA axis affect this matrix, making it a significant cofactor in many types of disease. If not corrected, stress can literally cause a person to burn out and die.

The HPA axis feedback loop system starts with the hypothalamus, which regulates the many aspects of homeostasis through the production of neuropeptides. These chemical messengers affect functions that are necessary for survival such as appetite, body temperature, blood pressure, blood sugar levels, emotional reactions, heart rate, hormone balance, immune response, libido, metabolism, and sleep.

When a person feels stress, the hypothalamus produces a neuropeptide called corticotropin-releasing hormone (CRH), which is delivered to the pituitary gland, causing it to secrete a hormone in the form of a peptide called adrenocorticotropic hormone (ACTH). This circulates throughout the body, finally reaching the adrenal glands located just above the kidneys. ACTH stimulates the adrenal cortex to synthesize and secrete a group of steroid hormones called glucocorticoids. Cortisol, the most important of the glucocorticoids, regulates glucose metabolism and the body's response to stress by accelerating the breakdown of protein that provides fuel to regulate many important cardiovascular, immunologic, and other homeostatic functions.

When cortisol reaches various target tissues, it initiates a series of reactions known as the "fight-or-flight response." This stress response causes hormones such as adrenaline, noradrenaline, glucocorticoids, and mineralo - corticoids to be secreted by the adrenals to prepare the body to cope with stress. The feedback loop is completed when the electrochemical information from these target tissues is monitored by the hypothalamus. If these stress responses tell the hypothalamus that more help is needed, more CRH is released, triggering the pituitary gland to secrete more ACTH, which, in turn, stimulates ever-higher secretion of cortisol. When cortisol rises to the level needed to deal with the stress, the stimulus for the production of more cortisol is inhibited, and the system returns to normal. However, when there are chronically high stress levels, cortisol levels may remain high indefinitely, causing adrenal fatigue and exhaustion. This results in chronic hypercortisolemia, which may be a significant cofactor in depression, nutritional deficiencies (B vitamins, vitamins C and E, calcium), and many chronic degenerative conditions.

Various forms of stress fatigue the adrenal glands and contribute to emotional and neurological problems. For instance, depression results from elevated levels of cortisol, which increase the activity of enzymes that destroy tryptophan, a precursor to serotonin[11] (see Chapter 15). There is also increased risk for neurodegenerative disorders like Alzheimer's disease[12], multiple sclerosis[13], brain aging, and cognitive memory decline.[14] Adrenal stress can also exacerbate or cause new hormonal problems such as reducing DHEA levels (adrenals), increasing insulin resistance (pancreas), decreasing TSH and T3 production (thyroid) and growth hormone (hypothalamus), and suppressing pituitary function. It can also decrease the capacity of the liver to detoxify and increase the risk of ulcers, heart attack, and stroke. Linda commonly channels that stress/cortisol imbalances are a frequent component in complicated health issues.

Stress and Obesity

Many women who are stressed out when they come to see Linda obsess about being overweight. What women will be interested to know is that Linda channels a clear cause-and-effect relationship between stress and obesity. *Stress is a major factor in one's inability to lose weight. When one is continuously stressed out, the stage is set, from a biochemical perspective, for rapid weight gain.* One of the harmful effects of chronic stress on the adrenals is that excess cortisol levels decrease your cells' sensitivity to insulin, the hormone that delivers blood sugar to cells. The result is insulin resistance, a precursor to type 2 diabetes.

Prolonged levels of elevated cortisol also promote the storage of fat in the abdomen. With client after client, Linda channels that excess cortisol from chronic levels of stress has a profound impact on leptin, a protein hormone produced by fat cells that helps regulate fat storage. Leptin acts on the brain as an intercellular messenger, signaling the body to decrease food intake and increase metabolism. However, insulin resistance causes the receptors for leptin, located in the hypothalamus, to shut down. When these receptors do not respond to leptin, the likelihood of obesity greatly increases. This, in turn, creates a vicious cycle of more elevated cortisol levels, insulin resistance, leptin resistance—and depression. Linda often channels that herbal support to control cortisol levels and/or adrenal glandular supplements is helpful in counterbalancing this.

LINDA'S APPROACH TO PROBLEMS WITH THE ENDOCRINE SYSTEM

In putting together the endocrine database for Linda some years ago, I realized that it was not as cut and dry as simply assembling lists of information that covered the structure/function and imbalances of each gland. The endocrine database had to deal with layers of complexity involving neurotransmitters, peptides, and hormones coupled with years of clinical observations by leading endocrinologists. The resulting database gives Linda a detailed set of variables that enable her to diagnose and solve complex hormonal issues.

Thanks to the very thorough endocrine database, Linda can identify toxins, design detoxification programs, and address specific hormonal imbalances through orthomolecular nutrients, herbs, glandulars, and homeopathy. For example, Linda has had real success treating PMS using a synergistic cocktail of nutrients that includes B_6, zinc, magnesium, and evening primrose oil (an essential fatty acid). These are useful in reducing nervousness, headaches, breast tenderness, and weight gain so commonly found in women with PMS. Linda can correct a hormonal imbalance outright or, in more challenging cases, prep the body for working with a holistically oriented gynecologist or endocrinologist who can then prescribe effective bioidentical hormones (described later in this chapter).

Here are the most important observations Linda has channelled when assessing hormonal issues.

1. **Inflammation affects endocrinology.** Linda consistently channels that inflammation is the most common cofactor in a malfunctioning endocrine system. Heavy metal toxins, infections, stress, and allergens promote the pre-

mature aging process by increasing cytokines—destructive protein messengers that set off inflammatory autoimmune responses implicated in many forms of chronic and/or neurodegenerative disease. Just as one can experience inflammation in the form of swelling anywhere in the body, new evidence points to the link between inflammatory cytokines and inflammation in the brain. This can overstimulate the HPA axis or increase the function of an enzyme that breaks down tryptophan, lowering serotonin levels; both are hallmarks of depression. This also explains why depression is more common in people with such inflammatory conditions as heart disease and autoimmune diseases like chronic fatigue syndrome.[15]

Another undesirable cause of inflammation is food sensitivities or allergies, which trigger an inflammatory response. These often involve certain types of proteins such as casein, gluten, egg, and soy. Linda channels the culprits so the client can then eliminate them from the diet. Quite often she channels that essential fatty acids such as fish oil also need to be taken to decrease the inflammatory response. A normal metabolic response can usually be restored.

2. Blood sugar disorders must be corrected when attempting to balance metabolic and endocrine disorders. Linda channels that it is difficult to normalize hormonal imbalances if blood sugar and adrenal disorders are not addressed and managed. This is because many hormonal disorders are initiated by blood sugar imbalances. Hypoglycemia, for example, can lead to adrenal exhaustion and altered cortisol levels. Insulin resistance in women may be associated with elevated levels of certain hormones, including testosterone and estrogen or decreased levels of sex hormone-binding globulin (SHBG).

When channeling any hormonal imbalance, Linda checks to see if a potential relationship exists with insulin and adrenal disorders. She may review the food list with this variable in mind to optimize a diet with the proper Glycemic Index. She also channels supplements that regulate insulin levels, such as cinnamon, fenugreek, chromium picolinate, vanadium, and gymnema sylvestre. For adrenal disorders, she channels from a list of Western, Chinese, and Ayurvedic herbs, as well as adrenal glandulars.

3. There is often a strong relationship between environmental or internal toxins affecting liver detoxification pathways and endocrine disorders. This refers to the damaging effects on the liver caused by a variety of toxins ranging from heavy metals and pharmaceutical drugs to the buildup of old estrogen. In cases where a woman has symptoms of hormonal imbalances which do not correlate with lab results or where the patient is unable to handle drugs or even bioidentical hormones, it is important to detoxify the phase I and phase II metabolic pathways of the liver. Linda channels various herbs, amino acids, and antioxidants to detoxify these pathways, which is vital to restoring normal metabolic functioning.

A Word on Bioidentical Hormone Replacement Therapy

We are impressed with the crusading efforts of actress-turned-medical-researcher Suzanne Somers to raise the bar on hormone consciousness for both women and their doctors. Somers is a staunch advocate of bioidentical hormone replacement therapy (BHRT), which involves oral, injectable, or transdermal application of natural sex hormones processed from precursors found in yams or soy plants. Bioidentical hormones are designed to alleviate symptoms caused by the natural decrease in the production of sex hormones as well as provide the protective benefits originally supplied by naturally occurring hormones. Bioidenticals are molecularly identical to hormones made in a woman's body, which cannot distinguish any difference between them.

The pharmaceutical HRT approach uses hormones derived from pregnant mare urine or synthesized in a laboratory and are not identical to the hormones produced naturally in a woman's body. *Therein lies the core of the problem with the pharmaceutical approach.* As the Women's Health Initiative and other studies amply demonstrate, the use of pharmaceutical estrogen and progesterone is associated with the risk of breast cancer, heart attack, and stroke.[16] Amazingly, a large-scale European study showed that women using bioidentical progesterone in combination with estrogen experienced a significant reduction in breast cancer risk compared with those using HRT progestins.[17]

Linda agrees with Suzanne Somers that hormone replacement drugs such as Premarin, Provera, and Prempro are of limited value for many women due to unacceptably high levels of serious side effects. As for BHRT, we find ourselves agreeing with her—with certain reservations. Linda has channeled that there is no universal approach. BHRT may help many women, but by no means all. Although it has tremendous potential, the truth of the matter is that BHRT is a relatively new field. A woman should only work with a doctor who is experienced in the field and belongs to organizations or societies of doctors conducting ongoing research.[18]

Linda's Mantra Is Safety First:
An Innovative but Common Sense Nutritional Approach

Hormone replacement therapy in general does have potential risks. As women age, their bodies have a diminished capacity to repair or remove damage to cells and tissue. This is because cell growth regulatory genes in their DNA accumulate mutations. In a worst-case scenario, this can result in uncontrolled cell propagation that leads to cancerous tumors. That puts women at greater risk for breast cancer as they age, regardless of their estrogen levels. But for menopausal women, changes involving estrogen in breast tissue cells also heighten the potential risk of breast cancer.

That is why Linda is excited that the complementary nutritional supplements and dietary suggestions she consistently channels for her female clients who are candidates for BHRT are scientifically in sync with the latest scientific research. A white paper entitled "Bioidentical Hormones: Why Are They Still Controversial?" published in the October 2009 issue of *Life Extension* magazine examined every significant scientific study related to estrogen and progesterone replacement therapy. It highlighted research studies showing that specific complementary anticancer nutrients can make BHRT or even synthetic HRT significantly safer by preventing and even repairing gene mutations. Anticancer nutrients include vitamin D[19], indole-3-carbinol[20,21,22], fish oil[23,24], soy isoflavones[25,26], flax lignans[27,28,29], green tea[30,31,32], and D-glucarate.[33,34,35] Dietary suggestions include a vegetarian-oriented diet with high levels of cruciferous vegetables such as broccoli, cauliflower, cabbage, and kale.

Linda also channels that other less expensive natural approaches may work well in less severe cases. These include plant-based phytoestrogens (black cohosh, genistein, maca root, chasteberry, and dong quai) and homeopathic forms of sex hormones, which also offer real solutions either by themselves or in conjunction with BHRT.

In the final analysis, *unless a woman addresses the underlying toxins that compromise her endocrine system, no natural approach is a slam dunk.* In fact, Linda often channels that BHRT will achieve far more meaningful results if the underlying toxic burdens affecting the endocrine system are detoxified ahead of time. This is why she focuses on detoxification of the endocrine system and the proper nutritional support before referring a client to a medical doctor who specializes in BHRT.

PART THREE

Spirit, Metaphysics, and Reincarnation

CHAPTER 17

Sigmund Freud Speaks: A Preamble to the Metaphysical Database

Sometimes a cigar is just a cigar.
—SIGMUND FREUD

Sometimes a cigar is not a cigar.
—SIGMUND FREUD
(*CRYPTIC NEW PROCLAMATION FROM THE SPIRIT WORLD*)

TO GIVE THE READER INSIGHT into the level of personal growth that Sigmund Freud has achieved in the spirit world, here is a brief story that bespeaks of the man's personal integrity. In 2005 I took my family on a working vacation to Switzerland where Linda saw clients at the Kientalerhof Center of Wellbeing. Before that we stopped over in London where we vacationed for several days. While there, I took Linda and our son, Aryeh, to visit the Sigmund Freud Museum in the Hampstead district of London, which Linda had never visited before. On a previous trip decades earlier, I had the good fortune to meet Anna Freud, Sigmund's daughter, who continued to live in the house until her death in 1982, whereupon it was converted into the museum. She was a brilliant psychoanalyst in her own right.

The wonderful presentation of Freud memorabilia speaks volumes about the awe and admiration, bordering on worship, that the museum has for Freud and his work. After touring the house, we met with the directors of the museum who were most cordial to us. We told them about our communication with Sigmund Freud in the spirit world, which slightly startled them. Nonetheless, our visit with them was quite pleasant and much appreciated. As we were leaving, Linda started shaking. I pulled her aside and asked her to get out the pendulum. Sigmund had come to Linda to tell her what he thought of his museum.

Although he was touched by the love and admiration shown to him, he told Linda: "The continued glorification of my work as a springboard for future research is stale." Other than for the historical significance of his life and work, he wishes the museum could be transformed into a center of research to explore the new ways of thinking he has embraced from his perspective in the spirit world. Perhaps 20 Maresfield Gardens will become that place one day.

AN UNEXPECTED TWIST OF FATE—AND REVELATIONS

It was my original intention to allocate twenty-five pages of this book for Sigmund to use as a forum to expound on any aspect of his controversial life. I prepared a list of potential topics I thought he might want to discuss. Chief on the short list were interpretation of dreams, libido theory, rejection of the seduction theory, Oedipal complex, transference, free association, and the theory of superego, ego, and id. After Sigmund picked the topics he wished to discuss, Linda and I could formulate questions to ask him. Linda would then channel the information, which I would then transcribe. But as I went through the list, his response to each item was essentially the same: "No, it is interesting but we can talk about that in a future book." Only on *The Interpretation of Dreams* did he venture any information, volunteering that it was his favorite of all his books.

Linda then channeled that Sigmund was getting somewhat agitated and that he had "something that he very much wanted to get off his chest," as he put it. She then blurted out his words: "I want to talk about Carl Jung!" We were a bit surprised by this choice but also enthralled; this was also a great topic. After all, Freud and Jung collectively represent not only the two most important personalities in the psychoanalytical movement, but they also spawned its two most important schools of thought: Freudian and Jungian.

Freud's genius was as an original thinker who developed methodologies of dialogue between patient and therapist that brought subconsciously repressed thoughts and feelings into the conscious mind, thus helping to free the patient of neurotic behaviors. Some of these techniques included dream analysis, free association, and transference. He also stressed that sexual desires were the primary motivating factor behind much human behavior and repressed emotions. Jung's genius lay in the expansion and integration of psychoanalysis to include psychic and spiritual concepts derived from universal, unconscious archetypes found in the world's religions and cultures, including their myths, literature, and art.

I must confess that the writing of this book took a major left turn when Sigmund announced his intention to speak about C. G. Jung at length. While I was keenly aware that the primary focus of this book was to explore Linda's healing gift, *the revelations that Sigmund disclosed here are so shocking that I soon realized there was no way we could not include them in this book!*

Linda initially questioned Sigmund as to why he did not want to discuss any of the topics that I had suggested. After all, any student of psychology would be chomping at the bit to know how Sigmund Freud viewed his life's work in hindsight from the spirit world. His response was twofold: (1) Topics such as those could not be relegated to "sound-bite answers," which would be required given the number of pages allotted for this chapter in this book. (2) The revelations about his relationship with Jung cut across multiple fields, including religion, psychology, and literature, in addition to having major implications for Linda's work.

Sigmund also assured us that working through Linda he plans to be heard from in the future and believes his best work lies ahead of him. From his vantage point in the upper worlds, he is now able to assist humanity from an utterly unique perspective. For this book, he has specifically requested to speak about the metaphysical implications of his relationship and subsequent breakup with Carl Jung. We have a tacit understanding with him that another book, to be entitled *Sigmund Freud Speaks,* will offer a unique glimpse into the transformation that has occurred in Freud's thinking since he transitioned out of his physical body in 1939 and returned to the spirit world. That book will expound on a wide array of topics, ranging from the many controversial aspects of his life's work to an in-depth understanding of his views on the future of psychology. In addition, he will voice his opinions on the key issues facing humanity.

THROUGH THE METAPHYSICAL LOOKING GLASS: A BOLD NEW LOOK AT THE RELATIONSHIP OF FREUD AND JUNG

Our preparation for the actual interview process represents a fascinating look at how Sigmund communicated with Linda when dissecting his complex relationship with Carl Jung. I should point out that Linda actually hears Sigmund's voice when she goes into trance. From the beginning of this process, he made it quite clear that we first needed a deep historical perspective to grasp the complexity of his thought process. He therefore insisted we research his tumultuous relation with Jung so that the historical context of the most important relationship in the history of psychology could be presented in an accurate light. This required assembling research materials covering the linear progression of events as they occurred. Linda could then draw from existing commentary to ask Sigmund about specific chronological events that were written directly by him or Jung or were written about him or Jung. He told us to start our educational process by reading specific passages in books he recommended that pertain to his relationship with Jung. Only this much will I reveal now: It is a tale of misconceptions and bruised egos spinning out of control with startling parallels to their past lives from an ancient era. After I presented him with a list of books on the subject, he recommended the following:

- *The Freud/Jung Letters* edited by William McGuire (Princeton University Press, 1974). This correspondence of 358 letters documents the various phases of their relationship that lasted for eight years.[1]

- *On the History of the Psychoanalytical Movement* by Sigmund Freud (1914; W.W. Norton & Co., 1966).

- *The Interpretation of Dreams* by Sigmund Freud, standard edition (1899; Hogarth Press, 1963).

- *Memories, Dreams, Reflections* by C. G. Jung (Pantheon Books, 1963).

- *Psyche and Symbol* by C. G. Jung (Princeton University Press, 1958).

- *Freud: A Life for Our Time* by Peter Gay (W.W. Norton, 2006).[2]

- *The Life and Work of Sigmund Freud*, vols. I–III, by Ernest Jones (Basic Books, Inc., 1955; out of print).

- *Freud & Jung: A Dual Introduction* by Anthony Storr and Anthony Stevens (Barnes & Noble Books, 1998).

- *Freud and His Followers* by Paul Roazen (1975; Da Capo Press, 1992).

- *Sigmund Freud: His Personality, His Teaching, His School* by Fritz Wittels (Dodd, Mead & Co., 1924; out of print).

- *Kabbalah and Psychology* by Z'ev ben Shimon Halevi (Samuel Weiser Books, 1992; out of print).

- *The Mythological Unconscious* by Michael Vannoy Adams (Karnac Books, 2001).

I wrote the following history based on our research, which was then guided by Sigmund's insights.

Father and Son

Freud was fifty years old in 1907 when he met Jung, who was thirty (see Figures 17-1 and 17-2). Jung was quite taken by Freud's landmark book *The Interpretation of Dreams*, and had quoted from it in his own writings. In fact, in the Foreword of *The Psychology of Dementia Praecox*, Jung challenged a dismissive psychiatric establishment by lavishing praise on Freud. He declared, "Even a superficial glance at my work will show how much I am indebted to the brilliant discoveries of Freud."[3] In 1906 he sent Freud copies of this and *Studies in Word Association*, both of which extended ideas initially developed by Freud.

Recognizing a kindred spirit, Freud was sincerely impressed and invited Jung to visit him in Vienna. Jung reported that at their first meeting they talked virtually without pause for thirteen hours![4] So enthralled was Freud with the instantaneous intellectual connection with Jung that he reciprocated by sending Jung a collection of his latest published essays. In addition to professional conferences, personal meetings in Zurich and Vienna, and a trip to

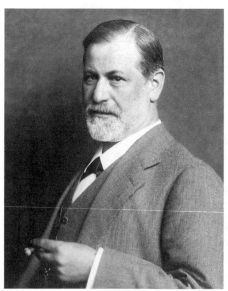

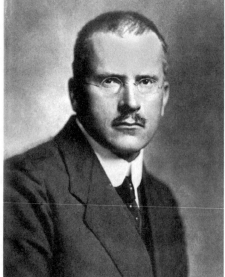

Figure 17-1. Sigmund Freud.
Used with permission of the Freud Museum, London. Photographer: Max Halberstadt.

Figure 17-2. Carl Jung.
Used with permission of Getty Images. Photographer: Imago. Collection: Hulton Archive.

America together, their blossoming intellectual infatuation was largely sustained by written correspondence that lasted for the next six years.

In *Freud & Jung* authors Storr and Stevens write, "[Jung's] desire for Freud's friendship was as much personal as professional. In the older, more experienced man, he found a mentor—a distinguished colleague who represented the intellectually courageous father that his own father, the doubting theologian, was not . . . 'Let me enjoy your friendship not as one between equals but as that of father and son,' " wrote Jung soon after their first meeting.[5]

Securing a line of succession was critically important to Freud, who viewed himself as the patriarch of the psychoanalytic movement. Freud treated Jung as if he were "formally adopted . . . as an eldest son" and anointed him as his "successor and Crown Prince" of the great intellectual movement he had founded.[6] His face beamed whenever he spoke of Jung, "This is my beloved son in whom I am well pleased!"[7] These patriarchal feelings are what led Freud to install Jung as president of the International Psychoanalytical Association (IPA) in 1910.

Another dimension to their relationship is worth noting. As of 1910, the Viennese psychoanalytic group was made up almost entirely of Jews. Freud was keenly aware that the fledgling field of psychoanalysis risked being labeled as a "Jewish science."[8] Freud was therefore eager to expand the ethnic and religious diversity of his core group to gain wider international acceptance within the scientific community. This is why Paul Roazen, author of *Freud and His Followers*, noted, "As a Jew, Freud keenly felt the need for help of the Gentile Jung."[9] And Jung, as the son of a Christian pastor, could hardly have had a more different upbringing than Freud.

At the time of their fateful meeting, Jung was already an assistant to Eugene Bleuler, head of the Burghölzli, one of Europe's most prestigious centers for psychiatric training in Zurich. Bleuler and Jung represented the best of academic psychiatry of their day. For Freud the period from 1906 to 1909 constituted a break with his past, as he emerged from the narrow sphere of Vienna into European psychiatry as a whole.[10] A few years following their fortuitous meeting, Jung broke with Bleuler in order to devote himself entirely to psychoanalysis. According to Ernest Jones, Freud's official biographer and closest confidant, Freud "came away rejoicing" as the inclusion of the well-regarded Jung within his movement boded well for the international acceptance of psychoanalysis.[11] That was the driving force behind everything Freud strove for.

It is important to know that Freud was fixated on the Jewish leader Moses throughout his career, sometimes writing about him with admiration, sometimes with disdain. In his relationship to the psychoanalytic movement, he aligned himself with Moses in that he foresaw a time when the people he led would turn on him with anger and disobedience. Ernest Jones, who perhaps knew Freud better than anyone else, wrote, "Jung was to be the Joshua destined to explore the promised land of psychiatry which Freud, like Moses, was only permitted to view from afar."[12] However, during this early father/son phase of their relationship, Freud could not fathom the possibility that Jung was even capable of turning on him. In fact, Freud said, "When the Empire I founded is orphaned, no one but Jung must inherit the whole thing."[13]

When Jung in correspondence in 1908 expresses partial disagreement over aspects of the libido theory, the fatherly Freud states: "I know it will take you time to catch up with my experience of the last fifteen years."[14] Eager to be accepted by the father as a faithful follower with his own ideas, Jung writes back: "I beg you to have patience with me and confidence in what I have done up till now."[15] However, as a result of deepening intellectual disagreements that centered on the libido theory, their bond began to weaken in 1909 for this very reason. In *Freud & Jung*, authors Storr and Stevens state, "Two of Freud's basic assumptions were unacceptable to Jung: (1) that human motivation is exclusively sexual; and (2) that the unconscious mind is entirely personal and peculiar to the individual. Jung found these and other aspects of Freud's thinking reductionist and too narrow. Instead of conceiving psychic energy [or libido as Freud called it] as wholly sexual, Jung preferred to think of it as a more generalized 'life force' of which sexuality was but one mode of expression. Moreover, beneath the personal unconscious of repressed wishes and traumatic memories, posited by Freud, Jung believed there lay a deeper and more important layer that he was to call the *collective unconscious*, which contained *in potentia* the entire psychic heritage of mankind."[16]

However, despite their disagreements, Jung still remained in awe of his "father." In November 1909, contrite about not writing more promptly after his return to Switzerland from a visit to Clark University in Massachusetts, Jung submissively confessed to his "father" that he had sinned: "*Pater peccavi.*" In the early years of their relationship before their breach became visible, Jung treated his disagreements on psychoanalytical theory with Freud as his own personal flaw. If he had some problem with them, this must be, "obviously," because he had "not yet adapted my position sufficiently to yours."[17]

The following story reveals another dimension of the father/son relationship. Freud was barely 5 feet 7 inches tall, while Jung was 6 feet 2 inches. Freud was sensitive about his stature, at least when it came to Jung. In psycho-

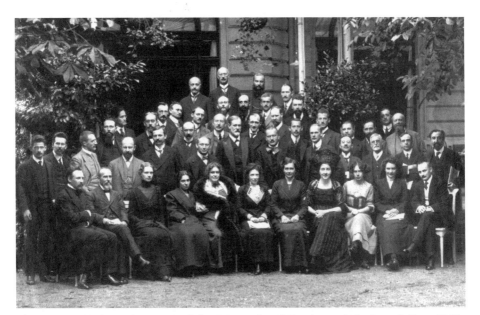

Figure 17-3. Weimar Congress of the International Psychoanalytic Association, 1911.
Freud is in the center, and Jung is the second person to Freud's left.
Used with permission of the Freud Museum, London.

analyzing the photograph of the famous early group portrait of Freud and his followers, taken at the Weimar Congress of the International Psychoanalytic Association in 1911, Freud appears to be taller than Jung, who is the second man to Freud's immediate left in Figure 17-3. Freud was not only standing on something to achieve this effect, but Jung was loyally crouching forward in order to permit Freud to stand out as the leader of the movement.[18]

However, the phase of their father/son relationship was coming to a close. According to Ernest Jones, "Early in 1912 the clouds began to darken on their relationship" and Jung was moving in a direction that would prove to be the undoing of their personal and professional relationship.[19] In 1913 Jung's behavior culminated in what Sigmund told Linda he considered to be nothing less than "an act of treason."

The Gathering Storm

Sigmund next directed us to *The Freud/Jung Letters.* He told Linda that he wanted to pick passages from specific letters in a particular linear sequence and then have me transcribe additional commentary that he dictated to Linda while she was in a trance state. The letters are numbered in chronological order as well as by author: F for Freud writing to Jung and J for Jung writing to Freud. He also requested "final cut" over the commentary.

Sigmund started this exercise with an excerpt from letter 318J written in June 1912. It concerns an irritating miscommunication between them that came to be referred to as the infamous "Kreuzlingen gesture." Jung fires the first salvo by accusing Freud of snubbing him when he does not find time to meet with Jung in Zurich when he is only forty kilometers away in Constance. Freud went there to visit their mutual friend and colleague Ludwig Binswanger, who had just undergone surgery for a malignancy. Jung wrote: "The fact that you felt no need to see me during your visit in Kreuzlingen [near Constance] must, I suppose, be attributed to your displeasure at my development of the libido theory."[20]

Freud begins letter 319F with a conciliatory gesture, stating, "There is no reason to suppose why this scientific difference will detract from our personal relations." However, he is clearly irritated by what he perceived as Jung's miscalculation regarding his motives for not visiting him, insisting that it was not "motivated by my displeasure at your libido theory." Due to scheduling issues brought on by an illness in his own family, he was simply unable to visit Jung in Zurich on that trip. Freud is annoyed that Jung did not accept the sincerity of that explanation and reminds him that in an earlier letter he had asked Jung to visit him and Binswanger in Constance.[21]

Sigmund next directed Linda to letter 323J dated Nov. 11, 1912. Earlier that year, Jung had given a series of lectures at Fordham University in New York entitled "The Theory of Psychoanalysis" in which he publicly distanced himself from Freud regarding the libido theory. Jung claims to have met with considerable professional acceptance because American colleagues were "put off by sexuality as the basis for neurosis."[22] Knowing that Freud resented any "pushing into the background of the sexual factor in psychoanalytic theory,"[23] Jung offers to send Freud a copy of his lectures, hoping that Freud will gradually come to accept his innovations, adding: "I regret it very much if you think that the modifications in question have been prompted solely by resistances to you. Your Kreuzlingen gesture has dealt me a lasting wound . . . Obviously, I would prefer to remain on friendly terms with you, to whom I owe so much, but I want your objective judgment and no feelings of resentment . . . [as] I have done more to promote the psychoanalytical movement than [key members of the IPA like] Rank, Stekel, Adler, etc. put together."[24]

Sigmund asked Linda to read letter 324F dated Nov. 14, 1912. Jung's verbal chafing is beginning to have its effect on Freud. He now declares that Jung has broken him of the habit of addressing him affectionately—a father scorned by his son. Nonetheless, Freud still expresses "considerable sympathy, interest, and satisfaction at your personal success" in America.[25] However, Freud feels that Jung's new-found resistance to addressing the objections of people who seemed incapable of understanding Freud's theories is nothing to boast of. They are, in terms of the big picture of psychoanalysis, ultimately misguided. Freud feels that if Jung would merely stay the course and fight for "the hard-won truths of psychoanalysis, the more you [would] see resistance vanishing."[26] He urges Jung not to put his recent success "in the credit column because . . . the farther you remove yourself from what is new in IPA, the more certain you will be of applause and the less resistance you will meet."[27] He tells Jung that he can count on his professional objectivity and again reminds him that their past intellectual differences have never gotten in the way of their friendship. He then adds, however, that "I find your harping on the 'Kreuzlingen gesture' both incomprehensible and insulting," but allows that "there are things that cannot be straightened out in writing."[28]

Munich Conference: A Turning Point

In November 1912, Jung arranged a meeting in Munich of key members of IPA where they discussed and agreed with Freud's plan to disassociate themselves from Wilhelm Stekel, editor of *Zentralblatt*, a monthly periodical of the psychoanalytical movement, and replace it with a new journal. Then during a two-hour private walk before lunch, Freud and Jung discussed the "Kreuzlingen gesture," Jung became contrite, apologizing for his oversight, and a reconciliation was reached. Toward the end of an animated discussion over lunch, Freud began to criticize the Swiss contingent, which included Jung, for omitting his name from their articles that appeared in Swiss psychoanalytical publications. He openly interpreted Jung's action as revealing a death wish against him. Suddenly, without warning, he fell on the floor in a dead faint.[29]

The fainting attack was significant as this was the second meeting with Jung that was marred by one of Freud's fainting spells. In fact, it was an exact replay of what had happened in Bremen three years earlier. At the end of a luncheon, there had been a spirited discussion between Freud and Jung that also centered on a disagreement about why Jung had published articles in various Swiss psychoanalytical journals without mentioning Freud's name.[30] He then suffered a fainting spell. As with the fainting attack in Munich, Freud chose to interpret what Jung had done as revealing a death wish against him.[31]

Freud put his own positive spin on what had transpired during his meeting with Jung in Munich. He expressed a strong desire to promote harmony within the group so as to allow psychoanalysis to flourish, while at the same time allowing room for individual intellectual disagreements, including his own. He wrote to another associate: "Everyone was charming to me, including Jung. A talk between us swept away a number of unnecessary irritations. I hope for further successful cooperation. Theoretical differences need not interfere. However, I shall hardly be able to accept his modification of the libido theory since all my experience contradicts his position."[32]

Sigmund then directed Linda to the following excerpt from letter 328J dated Nov. 26, 1912.

Dear Professor Freud,

I am glad that we were able to meet in Munich as this was the first time that I have really understood . . . how different I am from you. This realization will be enough to affect a radical change in my whole attitude. Now you can rest assured that I shall not give up our personal relationship . . . I hope that the insight that I have at last gained will guide my conduct from now on. I am most distressed that I did not gain this insight much earlier. It could have spared you so many disappointments.[33]

At this point, Jung goes on to express his concern about Freud's health from the fainting attack in Munich. Sigmund told Linda that while Jung's opinion of him at this point may have been "strictly professional," he nonetheless sensed a significant shift in Jung's demeanor in 1912. Jung had finally succeeded in compartmentalizing his feelings for Freud between "personal and professional." Yet he still felt the need to maintain a personal relationship with Freud. For Freud, however, this letter further inflamed an underlying tension that had been building between them.

In letter 329F dated Nov. 29, 1912, Sigmund refers Linda to a specific passage in his response to Jung regarding the fainting attack: "According to my private diagnosis, it was migraine, not without a psychic factor [emotional component] which unfortunately I haven't time to track down now. The dining room of the Park Hotel in Munich seems to hold a fatality for me. Six years ago I had a first attack of the same kind there, and four years ago a second. A bit of neurosis that I ought really to look into . . . "[34]

Freud goes to considerable lengths to build upon the friendship he felt was rekindled in Munich. He even entertains the idea of a future collaboration with Jung noting that, in spite of their differences, "our relationship will always retain an echo of our past intimacy." He offers a conciliatory olive branch to Jung regarding his lectures on the libido theory given earlier in the year at Fordham University. "I am gradually coming to terms with this paper [of yours] and I now believe that you have brought us a great revelation, though not the one you intended. You seem to have solved the riddle of all mysticism, showing it to be based on the symbolic utilization of complexes that have outlived their function . . . "[35]

However, a streak of paranoia seems to have infiltrated Jung's psyche. Jung was intent on being offended and chose to read compliments as insults.[36] As with the "Kruezlingen gesture," Jung *misinterprets* what was clearly a complement as a condescending insult— that Freud undervalued his work. In response, in letter 330J dated Dec. 3, 1912, Jung is beginning to come apart at the seams when he opens the letter with a verbal warning to Freud:

This letter is a brazen attempt to accustom you to my style. So look out!

Dear Professor Freud,

My very best thanks for one passage in your letter, where you speak of a "bit of neurosis" you haven't gotten rid of. This "bit" should, in my opinion, be taken very seriously indeed because, as experience shows, it leads "to the semblance of a voluntary death." I have suffered from this bit in my dealings with you, though you haven't seen it and didn't understand me properly when I tried to make my position clear. If these blinkers were removed you would, I am sure, see my work in a very different light. As evidence that you—if I may be permitted so disrespectful an expression— *underestimated* my work by a very wide margin. I would cite your remark that "without intending it, I have solved the riddle of all mysticism, showing it to be based on the symbolic utilization of complexes that have outlived their function."

My dear professor, forgive me again, but this sentence shows me that you deprive yourself of the possibility of understanding my work by your underestimation of it. You speak of this insight as though it were some kind of pinnacle, whereas actually it is at the very bottom of the mountain. This insight has been self-evident to us for years. Again please excuse my frankness. It is only occasionally that I am afflicted with the purely human desire to be understood *intellectually* and not measured by the yardstick of neurosis.

As for this bit of neurosis, may I draw your attention to the fact that you opened *The Interpretation of Dreams* with the mournful admission of your own neurosis—the dream of Irma's injection—identification with the neurotic in need of treatment. Very significant.[37]

Jung then goes on in this letter, as well as in his book *Memories, Dreams, Reflections,* to recount where the seeds of his doubts about Freud originated, which would lead to their breakup in 1913. This involved an event during the trip that he took with Freud to America in 1909 where he and Freud analyzed each other's dreams every day. "Freud had a dream. . . I interpreted it as best I could, but added that a great deal more could be said about it if he would supply me with some details from his private life. Freud [essentially responding that he could not submit to that analysis] replied: 'I cannot risk my authority!' . . . That sentence burned itself into my memory; and in it the end of our relationship was already foreshadowed."[38] Jung judged Freud, the self-proclaimed apostle of scientific candor, as having placed personal authority above truth.[39,40]

There is a secondary subplot in the final schism between Freud and Jung involving insubordination in IPA ranks of two other members of the core group in Vienna, Wilhelm Stekel and Alfred Adler. In letter 338J dated Dec. 18, 1912, Jung adds a new dimension to their war of words:

> Your technique of treating your pupils like patients is a *blunder.* In that way you produce either slavish sons or impudent puppies . . . I am objective enough to see through your little trick. You go around sniffing out all the symptomatic actions in your vicinity, thus reducing everyone to the level of sons and daughters who blushingly admit the existence of their faults. Meanwhile, you remain on top as the father, sitting pretty. For sheer obsequiousness nobody dares to pluck the prophet by the beard and inquire for once what would you say to a patient with a tendency to analyze the analyst instead of himself. You would certainly ask him: "Who's got the neurosis?"
>
> You see, my dear Professor, so long as you hand out this stuff, I don't give a damn for my symptomatic actions; they shrink to nothing in comparison with the formidable beam in my brother Freud's eye. I am not the least neurotic—touch wood! . . . You know, of course, how far a person gets with self-analysis: *not* out of his neurosis—just like you. If ever you should rid yourself of your complexes and stop playing the father to your sons and instead of aiming continually at their weak spots took a good look at your own for a change, then I will mend my ways and at one stroke uproot the vice of being in two minds about you . . . Adler and Stekel were taken in by your little tricks and reacted with childish insolence. I shall continue to stand by you publicly while maintaining my own views, but privately shall start telling you in my letters what I really think of you.[41]

Freud responds in letter 342F on Jan. 3, 1913, by pointing out Jung's penchant for erroneous assumptions before lowering the boom on their relationship:

Your allegation that I treat my followers like patients is demonstrably untrue. In Vienna, I am reproached for exactly the opposite. I am held responsible for the misconduct of Stekel and Adler; in reality I have not said one word to Stekel about his analysis since it was concluded some ten years ago, nor have I made any use of analysis with Adler, who was never my patient . . . In building your construction on this foundation you have made matters as easy for yourself as with your famous "Kreuzlingen gesture" . . . It is a convention among us analysts that none of us need feel ashamed of his own bit of neurosis. But one who while behaving abnormally keeps shouting that he is normal gives grounds for the suspicion that he lacks insight into his illness. Accordingly, I propose that we abandon our personal relations entirely. I shall lose nothing by it, for my only emotional tie with you has long been a thin thread—the lingering effect of past disappointments . . . I therefore say, take your full freedom and spare me your supposed "tokens of friendship."[42]

As for the content of letter 338J and his overall feelings about the breakup, Sigmund told Linda that he was misjudged by Jung. In fact, he still views the departures of Adler, Stekel, and most of all Jung as treasonous. Freud devoted his entire professional life to promoting psychoanalysis. This, he explains, was bigger than any individual member of IPA including himself. Because of its revolutionary nature, unity in the group was essential for it to move forward. Sigmund does not deny that the psychoanalytical movement was his "baby," or that he had paternal feelings toward the other members of the group. However, he steadfastly maintains that Jung confused differences of opinion, which were tolerated, with lack of intellectual honesty. He also strongly denies Jung's assertion that he treated his pupils like patients or like fault-infested sons and daughters who must acquiesce to the will of the father.[43]

OUR INTERVIEW WITH SIGMUND

In October 2008, Linda and I interviewed Sigmund for several days about his relationship with Jung. We could never have imagined the magnitude of metaphysical revelations that would follow. I opened the conversation with the following:

David: From an astrological perspective, there was an astonishing confluence of astrological correspondences between you and Carl Jung that governed the various phases of your complex connection, beginning as a close father-son relationship in 1907 and ending in an acrimonious breakup in 1913. I will read an excerpt from a book entitled *Psychology and Kabbalah* by Z'ev ben Shimon Halevi:

> Carl Jung was born in 1875 and died in 1961. His horoscope had Sun (*Tiferet*) in Leo, a fiery fixed sign, and Moon (*Yesod*) in Taurus, an earthly fixed sign. Thus his Moon corresponded with Freud's Taurus Sun, which encouraged a close relationship as long as Jung's ego reflected the light of Freud's self. However, as their Suns were squared, conflict would be inevitable among equals. This is exactly what happened when Jung went his own way and ceased to be, as Freud called him, "his crown prince." The split, it is interesting to note, as an event in Freud's pattern of fate, occurred in 1913 when Uranus, the planet of illumination and sudden change, with Mars the planet of confrontation and decision, were exactly opposed to Jung's Sun, precipitating a revolution in the House of Partnership. Their relationship, moreover, was not helped by Saturn, the weighty planet of law, conjuncting Freud's Moon later that year, as Mars did likewise to his Sun. The combination of these cosmic aspects could only bring about a fatal parting, as the principles, represented by the planets, reflected in their psyches brought their differences to a crisis head. Jung, having a fiery and equally fixed Sun or Self, would inevitably turn away from Freud's earthy approach and follow the more inspirational standpoint. This has been borne out by his life and work. This does not mean that he was Freud's superior. *They simply perceived different levels of reality.*[44]

David: Do the astrological configurations of your and Jung's birthdays have any significance to you regarding your relationship with him?

Sigmund: *As to the significance that you speak of in this book, yes, there is a definite relevance to it, not so much as a "cause" of the issues between me and Jung, but as an "effect" of a still deeper cause—that of our unresolved and primordial dysfunctional pattern that has existed in lifetime after lifetime. Therefore, playing itself out in our lifetime as Freud and Jung dictated by necessity that I had to be born on May 6, 1856, and that Jung had to be born on July 26, 1875. Our birthdays and their corresponding astrological signs were the necessary divine setup to allow our relationship to play itself out in accordance to the year that we met, 1907, as well as the year of our professional and personal breakup, 1913. These are* *"markers" to delineate the tendency for certain events to occur during specific passages of time.*

Were Jung and I to be of sufficient consciousness, it was not necessarily "set in stone" that what did happen actually had to occur. Consciousness can certainly overcome negative astrological markers. That's precisely the point! Alas, neither Jung nor I possessed the rarefied level of consciousness that was divinely required at that particular juncture in our soul journey together. This would have allowed us to rise above our sad and pathetic "repeating karmic pattern" and achieve a better, corrected result. Will Jung and I have to go through this dance again in another time and place as other people to rectify our primordial imbalance? God only knows, although it would not surprise me.

I will now explain to you a higher truth regarding what was really behind the breakup between Jung and me. The setting for the unfortunate outcome between us is deeply rooted in our past-life relationships together. Our coming together to again attempt to sort through our issues in our last incarnation as Freud and Jung was yet another failed effort to fully correct a primordial imbalance that has perpetually played itself out in previous lifetimes. However, before I get into specifics, I must provide you with information regarding the transmigration of souls that I have learned in the spirit world. You may think of it as a metaphysical background check.

First of all, it is important, when one is trying to understand the nature of the soul, to know that while your society today operates from the premise that "all men are created equal," from an upper world perspective, no two souls are created exactly "equal." Every soul has its own unique set of strengths and weaknesses that it copes with as it makes its way from lifetime to lifetime. Some souls are simply older than other souls and have reincarnated more times. There is a reason why Shakespeare was Shakespeare and why a common laborer is more likely to have been a common laborer in a past life than say . . . Shakespeare. Please do not construe from this that I do not have an egalitarian point of view, God forbid. Through hard work, any soul could theoretically raise his or her lot in life to become something quite different from what he or she was in a past life. It is just that there is a far greater likelihood for one to excel at the same skills or possess the same innate talents from lifetime to lifetime that are truly "God given." As I have since learned in the spirit world, one's God-given capabilities are in large part dependent upon where the "root of one's soul" on a reincarnated level originated from on the Tree of Life as described in Kabbalah.

If we take this one step further, it is also a simple fact of metaphysical life that powerful or famous people tend to have a far greater likelihood of having been powerful or famous souls in multiple past lifetimes. They tend to be older and more advanced souls that have more complicated tikkuns than other people. That is not to say that one could not be born into more humble origins and overcome many hardships as one ascended to become that powerful or famous soul. In fact, this very ability to overcome adversity is a common attribute of such souls.

Now that this is understood, I will now divulge the most important of these lifetimes and discuss its inner meaning as it relates to Jung and me. The revelation is as follows: The breakup between Jung and myself needs to be viewed as the continuation of an ancient Greek tragedy because, well, that is exactly what it is. I am the incarnation of the ancient Greek king Agamemnon and Jung is the incarnation of his antagonist, Achilles, the greatest of Greek warriors, as described in The Iliad *by Homer.* (See Figures 17-4 and 17-5.)

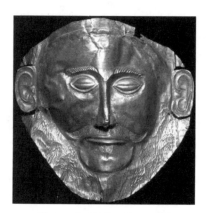

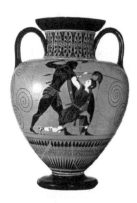

Figure 17-4. Death mask
of Agamemnon.

Figure 17-5. Achilles slaying
Penthesilea.

David: As Linda sat in trance, words spilling forth from her mouth, she started to convulse violently, shaking back and forth and from side to side. I have been blessed to witness this sort of physical outburst whenever a metaphysical bombshell like this has been dropped on us. Those who know me know I am rarely at a loss for words. However, I was speechless as I silently contemplated *the sheer historical importance of this revelation.* After regaining my composure a minute or two later, I spoke to Sigmund: "This is an astonishing revelation that will no doubt have serious implications for the fields of religion, psychology, and literature. We are stunned."

Sigmund: *This is precisely why I chose to discuss this story in this book instead of the other subjects you offered. I now understand the deeper meaning of the self-confession I wrote in* The Interpretation of Dreams *in 1899 where I stated that "an intimate friend and a hated enemy have always been necessary requirements of my emotional life."[45] My soul must have later recognized that I had found both* *of these opposite qualities in one person—Jung—because I had experienced just this phenomenon with him in our past lives as Agamemnon and Achilles and felt compelled to play it out again, hopefully with a better outcome. His soul must have felt the same way. Without knowing that he was talking about us, Jung was brilliantly prophetic when he stated, "When an inner situation is not made conscious, it happens outside as fate."*[46]

The implications of this revelation also have bearing on your healing work and bespeak of the importance of reincarnation and past-life research as well. Jung was essentially right about synchronicity[47]*, but we now need to carry it to the next level. Do you think for one moment that it is mere coincidence that both Jung and I were fascinated by mythology and its implications for psychoanalysis? Both of you visited my museum. Did you not see my wonderful collection of antiquities that are so connected to mythology? I am sure that you can imagine the time and money I spent collecting these pieces. I was mesmerized by their energy, although I myself did not truly understand why.*

When I received this information about Jung and myself when I went to the other side, I looked back on my recently completed life and all of a sudden, it all made an elegant sense. All my life I knew that I was different, even from my other siblings. My dear mother used to refer to me as "mein goldener Sigi" [my golden Sigmund], and although she loved all of her children, I was clearly her favorite. In fact, I attributed her special love as the source of my strength and inner confidence. However, as it turned out, there was more to it than that. I have never exactly said this in my writings, but as a boy I always felt as though I were royalty, anointed to do something truly important in my life, although I did not yet know what that would be. I did not want to appear to my siblings whom I loved as being haughty like the biblical figure Joseph appeared to his brothers, although in hindsight, I probably was a bit anyway.

In Search of Corroborating Evidence: Our Path to Verification

Freud's message was clear: As the two leading explorers of the conscious and unconscious mind, Freud and Jung were unable to achieve the transcendent awareness needed to understand that their expanding personal woes were directly tied to their own intense past-life connection. After the Agamemnon/Achilles revelation, Linda and my task was to research all aspects of the Freud/Jung relationship to determine if any historical or past-life clues existed that would corroborate this astonishing metaphysical detective story—clearly a higher level of reality—that Freud had just revealed to us. What followed were a series of tantalizing clues that revealed their connection to Greek history and mythology.

I must confess that the very first thing I did was Google the phrase "Jung and Achilles." What came up floored me. The full name of Jung's father, a Swiss pastor, was Paul *Achilles* Jung, as if to subliminally suggest that the metaphysical origin of his offspring Carl was "veiled" within his father's name! What makes this all the more amazing is that Achilles is a Greek name, not a Swiss or a German name. Although this, in itself, is not "proof" that Jung is the reincarnation of Achilles, I ask: *What are the statistical odds of this occurring?*

Sigmund next revealed one of several metaphysical "links" between him and King Agamemnon. He instructed Linda to locate a specific passage describing his feelings of being like royalty from *Freud & Jung: A Dual Introduction*, which was confirmed by a fast rightward swing of the pendulum.

> From his earliest years, Freud was a serious, dedicated student who was evidently expected by his teachers to make his mark in the world, and who himself acquired a conviction that he was destined to make some important contribution to knowledge. Family life revolved around his studies. He took his evening meal apart from the rest of the family and, because the sound of her practicing disturbed him, his sister Anna's piano was removed from the apartment by his parents.[48]

Freud then led us to what he states is a most important piece of corroborating evidence. In letter 87F from May 3, 1908, Freud asks a favor of Jung. After attending the First International Psychoanalytical Congress in Salzburg a week earlier, he observes that a rift is developing between Jung and another psychoanalyst, Karl Abraham, a man whom Freud regarded as being "of great worth." When Abraham presented his research on dementia at the Salzburg Congress, he neglected to mention or credit Jung for his earlier research. This oversight was highly irritating to Jung. Nonetheless, Freud urges a peaceful resolution, declaring that "there are so few of us that we must stick together." He then goes out of his way to comfort his anointed son and crown prince by declaring, "There can be no question of him replacing you in my eyes" and "you have every advantage over him."[49]

As if planning a strategic move on the battlefield, with a wink and a nod, he calls upon Jung to help him smooth over a potentially disruptive situation. Jung should set aside any ego issues and let Abraham take credit in his pronouncements about dementia. Jung should be helpful and consult with Abraham regarding their philosophical differences before Abraham's article is published in a peer journal. In essence, Freud is saying: Acquiesce now and real future merit will come to you in the "details" that will follow. In what can only now be described as the single most important Freudian slip ever made in history, Sigmund unmasks their true past-life identity when he declares to Jung, *"We mustn't quarrel when we are besieging Troy."*[50]

From these initial clues, we will now systematically build the case for this shocking revelation that confirms the existence of reincarnation.

Myth and the Dream State: The Forgotten Language of God

Sigmund next instructed Linda to look at his masterwork *The Interpretation of Dreams* as we searched for more clues to connect the metaphysical dots to this epic Greek tragedy. This book inaugurated the theory of dream analysis, which Freud called "the royal road to the understanding of unconscious mental processes."[51] As sleep dims our conscious mind, we enter various sleep cycles that lead to the dream state. Here, our imagination roams freely without interference from the conscious mind. While the significance of a particular dream can vary from person to person or even from culture to culture, Freud's stunningly original efforts to codify this knowledge into a universally accepted science remain one of the crowning achievements of his career.

In spite of their contentious breakup, Jung, in his obituary about Freud in 1939, called this work "epoch making" and "probably the boldest attempt that has ever been made to master the riddles of the unconscious psyche upon the apparently firm ground of empiricism."[52] Later he adds, "By evaluating dreams as the most important source of information concerning the unconscious processes, he gave back to mankind a tool that had seemed irretrievably lost."[53] Linda channeled the table of contents of *The Interpretation of Dreams* until Sigmund directed her to the following passage:

> I recognized the presence of symbolism in dreams from the very beginning. But it was only by degrees and as my experience increased that I arrived at a full appreciation of *its* extent and significance . . . Advances in psychoanalytic experience have brought to our notice patients who have shown a direct understanding of dream-symbolism of this kind to a surprising extent . . . This symbolism is not peculiar to dreams, but is characteristic of unconscious ideation . . . and it is to be found in folklore, and in popular myths [and] legends . . . to a more complete extent than in dreams.[54]

Sigmund: *There existed in many ancient cultures including the Hebrews, a belief that a dream could be a direct message from God that offered advice and instruction. I can assure you that the phenomenon of receiving divine or prophetic infor-*

mation in a dream is obviously so. As you know, the Hebrew patriarchs and prophets often received their information in a dream state. This practice was also common in ancient Egyptian and Greek royal society. There were specific temples where one could go to sleep and then have dreams where specific instructions or even a healing could come from the gods. You should know, Linda, that even Hippocrates used dreams as a means of diagnosis.

Sigmund then instructed Linda to look at *The Iliad*. When she channeled the table of contents, she was instructed to go to Book 2, where we stumbled upon what would prove to be a most unusual revelation. There, it is revealed that Zeus fulfills his promise to Thetis, mother of Achilles, to avenge the humiliation that Agamemnon has bestowed on Achilles by sending Agamemnon a false dream to bring about the false hope that he will shortly achieve a great victory over the Trojans. After we read the passage, Sigmund shook Linda, indicating she should go into trance and directly channel him as he had something else to communicate.

Sigmund: *The reason I had you look at that quote from* The Interpretation of Dreams *and Book 2 of* The Iliad *is that I now understand the reason I was able to have recognized this phenomenon "from the beginning." It was because it was so familiar to my soul. I had interpreted dreams before—as Agamemnon!"*

The deep fascination both Freud and Jung had for mythology as well as a direct connection to *The Iliad* can be found in their early work. A prime example is Freud's theory of the Oedipus complex. *Oedipus Rex* is a Greek tragedy by Sophocles involving the mythical character Oedipus who unknowingly fulfills a prophecy given to his father, King Laius, by an oracle. Oedipus would one day kill him and marry his mother Queen Jocasta of Thebes. In *The Iliad*, Homer briefly summarizes the story of Oedipus, including the patricide, incest, and Jocasta's subsequent suicide. In psychoanalytic theory, Freud uses the Oedipus complex to refer to the unconscious—often repressed emotions which center on the young boy's desire to possess his mother and eliminate the father during the "Oedipal phase" of libidinal and ego development. Our further research also revealed that Carl Jung believed that as females experienced desire for their fathers, they exhibited aggression toward their mothers. He named his theory the Electra complex after Electra, *the daughter of King Agamemnon!* In *The Iliad*, Electra wanted to kill her mother, who had helped plan the murder of her father.

Jung wrote more extensively about mythology than Freud. Early in his career, Jung came to the realization of the importance of myth in the psychoanalytical process. Sigmund directed us to letter 170J written in December 1909: "It has become quite clear to me that we shall not solve the ultimate secrets of neurosis and psychosis without mythology and the history of civilization."[55] In fact, the framework was already emerging for a "psychomythological" method to comprehend the mysteries of the unconscious mind. In letter 163F in November 1909, Freud writes encouragingly: "I am delighted with your mythological studies." He envisions a time when both Jung and he will apply the tenants of psychoanalysis to the study of mythology. "These things cry out for understanding and as long as the specialists won't help us, we shall have to do it ourselves."[56] He implies that psychoanalysts are better equipped to interpret the inner meaning of myths on the unconscious level than historians or mythologists.

Jung's Theory of Myth, Archetypes, and the Collective Unconscious

> **Sigmund:** *One of Jung's greatest accomplishments was showing us the importance of the mythological archetype and the collective unconscious as it relates to the practice of psychoanalysis. As Achilles was the greatest warrior of his era, so Jung was the greatest warrior for this aspect of psychoanalysis.*

In *The Mythological Unconscious*, author Michael Vannoy Adams underscores Jung's fascination with mythology and the impact it had on Jungian analysis with this example: "As he strove to complete *Transformation and Symbols of the Libido* in 1912, Jung compared himself to Hercules, trying to behead the Hydra: 'I am having grisly fights with the hydra of mythological fantasy and not all of its heads are cut off yet.' This is an example of what Jung was eventually to call his technique of *amplification,* the comparative method that establishes archetypal parallels with ancient myths and, on that basis, to interpret modern dreams and fantasies."[57] In this case, he is amplifying himself as the archetype of a monster-slaying hero.

> These mythological motifs are the structural elements of the unconscious that Jung called 'archetypes of the collective unconscious.' They appear in individuals with no prior knowledge of mythology. He believed that there are two dimensions of the unconscious, personal and collective, which could be studied either through mythology or through Jungian analysis.[58]

In fact, Freud biographer Peter Gay reveals Jung's interesting choice of language using this amplification technique to describe his feelings toward

Freud in the early years regarding the libido theory. "Despite his intellectual reservations, Jung . . . masked his true feelings for several years, even to himself. Freud remained 'like Hercules of old,' a human hero and higher god."[59]

Sigmund Freud's revisionist psychology of the 21st century has now come full circle. His newfound knowledge in the spirit world represents a radical departure from previous Freudian and Jungian thought. He now understands that an awareness of reincarnation, specifically that of his and Jung's reincarnation, was the critical missing link. *They themselves are the personification of psychic forces! They themselves are the archetypes! This is why these two souls had the God-given ability to be the world's two leading researchers of the conscious and unconscious mind. It was their karma to be brought together to attempt to rectify their complex soul connection.*

A Summary of Homer's Iliad as It Relates to Freud and Jung

Since they were written nearly 3,000 years ago by the Greek poet Homer, *The Iliad* and *The Odyssey* remain two of the most celebrated and popular stories ever written. (See "The Historical Accuracy of Homer's Iliad.") In the introduction to his recent translation of *The Iliad*, author Martin Hammond states: "*The Iliad* is the first substantial work of European literature, and has fair claim to be the greatest. The influence of *The Iliad* determined much in subsequent Greek literature, thought, and art, and thereby much that is central to the European tradition: it may fairly be described as the cornerstone of Western civilization."[62] The story of *The Iliad* is a long, complicated story interlaced with several subplots, involving gods, mortals, warrior combatants, and empires, that contain many subtle levels of historical, emotional, and metaphysical meaning. Our discussion here provides only the briefest outline of the story as it relates to the past life and historical relationship between Freud and Jung.

Book 1 of *The Iliad* begins in the tenth year of a protracted war with Troy. The cause of the war is the seduction and abduction of the beautiful Helen, the wife of King Menelaus of Sparta by the Trojan warrior named Paris, son of King Priam of Troy, while he is a guest of Menelaus. Homer implies that Helen is a willing accomplice in her abduction, which occurs while Menelaus is on business in Crete. She went on to become Helen of Troy, the woman whose face launched a thousand ships.

When word of Helen's abduction reaches Menelaus, he enlists the support of his brother, King Agamemnon of Mycenae. After diplomacy fails, the two brothers raise an expedition to conquer Troy by securing the support of

smaller Greek (Achaean) kingdoms. Their mission begins with great cama-
raderie, operating under an assumption that in exchange for their cooperation, they will receive a share of the spoils of war resulting from the
destruction of Troy and the cities surrounding it.

When the Greek troops under the leadership of Achilles raid the neighbor-
ing Trojan city of Thebes, a beautiful maiden named Chryseis is captured. As
part of the spoils of war, she is turned over to Agamemnon to serve as his concubine. The troops then raid another town, Lyrnessus, where another beautiful maiden named Briseis is captured and turned over to Achilles. Homer
places particular emphasis on the division of the spoils after such raids. He
describes how Achilles harbored deep resentment toward Agamemnon, feeling
that the prizes of war he received were never equal to those of Agamemnon.

The Historical Accuracy of Homer's Iliad

Much has been made of the fact that there is no way to scientifically validate the historical accuracy of events in the story of Agamemnon and Achilles in *The Iliad.* According to historian Barry Strauss in *The Trojan War,* "Spectacular new evidence makes it
likely that the Trojan War indeed took place. New excavations since 1988 constitute little less than an archaeological revolution, proving that Homer was right about [his
description of] the city . . . The recently discovered urban plan of Troy looks less like
that of a Greek [city] than of an Anatolian city . . . New documents suggest that most
Trojans spoke a language closely related to Hittite and that Troy was a Hittite ally. The
enemy of Troy's ally was the Greeks." Although Homer lived around five hundred years
after the Trojan War, Strauss observes, that these new archaeological "discoveries vin-
dicate the poet as a man who knew much more about the Bronze Age than had been
thought."[60]

Archaeological evidence shows that the Trojan War probably took place around
1200 BC. In describing Homer's depiction of the war, Strauss states: "He tells the story
in two long poems, *The Iliad* or Story of Ilion [Troy] and *The Odyssey* or Story of
Odysseus. According to Homer, the Trojan War lasted ten years [and] pitted the wealthy
city of Troy and its allies against a coalition of all of Greece. It was the greatest war in
history, involving at least 100,000 men in each army as well as 1,186 Greek ships. It
featured heroic champions on both sides. It was so important that [it is said that] the
Olympian gods played an active role. Troy was a magnificent city and impregnable
fortress . . . "[61] Linda consistently channels that there indeed was a Troy, a Mycenaean
king named Agamemnon, and an Greek (Achaean) warrior named Achilles.

An old man named Chryses, who is father of Chryseis and priest of the god Apollo, appears before Agamemnon and begs for the release of his daughter, offering to pay an enormous ransom. He is the archetype of an innocent whose life has been ruined by war or who has suffered the loss of a son or a daughter while maintaining his dignity. Agamemnon, however, rejects his appeal and dismisses him with deliberate cruelty. Following this, Chryses prays to Apollo for help. Apollo's response is swift revenge; a plague is brought upon the Greek army that results in the death of many soldiers.

After ten days of suffering, Achilles can no longer wait for Agamemnon to act to end the plague and risks usurping his authority by calling for an assembly of the army. He asks a powerful soothsayer, Calchas, to determine the source of Apollo's anger. Calchas fears retribution from Agamemnon and asks Achilles to guarantee his safety, which he does. Calchas then reveals that by virtue of Agamemnon's refusal to return Chryseis to her father, Apollo brought the plague as a strategic and vengeful move against the Greek forces. Agamemnon flies into a rage, furious that he has been publicly named as being responsible for the deadly pestilence. In a bout of irrational, self-obsessed arrogance, he insists that he will surrender Chryseis, his rightful prize of war, but only in exchange for Briseis, the war prize of Achilles.

The Greeks are aware that they can never hope to conquer Troy without the help of Achilles, the greatest warrior in the world. The situation is compounded, however, by the fact that Achilles had been warned earlier by the oracle that if he participated in the Trojan War he was fated to live a short life. The incredible intensity of his life was due, in part, to the fact that he knew he had little time in which to earn eternal fame.

This, along with Agamemnon's ultimatum, is enough to push Achilles over the top. Known for his quarrelsome temper, Achilles threatens to abandon the army and take his people, the Myrmidons, back home to Phthia. In Book 1, verses 149–171, Achilles sets forth his grievances, claiming that while he is fighting for the honor of Agamemnon and Menelaus, the Trojans have never harmed him. In addition, while he does all the fighting, Achilles is given an unfair split of the rewards, which Agamemnon now threatens to take away from him. In response, Agamemnon announces before the whole Greek army that the services of its greatest warrior are no longer needed and that as king he will do as he wants with Achilles' hard-won property.

This humiliating public attack on Achilles' importance to the Greek army, following Agamemnon's seizure of what is rightfully his, drives Achilles to announce the withdrawal of all his troops from battle. He not only refuses to fight but also is determined to return home with his troops as soon as possible. He contemplates killing Agamemnon with his sword if he should come and take Briseis, but the Goddess Athena is able to restrain him. What is significant is that no Greek soldiers object to Achilles walking out. It is obvious to all that Agamemnon is clearly wrong.

By the time *The Iliad* progresses to Book 9, the tables have turned considerably. With Achilles on the sidelines, the Greek army has sustained heavy losses. Agamemnon, ever the strategic pragmatist when necessary, relents and agrees to offer financial compensation to Achilles if he will return to the battlefield. However, by this time Achilles has also hardened his position, and no incentive will induce him to fight. He repeats his original accusation to the Greek embassy—that he does all the fighting while Agamemnon reaps the lion's share of rewards. Now, however, he goes even further. No amount of material compensation that Agamemnon can offer is enough to overcome his public humiliation. Even a visit from his closest friends and advisers cannot get Achilles to budge from his position. Unaccustomed to such insolence, Agamemnon is stunned by this rebuff. The Greek warrior Diomedes observes that Achilles has never been anything other than his own man; he will fight when he wants, and nothing can be done about it.

Even Patroclus, Achilles' closest friend and confidant, reminds him that a hero is supposed to benefit his people. Achilles has let anger, pride, and selfishness overwhelm his judgment. His absence from the battlefield serves no purpose. "You and your disastrous greatness—what will future generations have to thank you for if you do nothing to prevent the Greeks' humiliating destruction?" Seeking full revenge is now his only motive, as "Agamemnon must pay back the whole heart-rending insult." This is why the Greek philosopher Aristotle called Achilles "a good man, but a paradigm of obstinacy."[63] While the karmic consequences of this obstinacy are bad for the Greeks, they are soon to prove catastrophic for Achilles.

In Book 11, Achilles miscalculates that the Greeks will beg him to come back, which they do not. In Book 14, after the Trojan warrior Hector sets fire to a Greek ship, Achilles clearly understands that his presence is needed to turn the tide of battle. Torn between this understanding and his stubbornness, he opts to send Patroclus to fight in his place, where he is tragically killed in battle. At his burial, Achilles has a tentative reconciliation with Agamemnon.[64] In Book 18, a thoroughly grief-stricken Achilles not only avenges Patroclus' death by brutally slaying Hector, but then proceeds to mutilate his body in a grotesque manner.

Achilles realizes that his decision to kill Hector amounts to signing his own death warrant. The oracle's prophecy of his early demise will now be fulfilled, although that does not actually occur in *The Iliad*. Subsequent Greek myths describe the death of Achilles. This occurred in spite of the fact that, according to legend, Achilles was invincible as a warrior because his mother had dipped him in the River Styx, rendering him immortal except where she held him by the heel. Later Paris, the brother of Hector, discovers this vulnerability and shoots a poison arrow into Achilles' heel, leading to his death. This is the origin of the expression "Achilles heel," which refers to a person's vulnerability.

Achilles stands by his belief: It's worth sacrificing his life to take revenge on the person who killed his beloved companion. In the end, he forsakes everlasting glory, choosing death as he holds himself responsible for Patroclus's death. Homer goes out of his way to emphasize how far Achilles has plunged off the scale of normal human behavior. Achilles' excessive rage and desire for revenge are more important than his own life or the everlasting glory he had earlier desired.

As part of his self-serving desire to avenge the death of Patroclus, Achilles ends his refusal to fight. In order to lead a united Greek army into battle to destroy Hector and Troy, he accepts an uneasy truce with the pragmatic Agamemnon, who still needs Achilles to wage war against the Trojans. For his part, Agamemnon returns Briseis to Achilles, along with other numerous gifts. However, excessive pride and anger at Agamemnon still permeate Achilles' psyche. Their issues with each other remain unresolved, but not enough so they cannot get on with the war effort. Though not perfect, this reconciliation dissipates the negative energy between them so Achilles and Agamemnon can focus on their mutual enemy Troy. It also draws to a close the focus of *The Iliad* on their inner battles so that Achilles can focus on upcoming battles.

Agamemnon/Freud and Achilles/Jung Psychoanalyzed

In *The Interpretation of Dreams*, Freud revealed that the language of metaphor and allegory are important components in dream analysis. He now declares that these same components are essential in analyzing the higher abstract truths behind reincarnation. Using this same logic, his breakup with Jung closely parallels the deteriorating relationship between Agamemnon and Achilles. The struggles between them as Freud and Jung were an unsuccessful "karmic replay" needed to resolve the same type of interpersonal dynamics that existed between Agamemnon and Achilles. What is most astonishing is that these personality quirks and defects that plagued Agamemnon and Achilles have amazing parallels in Freud and Jung. Their attempt to achieve a mutual soul correction, which occurs through a process in Kabbalah called tikkun, was played out between 1907 and 1913 in line with their astrological predispositions.

Of course, the settings, occupations, and issues of the reincarnated participants are entirely different except for the fact that both sets of individuals exhibit similar personalities and are in positions of leadership. Clearly, they were powerful beings who left a lasting impression on the world stage in their respective lifetimes. Agamemnon and Achilles' world was one of conquest, justice, and survival, while Freud and Jung mined the psychic depths of the conscious and unconscious mind.

The manner in which their friendship ended was typical of both sets of lives. The unfolding of *The Iliad* reveals that both Agamemnon and Achilles had incredibly stubborn personality traits, which led to repeated catastrophes for the Greek army and ultimately themselves as well. The breakup of Freud and Jung in the early 20th century was a tragic loss for the fledgling psychoanalytical movement as its two most brilliant innovators chose to go their separate ways. Freud's self-fulfilling prophecy about not quarreling "when we are besieging Troy"—the archetype of ignorance of the human psyche—became a reality. To establish his case for the scientific validation of reincarnation, Sigmund now summarizes five extraordinary parallels between Agamemnon/Freud and Achilles/Jung.

Parallel 1. Interpersonal Dynamics. Of Jung's early years with Freud, Storr and Stevens state: "Freud needed a 'son' no less than Jung needed a 'father,' but the kind of son that Freud wanted was one who would be willing to defer unconditionally to authority and to participate, without modification, in the doctrines and principles of his rule . . . His belief in the correctness of his theories was absolute, and this made him so intolerant of dissent that he usually ended up provoking it. He was a strange amalgam of autocrat and masochist; as he once admitted to Jung, his emotional life demanded the existence of an intimate friend and a hated enemy, and not infrequently, he encountered both in the same person."[65]

A similar dynamic manifested in the relationship between Agamemnon and Achilles. The "father and son" dynamic paralleling Freud and Jung existed in the sense that Agamemnon was the king/father who formed a movement among other Greek nations to conquer Troy, which was how he came to meet Achilles, the famous, heroic warrior. Agamemnon knew that he could never capture Troy without Achilles' help. In the early years of the Trojan War, Achilles was his greatest warrior/son, loyally committed to the cause.

However, Achilles became increasingly frustrated over what he viewed as the inequitable division of the spoils of war between Agamemnon and him.

As the founder and leader, Freud devoted his life to perpetuating the idea that his psychoanalytical movement (Greek army) must be regarded as the leading scientific approach to understanding human behavior. Freud sensed early on that Jung was a kindred spirit, a superior intellectual warrior who would work under the watchful father/king in accord with Freud's basic theories to achieve victory and immortality in the battle over ignorance of the human psyche (Troy). When Freud appointed Jung president of the International Psychoanalytical Association, Ernest Jones wrote: "Jung, with his commanding presence and soldierly bearing, [initially] looked the part of a leader."[66]

However, according to Storr and Stevens, "Although Jung basked in Freud's approval and was flattered to be a worthy successor to him, he knew that he could not endorse Freud's ideas in their entirety. Nor could he sacrifice his intellectual integrity to a set of dogmas in the way that his father had done."[67] Nevertheless, in the early years he acquiesced to Freud's desire that he should take on the responsibility of being the first president of the IPA, all the while affirming his loyalty to Freud and his theories. As his loyal follower, Jung crouched in the famous Weimar photo, deferring to the shorter Freud and showing respect to his father/king.

In the same way, in the early years of the Trojan War, Achilles acquiesced and deferred to Agamemnon's decisions about splitting the spoils of war. However, Achilles quietly harbored feelings of not being sufficiently appreciated for his efforts as a warrior and felt shortchanged by what he perceived was an unfair split. As the loyal warrior, he had been trained to defer to the king until the arrogance exhibited by Agamemnon over the incident with Chryseis and Briseis pushed him over the top.

Like Achilles with Agamemnon, Jung was frustrated by Freud's unwillingness to accept the validity of his version of the libido theory. This was further inflamed by resentments aroused by the infamous "Kreuzlingen gesture" and his misinterpretation of Freud's understanding of Jung's version of the libido theory (letter 329F). Although Jung did apologize to Freud at the Munich Conference in 1912, this reconciliation was short-lived. Letter 330J shows that Jung had paranoid feelings that paralleled Achilles' feelings when he writes that Freud "undervalued his work by a very wide margin," making him incapable of understanding it.[68] Achilles/Jung suffered from a growing paranoia that made him jump to conclusions and misinterpret the intent of Agamemnon/Freud.

Parallel 2. Similar Personality Attributes as Leaders. Both sets of figures exhibited similar strengths and weaknesses in their respective leadership roles. Like Agamemnon, Freud had the skills required to run an organization. Neither of them ever lost sight of the big picture, whether it was establishing a network of smaller Greek kingdoms to collectively fight Troy or establishing an international organization of like-minded individuals to further the cause of psychoanalysis.

As Storr and Stevens note in *Freud & Jung,* "To Jung, the purpose of life was individuation—that the realization of one's own potential was obtained by following one's own perception of the truth to become a whole person. If he was to keep faith with himself, he had to go his own way: it would have been impossible for him to spend his life playing second fiddle in a two-man band."[69] But the characteristic of wanting to go it alone translated into a skill set that was different than Freud's.

As Roazen observes in *Freud and His Followers,* "Jung did not try to be the organizer that Freud was and did not really like organizations, his own or anyone else's . . . Jung repeatedly felt burdened by the organizational demands Freud put on him . . ."[70] Freud repeatedly chided him for neglecting his responsibilities as president of IPA. After their falling out, Freud described Jung as "a person who was incapable of tolerating the authority of another, but who was still less capable of wielding it himself, and whose energies were relentlessly devoted to the furtherance of his own interests."[71]

Achilles' strong suit was as a warrior in the trenches; he was not a man of diplomacy and nuanced negotiation. To Achilles, the purpose of life was to live by his principles and convictions, no matter what the consequences. His pride would not allow him to be induced by financial reward. Agamemnon's attempts to reason with him regarding the ultimate goal of the Greek army to defeat Troy fell on deaf ears. Although they eventually reconcile to fight against Troy, Achilles' marched to his own drummer. His obstinacy leads to the death of many Greek soldiers, his closest friend Patroclus, and ultimately himself.

Parallel 3. A Strong Temper. It is well documented that Jung had a strong temper. He embodied the astrological profile of Aries and Mars; his personality was governed by urgency so that he pursued all things with a self-righteous fury. His temper erupted whenever he perceived a slight or was crossed. He resented Freud's followers after his separation from psychoanalysis, claiming they ruined his practice for years, while he spread stories about Freud's neurosis.[72] Amazing, Jung's most serious character flaws were the

same as Achilles'—explosive anger and excessive pride rooted in his principles and convictions. The opening lines of *The Iliad* reveal his rage:

> Anger—sing, goddess, the anger of Achilles, son of Peleus, the accursed
> anger, which brought the Greeks endless suffering and sent the mighty
> souls of many warriors to Hades, leaving their bodies as carrion for the dogs
> and a feast for the birds; and Zeus' purpose was fulfilled. It all began when
> Agamemnon lord of men and godlike Achilles quarreled and parted.[73]

Achilles' anger so poisons his outlook that he is unable to act with nobil-
ity and integrity, blinding him to the bigger picture. As a result, he is willing
to endanger the lives of those closest to him as well as subvert the safety of the
entire army to achieve emotional blackmail over Agamemnon.

It is interesting to note a similar pattern that Freud/Agamemnon exhibited toward Jung/Achilles. In the later Freud/Jung letters, Freud is still
attempting to repair their relationship, repeatedly offering olive branches,
while the tone of Jung's letters is increasingly acrimonious. In Chapter 9 of
The Iliad, with the Greek troops suffering heavy losses, Agamemnon pragmat-
ically tries to reason with Achilles, offering him financial incentives to return.
Achilles angrily rejects the overture.

Parallel 4. Convictions and Principles. In *Memories, Dreams, Reflections,* Jung
reveals that the essence of his problems with Freud was twofold.

1. As mentioned earlier, during a period in 1909 where they analyzed each
other's dreams, Freud chose not to reveal the *nth degree of extremely private and
sensitive information about his private life because he felt it would risk his authority.
Jung dismissed Freud's perspective, claiming he "was placing personal authority
above truth."*[74]

> **Sigmund:** *While Jung may believe that certain details I refrained from sharing
> affected his analysis, these private details would not have led to any breakthroughs.
> Additionally, the potential damage to me as leader of the psychoanalytical move-
> ment if certain information was revealed outweighed all other considerations.*

Given all they had done together, Freud, whose life was otherwise an
open book, still feels that Jung completely overreacted, using this as an excuse
to jump ship.

2. This concerns their ongoing disagreement over the libido theory. Jung
writes, "I can still recall vividly how Freud said to me, 'My dear Jung, prom-

ise me never to abandon the sexual theory. That is the most essential thing of all. You see, we must make a dogma of it, an unshakable bulwark.' In some astonishment I asked him, 'A bulwark—against what?' To which he replied, 'Against the black tide of mud . . . of occultism.' [Jung's problem with Freud's position is that it] no longer has anything to do with scientific judgment; only with a personal power drive."[75]

Jung continues, "This is the thing that struck at the heart of our friendship. I knew that I would never be able to accept such an attitude. What Freud seems to mean about 'occultism' was virtually everything that philosophy and religion, including the rising contemporary science of parapsychology, had learned about the psyche. To me the sexual theory was just as occult, that is to say, just as unprovable a hypothesis . . . Sexuality evidently meant more to Freud than to other people. For him it was something to be religiously observed . . . One thing was clear: Freud, who had always made much of his irreligiosity, had now constructed a dogma. . . ."[76]

Sigmund: *I do not deny Jung's accusation about me, but regrets will not change the past. The more important point here is that the drive for power at the expense of what Jung considers to be a higher psychoanalytical truth is, in an abstract way, an affront that is similar to the righteous indignation that Achilles suffered at the hands of Agamemnon. Achilles' abandonment of the Greek army was due to his personal squabble with Agamemnon over women captives who became their respective booty as the spoils of war. The oracle revealed that the plague decimating the Greek army was due to Agamemnon's refusal to return his female captive Chryseis back to her father Chryses. For the good of the mission, he finally relented, but only on the condition that Achilles would have to give his concubine Briseis to Agamemnon in exchange. I now recognize that Chryseis represents the archetype of my libido theory of sexuality as the key driving force behind all forms of human neurosis and Briseis represents Jung's concept of a libido theory, which was both an expansion of and a departure from my perspective. By taking Breseis, metaphorically, I isolated Jung and his theories from IPA.*

However, our lives had to move forward. In the same way that the core focus of The Iliad *after Chapter 19 shifts from the conflicts of Agamemnon and Achilles to the upcoming battles of Achilles in the continued war effort against Troy, by 1914 Jung was no longer the central irritant of my professional life. Though professionally and personally painful to Jung, he thankfully saw the wisdom of resigning from IPA, which then became the sounding board with faithful adherents I had always desired for my vision of psychoanalysis. Though our issues remained unresolved, the severity of the negativity between us waned, and we got on with our lives. From a metaphoric perspective, I released Briseis back to him so he could pursue his own version of psychoanalysis.*

A parallel situation occurred between Agamemnon and Achilles following the death of Patroclus when a reconciliation occurred and Briseis was returned to Achilles. The next chapters of Jung's and my professional life found us moving away from each other on divergent paths, although our common goal was the same—battling Troy (ignorance of the human psyche), albeit in our own separate ways. In the final analysis of how this relates to our earlier incarnation, the astrologically based observation of what Halevi wrote is true: Jung and I perceived different levels of reality.

Parallel 5. A Willingness to Go Down with the Ship. In his book *Memories, Dreams, Reflections,* Jung states, "When I was working on my book about the libido [*Transformation and Symbols of the Libido*] and approaching the end of the chapter 'The Sacrifice,' I knew in advance that its publication would cost me my friendship with Freud. For I planned to set down in it my own conception[s] . . . in which I differed from Freud . . . After the break with Freud, all my friends and acquaintances dropped away. My book was declared to be rubbish; I was a mystic, and that settled the matter. But I had foreseen my isolation and harbored no illusion about the reactions of my so-called friends . . . I had known that everything was at stake and that I had to take a stand for my convictions. I realized that the chapter, 'The Sacrifice,' *meant my own sacrifice.*"[77]

> **Sigmund:** *Writing the chapter entitled "The Sacrifice" is the metaphysical equivalent of fulfillment of the prophecy that the oracle told to Achilles: If he went to war, he would gain great glory, but he would die at a young age. When Achilles killed Hector to avenge the death of Patroclus, he was well aware that the consequences of this action would ultimately result in his own death.*

According to Storr and Stevens, "For Jung, the consequences [of the breakup with Freud] were almost as dire, for he fell into a protracted 'state of disorientation,' at times verging on psychosis, which lasted four or five years."[78] According to Sigmund, this parallels the intense despair that Achilles felt following the death of Patroclus that caused him not only to avenge his death by slaying Hector, but then to mutilate Hector's body.

Jung's "Achilles heel" is his overly inflated ego that manifests through blistering indignation and excessive pride when he perceives his honor has been slighted. This causes him to abandon the Greek army/psychoanalytical movement and go his own way despite unfortunate consequences for the movement, Freud, and himself.

Clash over Public Perception of Personal Honor

The clash between Agamemnon and Achilles highlights one of the most dominant aspects of the ancient Greek system of values: the vital importance of public perception of personal honor. Both Agamemnon and Achilles believed that their honor was compromised by their having to forgo their war prizes, the female captives. Their immature and selfish decisions blinded them to a greater good, forcing them to prioritize their respective individual glories over the well-being of the Greek forces. Although their pride started with noble intentions, it became sabotaged by emotion and degenerated into pettiness and irrationality.

The clash between Freud and Jung was also largely over public perception of personal honor. Freud like Agamemnon displayed arrogance toward Jung when his libido theory (his woman) was disputed first by the prevailing scientific community and ultimately by Jung. As his final letters to Freud demonstrate, Jung, like Achilles, flew into a rage and jettisoned the entire Greek army/psychoanalytical movement that Freud had created. At various times in their relationship, they both chose to prioritize their individual glories (their theories) over the well-being of the Greek army/unified psychoanalytical movement.

Sigmund: *The ultimate point to be learned from the Freud/Jung breakup concerns the incredible significance of reincarnation and the tikkun process in shaping not only the personalities but in resolving deep-seated conflicts within personal relationships. Clearly, from the beginning both Jung and I had mutually vested interests to be close professional associates. In him I found an intellectual giant and the heir apparent/prodigal son to take over psychoanalysis when I retired. In me he found an intellectual equal and totally original thinker who fulfilled the needs vacated by his own father who did not share his son's enthusiasm and passion for the same things.*

When two people give forth their best intellectual and emotional efforts to resolve a conflict and they reach an impasse, as did Jung and I, the principal blockage is often due to an unresolved past-life issue that is rearing its head, crying out for resolution. In both sets of past lives, as the unresolved negative energies waned due to life circumstances, the metaphysical window of opportunity to rectify those negative emotions did as well—to be continued in the spirit world and/or another lifetime. I hope that I am speaking for Jung when I candidly admit that our mutual massive egos blocked our ability to achieve a higher consciousness needed to resolve those negative emotions that originated from that tumultuous lifetime.

THE NEWFOUND SPIRITUAL LIFE OF SIGMUND FREUD

Sigmund has asked us to convey that his principal misunderstandings revolved around his lack of awareness about the pervasive influence that God has over the development of the psyche. While acknowledging that he did make an important contribution to the understanding of the human psyche, Sigmund prefers, these days, to stress the level of spiritual disconnect that one endures when unhealthy thinking from the dark side overwhelm a person's emotions. This admittedly is a radical departure for him, as he showed very little inclination toward spirituality within the context of Judaism in his lifetime. He has also stressed to us that the study of reincarnation is vital to understanding the healing of the psyche. His growth and personal transformation in the spirit world have been nothing less than extraordinary. His view of the future development of the human psyche is focused on the spiritual revelations derived from the spiritual science of Kabbalah. This extraordinary channeled exchange between Sigmund and Linda sums up his principal regrets:

> **Sigmund:** *In particular, I have a very strong regret that I lived my life as an agnostic.* [Linda saw him wringing his hands in a gesture of despair when he said this.] *Humans do not understand just how important it is to receive divine light. This is a necessary component to alleviate human suffering. This is an issue that I am still repairing after all this time.* [In a despondent mood he turned to Linda and asked:] *How can you repair that which has been lost? When you haven't utilized prayer in your life, you must literally begin anew in the spirit world.*

David: I have a follow-up question regarding any negative repercussions that have occurred in the spirit world arising from your agnostic beliefs that bordered on atheism. It is known that you had to endure more than thirty operations during your life due to cancer of the jaw and mouth. It is reported that at the end of your life, you asked your personal physician, Dr. Max Schur, to help end your suffering, which he did when you were in great pain and close to death. Linda has channeled that in your case this was ethically correct because the cancer was so advanced that to endure more suffering would have served no purpose, as you were close to death. What are your feelings about assisted suicide if a person is sick or merely unhappy over his or her life but not close to death?

> **Sigmund:** *I do not deny that I reached such a low point toward the end of my life where I sought to just put an end to it all by exploring the option of assisted*

suicide with my doctor. I had experienced extreme physical discomfort and pain for a considerable period of time, and frankly, I was very tired of it. Let me state that I clearly understand how people can be so racked with pain that they seek what they perceive as an easy way out. However, as I have learned in the spirit world, people don't have the right to "play God" with their own or another person's life. I also learned the hard way that sometimes, as part of a soul's correction process, a person has to physically suffer in accordance with the sins and ethical blunders he or she made in life. However, if people are only suffering physically, but not in the actual process of dying, they or their physicians do not have the spiritual right to take their own life. The medical ethics behind assisted suicide are really a question of timing.

In my case, thank God, the decision of Dr. Schur, my daughter Anna, and me to end my life by morphine injection was prolonged until I was near the moment of death. What he did by injecting me at that point did not cross a line where the doctor was playing God with my life. Having said that, I am very relieved that Dr. Schur did not inject me weeks earlier when the thought had crossed my mind. Linda, I have had enough to rectify in the spirit world, thank you, without adding the additional burden of the terrible tikkun of suicide.

A FINAL REVELATION: CARL JUNG APPEARS

I must report an amazing channeling session with Linda as we reviewed the final editing of Chapter 16 in late October 2009. As mentioned earlier, with really important information, such as the revealment of the Freud/Jung parallel relationship to that in *The Iliad*, Linda can actually hear Sigmund speaking to her. However, this process involves tremendous concentration and is a bit exhausting for her. When asking for guidance on other sorts of information where a yes/no answer suffices, she uses the pendulum, as it is easier on her nervous system. For the chapters that involved Sigmund, Linda called on him to assist in reviewing the manuscript paragraph by paragraph before it was turned in to the publisher. When we got to the section on B vitamins, Linda asked Sigmund what he thought of it. The pendulum started moving in a familiar but unusual pattern, indicating an answer other than yes or no. Suddenly Linda got a small shake, and she blurted out that another spirit had come to speak.

It was Carl Jung himself! Linda had previously asked Sigmund to discuss his relationship with Jung in the spirit world, but he seemed reluctant to talk about him. As odd a theatrical entrance as it may seem, Jung had come to offer advice on how to improve aspects of the B vitamin section! After getting over the initial shock of his arrival into our world, I asked him what he thought about nutraceutical approaches to dealing with emotional issues. He said he "found the whole subject fascinating." (Therefore, both Freudians and Jungians can unite behind the subject matter in the previous two chapters as it is wholeheartedly endorsed by their respective leaders!) Jung also volunteered that he endorsed the information contained in this chapter. And he expressed remorse for the psychotic behavior of Achilles and for the excessive temper he exhibited as Jung.

I then asked Jung if he and Freud had "patched things up" in the spirit world. He responded by saying it was "a work in progress." He and Sigmund were "communicating with each other in a cooperative manner, but that issues between them still remained!" This startling revelation opens up a whole can of metaphysical worms that we will explore in the future, but it certainly indicates that issues, at least between these two souls, continue to be worked on in the spirit world. Linda and I came away with the impression that the two of them have a certain timeframe within which they must resolve their issues in the spirit world; otherwise they will have to reincarnate and try again on earth.

CHAPTER 18

The Metaphysical Database

I don't want to achieve immortality through my work.
I want to achieve it through not dying.

I do not believe in an afterlife,
although I am bringing a change of underwear . . .
—WOODY ALLEN

THE METAPHYSICAL DATABASE CONTAINS information that further differentiates Linda's gift from that of other medical intuitives or psychics of whom we are aware. She uses it as a framework to communicate with archangels, angels, and spirits on a variety of subjects, including reincarnation and past-life research, clearance of earthbound spirits, and identification of one's guardian angel, a concept discussed in Chapter 19.

Linda's work in this area is, in my opinion, even more fascinating than medical channeling, although if one is sick, putting out the fire is always the first order of business. Nevertheless, when clients experience the miracle of healing based on information derived from angels and spirits, they invariably wish to continue receiving spiritual and emotional guidance in other areas of their life. Through astral traveling into the angelic realms, Linda is able to receive information on the soul journey of her clients. This often provides a more satisfying explanation of the unconscious drives and motivations behind a person's behaviors. It may also reveal the source of his or her strengths, weaknesses, and aptitudes. This sometimes surreal information may provide answers to illogical feelings that have haunted an individual for his or her entire life.

REINCARNATION: THE SCIENCE OF SOUL SURVIVAL

In spite of the overwhelming preponderance of evidence showing the validity of the Agamemnon/Freud and Achilles/Jung past life connection in the
previous chapter, some readers may still find the concept of past lives hard to
fathom. The fact remains that the greatest advances in science have failed to
answer the question of whether a soul exists. And if so, the paramount question remains: Do any aspects of one's soul or personality survive death? My
desire to explore this spiritual issue stems from my belief that Linda's gift is an
extraordinary research vehicle that can lead to the acceptance of reincarnation
as scientific fact. If society reaches the point where the medical information
that Linda channels is deemed to be completely objective, then our hope is
that information she channels on reincarnation will be taken seriously as well.

The angels have revealed that we have reached a linear timeframe and
spiritual juncture in human history where our knowledge of reincarnation is
set to expand exponentially. When Linda gets information on past lives, it is
important to realize that this comes from the same "spigot" as the medical
information. This makes Linda invaluable not only as a medical researcher,
but also as a metaphysical researcher revealing past-life information. Never
before in our modern era have we had such a unique opportunity to pierce
the veil of what lies just over the rainbow of our physical world. What is clear
from her work is that there is compelling evidence for the existence of nonphysical dimensions outside the normal spatial realities for what is commonly
referred to as an afterlife.

The term "afterlife" in traditional Western religious terms implies a place
where souls ostensibly go for all eternity. Reincarnation, however, asserts that
a soul experiences an "interlife," meaning that it goes somewhere and has
additional growth experiences between lives before returning to earth in
another body. Until now this type of information has primarily been the
province of the Eastern religious traditions of Buddhism and Hinduism. However, many people are unaware that reincarnation is also central to the esoteric philosophy of Kabbalah, the religion within a religion of the Jewish faith.
The spiritual discoveries that have been revealed to Linda, coupled with our
research in Kabbalah, have convinced us that we are on the cusp of expanding
the understanding of reincarnation—a new science of soul survival where the
knowledge of past lifetimes will reveal with clarity the roles and purposes of
our specific souls.

The message from the angels is clear: The prevailing philosophical framework through which we view the cycles of life and death must undergo a thorough overhaul as a necessary prerequisite for the coming new spiritual

consciousness. Linda has channeled that the gateway to this new understanding of reincarnation as a science will come in two parts. One part is through Kabbalah, the oldest spiritual doctrine that God taught His angels before creating humanity. The other is through a new, evolving, spiritual genetic science, still in its infancy, that explores the metaphysical and physical relationships between the name *Yahweh,* made up of the four Hebrew letters that are transliterated as *yud, heh, vav,* second *heh,* and the four building-block organic compounds called nucleotides—adenine (A), cytosine (C), thymine (T), and guanine (G) that make up DNA.

Why Understanding Reincarnation Is Critical to the Coming Consciousness

A belief system that is closed to the possibility of reincarnation only allows for a limited present-tense existence. Religions have been unable to provide completely soul-satisfying explanations as to why bad things happen to good people. Clergy may offer inadequate platitudes that dance around the issue, actively discouraging a deeper investigation for bewildered and disheartened parishioners. This, in turn, leads to spiritual dissatisfaction that compels many to seek answers outside religion, often in the realm of psychology. While this pathway to the unconscious mind can provide meaningful answers in certain areas of human existence, it falls short of explaining inexplicable human tragedies that are outside the realm of its theories.

Psychology cannot explain why a child is born with birth defects or why siblings who were born from the same parents and raised in the same environment with the same values could turn out so differently. It is of limited value in explaining why certain evil people can flourish and why certain righteous people endure lives of hardship. Psychology only provides marginal help in explaining why certain people get cancer or repeat the same patterns of negative behavior for no apparent reason. Nor can it fully explain how someone of humble origins could grow up to be a famous talk show host or even President of the United States.

How can that married couple, so seemingly opposite, possibly stand being married to each other? Or why does your best friend, so talented in certain aspects of life, exhibit self-destructive behaviors with predictable and disappointing outcomes? Why did your Uncle Jerry admit that he has had homosexual feelings for as long as he can remember? Does genetics or psychology hold the only answers in a family where that sexual preference was unknown? Many differing schools of thought within the field of psychology have flourished since Sigmund Freud developed his groundbreaking theories in the late 1800s. Can any of them explain, for example, why the Kennedy family has endured so much personal tragedy? The bottom line is that until humanity understands what happens to the soul following the death of the physical body, it will never be able to answer such questions.

THE PURPOSE OF REINCARNATION FOR THE SOUL

The soul is on a spiritual journey from lifetime to lifetime, descending periodically to earth to take on a physical body for the purpose of an ongoing correctional process of soul adjustment called tikkun. The soul is temporarily clothed in a body that it uses to continue its journey of spiritual development. The soul is a composite of all its past lives. In certain past lives, it may have accomplished certain righteous behaviors. In other lifetimes, the soul's actions may have been a mixed bag of good and sinful behaviors. In such cases, the successful behaviors have been filtered out and it is not necessary for those aspects of the soul to reincarnate. Only unrectified bad aspects must still be dealt with through reincarnation. Sometimes, when a soul who was involved in destructive behaviors in a past life reincarnates it may be necessary for that soul to be burdened with certain handicaps or negative attributes. That soul must overcome these burdens in order to rectify bad behavior or to learn lessons from a previous life or lives.

Life on earth is both a laboratory and a proving ground for the soul. Soul development is an evolutionary process that extends over multiple lifetimes. When a soul reincarnates into a new body, it is "on loan" from God to see if it can elevate its consciousness through self-mastery to merit a spiritual advance in its current or its next lifetime. In accordance with a divine plan for that particular soul, at some point it will have performed enough *mitzvahs* (good deeds) and lived a sufficiently righteous enough life(s) to completely rectify its shortcomings and sins. When the soul's corrections are completed, the soul merits the bliss of the world-to-come in the Garden of Eden where it cleaves to the Godhead in a state of enlightenment.

Of course, reaching this high bar of excellence is admittedly very challenging, and may require multiple lifetimes of trials and tribulations as well as a complete transformation of the personality that comes about through enormous personal difficulties. However, while God may test the limits of that soul's capacity, in His infinite mercy, He never gives a soul a spiritual assignment that it is not capable of performing.

So, at the end of its life in a particular body on earth, the soul is subject to one of two options. It can, metaphorically speaking, pass Boardwalk and Park Place and collect its $200 before going around the board again in a new body to work on a new spiritual assignment needed to complete its tikkun. Or it has to Go to Jail to repeat the whole sordid experience again in a new body, but with even more burdens or handicaps the next time around.

Sometimes God, with His upper world logic, deems it correct to give that soul certain deficiencies, physical or emotional handicaps, or difficult family circumstances to overcome in order to make the spiritual progress the Creator has assigned for it. This may be misconstrued by family members as some inexplicable and unjust tragedy for which there is no answer. How, for example, could a just and loving God allow their beautiful newborn baby to be born a hemophiliac? Perhaps it is a compensation for the fact that in a past life that person violated *God's law* and committed suicide by slashing his or her wrists. In this way the physical handicap is compensation for unacceptable behavior the soul committed in a previous life. Now it must work through this difficult tikkun with an additional handicap.

Three Spiritual Concepts

Linda has channeled three concepts the angels wish to reveal regarding reincarnation and the relationship between angels and humanity.

Concept 1. Free will is the most fundamental illusion that God bestows on humanity. God creates the illusion that one has free will over his or her behavior without consequences. With rare exceptions, great care is taken by the Creator not to interfere with one's free will. The burden is shifted to the unsuspecting soul that now bears full responsibility for making clear-cut moral decisions in his or her life. All reincarnated souls will make mistakes, but only some learn from them the first time around. For other, more stubborn souls, it may take multiple trial-and-error lifetimes.

The most important choice facing any person is the decision to turn to God and walk in His path. Fear of punishment may motivate one to refrain from sinful behaviors. However, if people do not believe the laws of karma—the sum total of their soul's moral legacy acquired from lifetime to lifetime—affect them in this world and after death, they succumb to temptations because they prefer them, believing they can get away with bad behavior. Free will allows us to choose between good and evil, enabling us to merit receiving reward or punishment, blessing or curse.

The battle for control over the soul is fought by the forces of light and darkness. In Hebrew, the dark angelic force is called the *yetzer hara,* or evil inclination. The yetzer hara does not give warning. Quite the contrary, its purpose is to tempt and seduce people toward the evil inclination. This force itself is an angelic agent of God, whose expertise is lulling human beings into thinking it doesn't exist—a world without consequences. However, a person has the power to overcome his or her yetzer hara by rousing another angelic force—the *yetzer tov,* or good inclination—to conquer it.

To experience higher consciousness, a person must come to his or her own conclusions regarding a moral code of conduct. In spite of occasional human failings of leadership, the world's religions offer a tried-and-true pathway for accessing spiritual light. Most people who attempt to navigate the road to spiritual knowledge with their own moral compass stumble and bumble along a morally circuitous path, learning the hard way to differentiate between right and wrong. However, by tilling the field of spiritual study and practice, a person can considerably shorten the process and activate the antidote to his or her yetzer hara. This focused study, the angels reveal, is often a necessary requirement to achieving enlightenment.

Concept 2. Many things we hold dear in this world are utterly insignificant in the angelic realms. Conversely, it is equally true that certain attributes and qualities that angels consider important are given short shrift by most of humanity. Most people are overly preoccupied with the material world, with little or no concern given to the *spiritual preparation for what lies ahead.* In the spirit world, where the cycles of life and death are viewed through a different spiritual lens, a person's soul is always before God. *In short, angels see divinity in almost everything, while humanity sees divinity in almost nothing.*

Money and fame represent power in this world, but not in the world where our souls wish to go. There are "no pockets in shrouds." Money and fame are useless in the world-to-come because they do not possess eternal value. The world-to-come is none other than the Garden of Eden, the state of spiritual perfection that Adam and Eve experienced before they were expelled because of their sin.

Concept 3. The importance of repentance. Sooner or later, the laws of karma invariably catch up with one who leads a life preoccupied with sinful behavior. And if that doesn't happen in the current lifetime, it occurs in the spirit world or in another incarnation. God has provided humanity with an antidote to recover from misuse of free will and reconnect to Him–the act of repentance, which in Hebrew is called *teshuvah.* Every religion provides opportunities for repentance, ranging from daily prayers of forgiveness to observance of holidays where this is stressed. Teshuvah is able to avert karmic consequences and transform consciousness. It is part of a continuous, lifelong process of refinement. Even a highly evolved spiritual being, ever mindful of his or her behavior, needs to do teshuvah to draw closer to God. The angels profoundly respect and appreciate anyone who performs sincere repentance. This attribute provides a shining example of what is taken much more seriously in the spirit world than on earth.

THE COMPATIBILITY OF REINCARNATION WITH JUDAISM AND CHRISTIANITY

Kabbalah is a religion within a religion for the Jewish people. However, most Jewish people remain clueless about the complex cycles of birth and death that exist at the deepest levels of their faith. Reform, Conservative, and even some Orthodox Jews are completely unaware of what Kabbalah teaches on the subject. Linda's clients who come from these backgrounds are often amazed, delighted, and relieved to find out their soul goes on for retraining and eventual return to earth. Death is not the end, just a transition, albeit with its own set of challenges. They are stunned to discover just how central reincarnation is to the Jewish faith. Indeed the most detailed account of how reincarnation works is in a recently translated book, *The Gates of Reincarnation (Sha'ar HaGilgulim)* written by the 16th-century Kabbalist Rabbi Yitzchak Luria. Frequently, Linda's Jewish clients reveal to her that although they personally believe in reincarnation, they have kept their feelings private out of fear of being ostracized by their friends, family, or synagogue.

Many Orthodox Jews know that reincarnation is real. However, their rabbis have told them that it is not necessary to know anything about the subject. All they need to do is perform mitzvahs (good deeds), practice *tzaddaka* (charity), and somehow everything else in their lives will magically fall into place. Well, since when is a Jew not supposed to know something? This cavalier attitude is both preposterous and astonishing to us! Why on earth would our religion want to keep us in the dark about something so basic and important? Why keep us ignorant about an issue that all of us will one day face?

In Kabbalah, the study of reincarnation was intended not only to gain insight into how one's soul reincarnates from one body to another, but, specifically, to answer questions regarding the metaphysical "lineage" of the key biblical figures in the Torah (Old Testament) and in the writings of the Hebrew prophets. In fact, reincarnation constitutes a whole "secret" level of Torah analysis within Kabbalah that has been conducted by religious scholars for thousands of years. It provides more soul-satisfying answers to biblical quandaries that otherwise make little or no sense. (A discussion of the Jewish understanding of reincarnation is beyond the scope of this book. We have, however, provided resources at www.thehealinggift.com for those interested in pursuing it.)

What does this mean for Christianity? Although the official position is that reincarnation does not exist, it must be stressed that all the original Christians were Jews. In fact, they did not consider themselves to be anything other than Jews who believed that Jesus fulfilled the requirements regarding the identity of the Messiah as laid out by the Hebrew prophets. Although there are important differences between the two faiths, a significant number of the key tenets of Christianity come from Judaism. Coupled with the fact that reincarnation is one of the great secrets of the Jewish faith and that Jesus and his disciples were all Jews, perhaps Christian theologians may one day reconsider reincarnation as a valid belief for Christians. Linda and I hope this book will help guide people of *all faiths* toward an understanding of the profound role of reincarnation in our secular and spiritual lives.

THE CENTRALITY OF REINCARNATION IN LINDA'S WORK

Linda channels different categories of past-life information that are important in clarifying underlying patterns behind dysfunctional emotional behavior. They may even reveal the deepest origins of stubborn health problems.

• **Unresolved health issues.** Past-life issues can play a significant role in determining disease etiology. The soul may have a memory of unresolved medical issues that affected it in another lifetime. In such cases that lifetime will "come forth" to be healed. Linda has identified certain negative physical ailments in some clients that were directly attributable to past-life physical trauma. In addition, cancer and other serious chronic degenerative diseases often have a metaphysical component. If a karmic correction does not occur by a certain point in a person's life, then cancer may be triggered through a variety of physical mechanisms in the body that force the individual to deal with his or her own mortality. This accelerates the urgency and necessity of making the karmic correction.

• **Inexplicable behaviors and phobias.** When a client is able to admit to Linda that certain negative emotional states are completely irrational or when the angels lead her to the negative emotions in the Emotional Database, Linda goes into trance to get specific past-life information regarding the origins of a specific pattern of behavior. Now, within the context of a particular past-life memory, that behavior begins to makes sense. A specific past life has come forth for emotional clarity and healing to help resolve similar issues in this lifetime.

• **Memories of death.** There are times when clients have past-life feelings or memories surface that allow them to remember in graphic detail the violent nature of their death in that lifetime. Often, this peak event has major consequences regarding a current unresolved health issue or irrational behaviors and phobias.

• **Marriages and romantic relationships.** Sometimes a stormy marriage or romantic relationship is a replay of unresolved issues from a past life relationship between the same two individuals—a new attempt to correct an old tikkun resulting from that lifetime. (One can only wonder what the tikkun was between Prince Charles and Lady Diana.)

• **Parents and children.** Reincarnations can, metaphorically speaking, stay in a family. Difficulty between parents and children or between siblings can sometimes only be explained by unresolved past-life issues and the ensuing tikkun. Sometimes a role reversal occurs where a previous parent is now the child or vice versa in order to correct a metaphysical imbalance from that lifetime. A child might have a very different personality from a parent or be a "one-timer," with no metaphysical relationship with that parent. In such cases, Linda can identify the reason why that particular type of parent had to be picked for the child to complete a tikkun and overcome a certain type of adversity.

• **One's life path and occupation.** Often a person's profession or particular talent or ability comes from what they did in certain past lives. For example, Linda channeled that one of her female clients, who is a staff piano accompanist and faculty member at a local music conservatory in the Los Angeles area, is the reincarnation of Clara Schumann, famed 19th-century concert pianist, composer, and wife of romantic era composer Robert Schumann. Linda has also channeled that spiritually oriented people such as priests, ministers, and rabbis were often involved in the same profession in past lives. More often, such individuals are continuing on their soul's path, albeit with newfound tools and knowledge of this modern era. A significant number of alternative medical healers appear to have done some sort of spiritual work in past lives. Linda has also seen cases where a person can harbor deep-seated resentments because they are, on a soul level, ill suited for their current occupation. This may have a negative bearing on the soul's tikkun.

• **Innate knowledge beyond life experience.** Linda has had cases where a client, for no obvious reason, exhibits a particular affinity or unusual knowledge about a particular culture or era. She sometimes goes into trance to reveal details about that person's lifetime in that society or era.

AN INTRODUCTION TO *DYBBUKS*

One area of metaphysical work where Linda has done extensive research is the phenomenon of earthbound spirits, which in Hebrew are called *dybbuks*. The angels have revealed that earthbound spirits can exert negative emotional, spiritual, and physical damage over an unsuspecting individual.

The concept of an earthbound spirit possessing or controlling a person's behavior and health exists in practically every religion and culture going back to prehistoric times. It has been understood by so-called primitive cultures and their shamans on every continent ranging from Australian aborigines, North and South American Indians, and African and Asian tribal peoples, as well as the primary Western and Eastern religious traditions. For centuries, priests and ministers of the Catholic and Protestant faiths, rabbis of the Jewish faith, mullahs of the Islamic faith, and priests of the Buddhist and Hindu faiths have relied on the traditions of ritualistic practice called exorcism to drive away "evil spirits" of one who is possessed. However, in recent years, this practice has been largely ignored by these religions because of fear of ridicule from the scientific and secular communities.

The Jewish faith has had a historic tradition of dealing with earthbound spirits. For centuries, Chassidic rabbis were trained in how to remove a dybbuk that afflicted a suffering parishioner. (This is described in an excellent book on the subject entitled *Dybbuk* by Gershom Winkler.) Today, however, these traditions are a lost art—largely ignored by most rabbis who instead refer troubled parishioners to mental health professionals. If the thought were ever to cross the minds of the very few rabbis capable of performing such rituals, even fewer would actually do them due to fear of ridicule.

With the onset of the Industrial Revolution in the late 18th century, the supremacy of rational scientific principles overwhelmed traditional spiritual reasoning. The concept of a spirit remaining earthbound after death, let alone affecting another human being, ran completely contrary to prevailing scientific wisdom. Such antiquated ideas were considered preposterous, superstitious, old wives' tales, unable to be substantiated by scientific methods. In modern times, the success of films such as *The Exorcist* hit a nerve in the collective unconscious of the movie-going public, reinforcing the collective unconscious archetype that a force completely beyond the scope of the rational mind could somehow impact human behavior or health.

From his vantage point in the spirit world, Sigmund Freud finds it unfortunate that the field of psychology is largely unreceptive to paranormal phenomenon. He himself admits to this error of omission due to his lack of understanding about this aspect of Judaism and his obsession with establishing psychoanalysis as a science. These precluded him from understanding this higher reality. Our mental institutions and prisons, he now claims, contain individuals who exhibit extreme behaviors due in part to being possessed by dybbuks. This lack of awareness results in incorrect diagnoses. Psychiatrists and psychologists misinterpret spirit possession as the psychotic, delusional ramblings of someone in the throes of severe mental illness. The field does not even dignify the subject with a response (let alone research dollars). The pathetic fate of such people is mind-numbing drugs or electroshock therapy that attempt to quiet such behaviors. Linda and Sigmund are interested in sharing our findings with sincere and open-minded mental health care professionals for what we believe could be game-changing treatment for difficult cases of addiction.

Linda's Research into Dybbuks

The angels have revealed spiritual techniques to Linda whereby she can banish these unwanted intruders from a client's body or auric fields and send them back to the light where they belong. (See "An Introduction to the Body's Energy Fields.") Since the mid-1990s when Linda started doing this work, this phenomenon has proved to be more common than either of us had previously believed. Linda estimates that approximately 6 to 8 percent of her clientele have at one time or another been possessed by a dybbuk. She has never seen it manifest in quite so dramatic a fashion as portrayed in movies like *The Exorcist*, although she allows that might be possible. Dybbuks, it turns out, usually affect people's physical or emotional health in far more subtle ways. Examples might include lingering and inexplicable negative behaviors that deviate from a person's inherent nature. Linda has also seen cases where natural therapies that should work do not—because a dybbuk is blocking the healing.

An Introduction to the Body's Energy Fields

In energy medicine, a field is defined as a vibration of energy at a particular band of frequencies that can also be a carrier of information. There are two broad categories of fields: *veritable* or *physical* fields that can be measured and *putative* or *subtle* energies that cannot be measured through conventional scientific instrumentation. The primary difference between the measurable and unmeasurable fields is their range of frequencies and the speed and type of information being transmitted. The veritable fields consist of seven types of electromagnetic radiation: gamma, x-rays, ultraviolet light, the full visible wavelength spectrum of visible light, infrared, microwaves, and radio waves. Solar, geomagnetic, sound, and Schumann waves (extremely low frequency electromagnetic waves that oscillate between the earth and certain atmospheric layers) are other types of veritable fields. The lower frequencies of the subtle energy spectrum relate to one's physical well-being, while the highest of these relate to nonphysical emotional and spiritual energies—the thought forms of such emotions as love, will, intention, and intuition.

Ancient cultures have long known how to sense certain forms of vital life energy. These multidimensional anatomy systems include *meridians, chakras, thought forms,* and *subtle energies* (also called bodies). In Chapter 1, we discussed EAV (Electroacupuncture According to Voll) that utilizes acupuncture meridians as a physical/etheric (higher realms) interface for the diagnosis of physical and energetic disturbances in the body. Traditional Chinese Medicine works with energy called *Qi* that is connected through meridians. Ayurvedic medicine works with a vital energy called *prana* that is connected through chakras. First described in the Upanishads in India approximately 3,000 years ago, chakras are centers of activity for the reception, assimilation, and transmission of life energies.[1] Homeopathy works through *resonances* derived from dilutions of various substances that carry information which may not be measurable on a mass spectrometer. *Miasms* are inherited resonances that manifest as various forms of camouflaged illness. In the 1920s, Austrian psychologist Dr. Wilhelm Reich pioneered a technique to release negative emotions and ease physical suffering through a universal energy he called *orgone.* Since cells, meridians, chakras, and thoughts generate their own subtle fields, it is impossible to quantify the number of subtle energy fields that exist. Undoubtedly, a great many have not yet been discovered.

In all these medical models, beneficial and discordant energies move through the skin and bodily tissue. Certain illnesses can be viewed as disturbances in energy flow that are like a computer virus, which distorts information. EAV, applied kinesiology (muscle testing), and dowsing with a pendulum or divining rods are methods that allow illness to be detected in the subtle fields before there is a physical response. Besides referring to meridians, Linda uses two other ancient subtle energy systems for collecting diagnostic information on physical, energetic, and emotional disturbances: auric fields and the chakra system.

Auric Fields

The main subtle energy field we will discuss here is the *human energy field* composed of an aura. An aura is a subtle biomagnetic energy field that surrounds the whole body of all living things. It contains multiple bands of energy called auric fields that graduate in frequency and color as they move outward from the body.[2] Auric fields, working in conjunction with their associated chakras, can convey different types of information about what is going on in the body. This may involve specific organs, organ systems, and glands or address specific emotional, spiritual, and metaphysical issues.

Although many ancient cultures professed a belief in auras, their existence was scientifically proven by the advent of Kirlian photography developed in the 1930s by Russian scientist Semyon Kirlian. His process used pulsed high-voltage frequencies to take pictures (small corona discharges that surround an object) of these radiating energy fields. A famous and still controversial example of this is his photograph of a leaf that was ripped in half and yet still showed the phantom form of the aura surrounding the whole leaf. A more recent advance in aura color imaging technology called gas charge visualization (GVD) allows the color spectrum and brightness of the energy fields to be observed. It is claimed that certain parameters (both positive aspects and distortions) of physical, emotional, psychic, and spiritual health and well-being of an individual are now measurable (see www.kirlianresearch.com).

Subtle energies are the province of medical intuitives, psychics, and clairvoyants and are discussed in theosophical literature. Individuals such as Linda have the capacity to view subtle energies from different vantage points of perception, each one vibrating at a progressively faster rate. These include the etheric body, astral body, mental body, and causal body. While different models of auras are proposed by different psychic channels and scientists, what is common to each approach is that when partnered with a chakra, each auric field or body exchanges information with the various gradations of the spiritual realms linked to specific areas or meridians inside the body.

Figure 18-1 shows the following higher subtle energy fields surrounding the body providing physical, emotional, and spiritual information that interfaces with our physical being. The central column pertains to the chakra system described below.

Etheric body. This is an energetic duplicate of the physical body. Made of frequencies that vibrate at a lower rate than the bodies that follow, the etheric body acts as a template for the growth and development of the body. Meridians are the interface between the physical and the etheric body.

Astral body. This is the nexus between the physical and spiritual realms which is above time and space.[3] The astral body is also an energetic replica of the body, but it is com-

THE HUMAN ENERGY FIELD

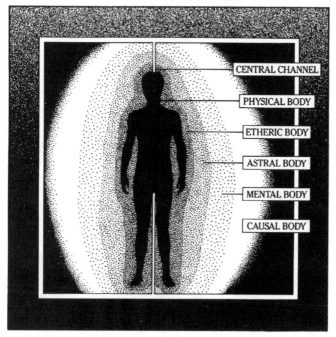

**Figure 18-1.
Auric fields.**

Used with permission of Dr. William Tiller. From *Vibrational Medicine* by Richard Gerber. Publisher: Inner Traditions.

posed of higher frequencies of astral matter that oscillate at a higher, supersensitive rate than those of the etheric body. It is associated with extrasensory perception and out-of-body experiences called astral projection. There is a correlation among the astral body, its related chakras, and emotional disturbances caused by neurochemical imbalances. The astral body is the primary domain of ghosts, dybbuks, and where astrology (the study of the astral) originates.

Mental body. This is information that comes from clairvoyant observation and involves the type of information that Carl Jung referred to as, and derived from, the collective unconscious and synchronicity.

Causal body. This information relates to reincarnation and the afterlife.

The Chakra System

The word chakra comes from the Sanskrit word for "wheels" because it is said to resemble whirling vortices of subtle energies.[4] There are different Hindu, Tantric, Chinese, Buddhist, and Western perspectives regarding the number and location of chakras as well as their physical, emotional, and spiritual correspondences. Linda uses the modern seven chakra system which is used by many other esoteric healers. Chakras are located along the main branches of the central nervous system. Six of the chakras are stacked in a column of energy that extends from the base of the spine to the middle of the forehead (the third eye), while the seventh one, located above the head (the crown chakra), is beyond the physical realm. Each chakra is associated with a major endocrine system gland and a major nervous system plexus or ganglia located near its region of the spine. Other correlations exist between emotions or states of enlightenment and various colors and sounds. In a manner similar to auric fields, the various chakras, from lowest to highest, are composed of varying degrees of matter, energy, and consciousness, which are transmuted in a usable form in the body.

The broad ramifications of these multidimensional subtle energies for the body/mind/spirit connection are beyond the scope of this book. For readers interested in studies confirming the scientific validity of auras and chakras, as well as a deeper understanding of spiritual correlations, see Suggested Readings.

Here is how Linda's process of discovery occurs. Although it does not happen often, Linda can receive a signal at the beginning of the pre-test alerting her to an abnormal energy or interference that needs to be immediately identified and addressed before she can proceed with the medical diagnosis. She calls upon Archangel Michael (whose role is discussed in Chapter 20) to ask for guidance about which database she should channel. Usually this leads to the part of the Metaphysical Database which Linda affectionately calls the "weird page." This may include any number of paranormal phenomena ranging from past-life issues and dybbuks to curses and spells.

Linda's research has shown that alcoholics, drug addicts, those abusing psychotropic drugs, or people under enormous stress can "blow out" their auric fields. This creates a hole in their auric field that becomes an opening for a dybbuk to enter the unwitting individual. The dybbuk may bring a "blueprint" of its negative emotional issues and even physical ailments. When her clients tell Linda they are not feeling themselves, *they may not be feeling themselves!*

When the angels alert Linda to a dybbuk, she channels what she calls a "blueprint of the dybbuk's physical health conditions" as well as a "blueprint of its negative emotions" that existed from a time when the spirit had a body. This allows her to differentiate between what is going on in the dybbuk and what is actually from her client. Sometimes, for no apparent reason, the client will suddenly take on the negative personality attributes or negative physical ailments of the dybbuk. In the latter case, this can sometimes manifest as a "phantom" pain, even though it cannot be detected by any known medical test. Unfortunately, a doctor may simply pass the problem off as psychosomatic.

Although Linda's research is ongoing, we are prepared to draw some tentative conclusions about what Linda has observed on the nature of dybbuks. We cannot, as yet, explain all the reasons why most souls ascend to the light, while a few unfortunate souls stay earthbound. However, it appears that certain alcoholics, drug addicts, and people who are overly sedated by morphine, alcohol, or recreational drugs at the time of death are prone to have their souls stay earthbound instead of returning to the spirit world from whence they came. Linda describes this damage to the soul as an energetic interference akin to static. It's almost as if when they were inebriated or incapacitated, they missed their "connecting flight" home. Likewise, there is a heightened level of mental and physical anguish for the unlucky recipients of such unwanted intruders. It is interesting to note that in each of the following three case histories, the dybbuk affected people either at the hospital or shortly after leaving the hospital.

Testimonial: Curing Tom's alcoholism

A client named Tom came to Linda with an unusual set of problems. Tom was a recovering alcoholic who had recently "fallen off the wagon" when his relationship with his girlfriend began to deteriorate, prior to their eventual breakup. He developed a throbbing ache in his heart that did not go away. After undergoing a battery of tests, all of which came back negative, his cardiologist gently suggested it might be psychosomatic. But there was other weirdness. Tom suddenly developed an insatiable appetite for chocolate, which he could not stop eating. This was remarkable considering that prior to this, Tom detested chocolate and never ate it.

In trance, Linda made an amazing discovery. Tom was possessed by a dybbuk that had taken up residence in his auric fields. The dybbuk admitted to being an alcoholic and understood his affliction had hastened his demise. He told Linda that he had recently died from a massive heart attack at a local hospital where, unable to ascend to the light, he quickly glommed onto the auric fields of a nurse who also had a drinking problem. When the nurse subsequently had intimate relations with Tom, the dybbuk transferred to Tom's dilapidated auric fields, which were in abysmal condition due to his drinking problem. The dybbuk recognized that Tom's reliance on alcohol to numb unpleasant experiences was similar to his own. He had found a match.

The pain in Tom's heart was actually not his—it was the dybbuk's! The dybbuk also related that he had been a full-blown chocoholic and was now satisfying that urge at Tom's expense. Linda then performed a ritual invoking angels and reciting various psalms of King David. Archangel Michael escorted the dybbuk out of Tom's auric fields to the upper worlds where his family was waiting for him. The pain in Tom's heart and his desire for chocolate immediately ceased. He was then able to rebound emotionally from his disappointment and swear off alcohol for good. (See "New Paradigm for Treating Certain Cases of Alcohol and Drug Addiction.")

New Paradigm for Treating Certain Cases of Alcohol and Drug Addiction

Sigmund Freud has told Linda the dybbuk phenomenon represents a whole new paradigm in understanding and treating certain cases of alcohol and/or drug addiction, which, from a metaphysical perspective, are conceptually the same thing. Alcoholism and drug addiction damage the body's auric fields and provide tears or openings for unsavory beings to intrude. The initial addiction is due to one's unwillingness to cope with stress in a less destructive manner. However, after their auric fields sustain damage brought on by alcohol, drugs, or extreme stress, the body and soul of an alcoholic or drug addict is vulnerable to unsavory metaphysical forces.

If the soul of an alcoholic or drug addict misses its opportunity to ascend to the light for future purification and probable reincarnation, it is trapped on the earth plane. It therefore seeks the illusionary comfort of booze or drugs because it is cut off from the normal metaphysical loop that controls a soul's ultimate destiny. Such a dybbuk is destined to wander the earth until it can find a host body that can satisfy the same destructive urges it experienced when it had a body. Reduced to a parasitic existence, the dybbuk occupies either the auric fields or, in some cases, the body itself. It is not in the least bit interested in helping the host body improve his or her lot in life. Quite the opposite, it is only interested in perpetuating the negative, selfish behaviors it indulged in while alive. Since it needs a host body to do this, it seeks out individuals with similar behaviors. This is why dybbuks hang out in hospitals or bars where they can always get another host body. They can also leave a host in the event that the addiction is cured or a better host comes along.

Organizations like Alcoholics and Narcotics Anonymous throw a lifeline to someone who is metaphorically drowning. Their Twelve Step programs are the best way to stay sober and clean because they give the alcoholic/drug addict the inner spiritual strength and emotional tools he or she needs to do battle with an unwelcome intruder. It is frightening to think that destructive behaviors of alcoholics and addicts not only result in misery in their current lifetime—it may not end there! Hopefully, Tom's testimonial will help to "scare straight" those caught in the snare of alcohol or drug addiction.

A particular scenario applies to certain chronic alcoholics and drug addicts who attend meetings, wanting to stop, but are unable to do so because they are possessed by a dybbuk. If you asked them, "Is that gin and tonic really good for you?" most will generally respond, "No, I know it's not good for me, but I can't help it." The reason for the illogical answer is that they are no longer "feeling themselves." They are no longer running their own show. Their critical thinking process, which under normal conditions would make them more susceptible to abstaining from alcohol or recreational drugs, has been taken over by a determined dybbuk who saw an opening in his or her victim's damaged auric fields and climbed in. The dybbuk eggs them on with doubts and insecurity to gain the upper hand for one very selfish reason—he or she wants a drink or a joint!

Testimonial: The source of Ben's exhaustion and depression

This story is an example of how excessive stress or trauma can wreak havoc on one's auric fields, with unforeseen and bizarre consequences. Several years ago, a highly respected surgeon at a local hospital came to Linda, complaining of "just not feeling himself" due, he assumed, to general exhaustion and an inexplicable depression. Ben maintained an incredibly busy surgical schedule, working long hours performing innumerable back-to-back surgeries day after day.

When Linda started channeling, she warned Ben that his workload was causing him to "burn the candle at both ends." She could see that his high levels of stress and anxiety had caused his auric fields to develop "holes that looked like Swiss cheese." She then revealed that Ben had picked up two dybbuks from people who had died in the hospital. As they wandered around the corridors, they saw the openings in his auric fields and climbed in. One of the dybbuks was a three-year-old child who had died in the hospital and appeared very lost, looking for her mama. For unknown reasons, she did not ascend to the light and attached herself to the first body she could find. A second dybbuk was an elderly gentleman whose blueprint of negative emotions caused the poor doctor to feel uncharacteristic waves of depression for no apparent reason.

As Linda completed the exorcism, the spirits were released from the doctor's auric fields and escorted to the upper worlds where their families were waiting for them. Ben immediately told Linda that an enormous physical and emotional weight had been lifted off his shoulders and he felt an "airiness" around him.

Testimonial: Rabbi Moshe's stress provides an opening for a dybbuk

This amazing story occurred when Rabbi Moshe (whose physical testimonial is in Chapter 10) rented an apartment in Los Angeles' Fairfax district, an Orthodox Jewish neighborhood, while paying us a visit. Although he was feeling better since the mercury and nickel dental materials were removed from his mouth, his cumulative health issues had been stressful. One day he started feeling a strong tachycardia (rapid heart beat) that would not stop. He frantically called Linda and came over right away. She asked him if he was upset about anything, and he said, "no." When she asked him if he had eaten any foods containing MSG (monosodium glutamate) that could also trigger such a reaction, again the answer was, "no."

Then Linda went into trance and clearly saw that a dybbuk had climbed into Rabbi Moshe's auric field, which prompted the tachycardia. When she spoke to the dybbuk, he related that he had been a local rabbi. At the time of his death, he had been given morphine to ease his considerable pain. However, when his soul separated from the body to begin its journey home, the morphine impeded the soul in such a manner that he missed the connecting flight taking him to the upper realms. He had walked around his old neighborhood for days until he spied Rabbi Moshe. He told Linda he could tell by the size of Rabbi Moshe's aura that the rabbi was a high soul. He hoped that Rabbi Moshe could somehow assist him in returning to the light. When Rabbi Moshe did not respond to his signals, the dead rabbi became highly agitated, thus prompting the tachycardia.

Linda again performed her dybbuk clearance ritual, causing the dead rabbi to be escorted by the angels out of Rabbi Moshe's auric fields and returned to the light. *What is most amazing is that only 30 seconds after the dybbuk left, Rabbi Moshe reported the tachycardia completely ceased and his heartbeat returned to normal! This phenomenon could not be faked, as there is no known medical approach that can so quickly achieve such results.*

The moral implications and issues of medical ethics raised by this story are mind-boggling. Although it would seem noble to take people out of physical suffering through the use of morphine or similar substances as they approach the moment of death, this story shows an unforeseen and spiritually undesirable consequence of this seemingly merciful act.

THE UPCOMING ASCENSION OF MICHAEL JACKSON'S SOUL

As Linda and I were reviewing the final edit of this chapter in November 2009, she again received a shake that someone from another realm or dimension wished to speak to her. It was pop singer Michael Jackson! He reported to Linda that his soul was still trapped and stuck on the earth plane, unable to ascend to the light since his death in June. As endlessly reported in the media, Michael was addicted to painkillers and was also receiving injections of propofol to help him with insomnia. This very powerful anesthetic is usually only administered in hospitals prior to surgery. At the time of his death, brought on by cardiac arrest, Michael had been heavily sedated with this and other drugs. As with the deceased rabbi in the previous testimonial, Michael's delicate soul was adversely affected by the medication, which blocked his ability to ascend to the upper realms. Michael had come to Linda for guidance and assistance in completing this process.

Linda found him to be a highly intelligent and amazingly kind and gentle man who has already recognized the errors he made in his most unusual life. She spoke to him about what has happened since he transitioned out of his body, and he seemed to have "a knowingness about the upper realms." But due to the blockage affecting his soul, he was not yet able to sense that. However, he was not afraid of that, and seemed eager to focus on the journey ahead to rectify his soul. Linda asked Michael if not being buried in a timely manner had caused any problems. He replied that it had "a bad effect on my soul." In a rather curious aside, Michael added, "I'm looking forward to reading your book!"

Linda asked Michael if the origin of his soul was human, and he replied, "no." Was he an angel? "No." He commented that he was "from a gentler and kinder place." Linda then received another shake, this time from Archangel Michael. He said that the ritual of sending Michael Jackson's soul to the light needed to be documented on film. As his life had been lived completely in the public eye, so shall his death and eventual ascension to the higher realms be played out in a similar fashion. In this case, however, the purpose is to glorify God by demonstrating the existence of His upper realms as well as to provide an example of how dangerous substances can damage the soul's ability to navigate its way home. Michael Jackson views this as his final parting gift to humanity. That is the inner meaning of "This Is It."

PART FOUR

The Source of Linda's Gift: Communicating with Angels

CHAPTER 19

Belief in Angels: A Common Bond of the World's Religions

Mightier than an army with banners
is an idea whose time has come.
—NAPOLEON

THE WORLD IS IN A TIME OF UNPRECEDENTED STRIFE and nervousness due to a global economic crisis, religious and territorial conflicts, nuclear proliferation, and environmental changes. Looming problems of such magnitude have not been experienced to this degree since World War II. We find it a bit surreal and disheartening to imagine that in a world with such abundant technology designed to ease many of society's fundamental problems, the possibility of a global conflict based mainly on old religious issues could loom so large. Various religions of the world are entrenched in dogmatic posturing that seems to preclude the possibility of peaceful, open dialogue. Does a common denominator exist between these religions that could serve as a basis for meaningful dialogue? Having scientific proof of the existence of angels would certainly be on our short list.

Although first discussed in the Old Testament (Torah) and by the Hebrew prophets, belief in angels is of real importance to Christianity and Islam. Stories abound in each faith regarding the angelic realms that are quite different from one another. For example, angels were said to have been key observers and participants at the birth and death of Jesus, as well as at other peak moments of his life. Similar stories about Mohammad exist as well. Christianity has been overt about the importance of an angelic presence in their religious doctrines. Although angels are of paramount importance in Judaism, their identity and true importance has been more concealed. While the Hebrew patriarchs and prophets communicated directly with angels, this ability mostly dissipated after the destruction of the Second Temple (the center of

Jewish worship in Jerusalem) a little under 2,000 years ago. Over the centuries, however, it was revived in a similar form by certain Kabbalistic rabbis. While not specifically referred to as angels, in Hinduism different types of spirit beings function in a similar manner. The Buddhist equivalent of angels is *devas*, which are celestial or enlightened beings. However, they do not normally interfere in human affairs.

Thus far, one of the goals of much of this book has been to establish a level of verifiable proof regarding the scientific accuracy of Linda's gift. As multiple testimonials show, clearly something astonishing is going on here. Assuming that we have established a "base camp" of belief where the reader accepts that premise, the next leg of our journey on the path of verification must be not only to prove, to the greatest extent possible, the existence of angels but also to show that Linda is indeed communicating with them. To support these claims, the problem must be addressed from two perspectives: 1) establishing angels as a universal unconscious archetype, and 2) examining the spiritual implications of thus-far-unanswerable questions raised by some of the most brilliant minds in quantum physics.

Linda claims that she receives all her information from angels and spirits. However, she does not say, as most other new age mediums do, that she is channeling "her higher self." As described in Chapter 1, Linda's form of communication bears a striking resemblance to the manner in which prophecy was received by the Hebrew prophets. As mentioned earlier, Linda's gift represents a unique opportunity for humanity to peer beyond the cosmic veil of hidden knowledge to grasp not only the higher angelic realms, but how angels function in our world. In this chapter and Chapter 20, we begin to explore angelology—the inner workings of God's angelic universe.

BEYOND CLARENCE: AN AMERICAN CULTURAL PHENOMENON

The question in our minds remains: Are people in our increasingly secularized and science-oriented society predisposed to believe in the existence of angels? In a 2008 book entitled *What Americans Really Believe*, Dr. Rodney Stark, Ph.D., reported a recent poll of 1,700 adult respondents, conducted by the Baylor University Institute for Studies of Religion, which showed that 55 percent answered the following statement affirmatively: "I was protected from harm by a guardian angel."[1,2] In addition, fully 61 percent believed "absolutely" that angels exist, and another 21 percent thought they "probably" exist.[3] The results were consistent regardless of religious denomination, region, or education, and indicate that a majority of the population engages in a kind of casual mysticism, independent of established religious doctrine.

A belief in angels is a cultural phenomenon that continues to fascinate and inspire our society. One of the most endearing angelic icons from the movies is Clarence, the angel who was able to "earn his wings" by assisting Jimmy Stewart's hapless character, George Bailey, out of a financially desperate situation. He continues to tug at the heartstrings of even jaded agnostics when the classic movie *It's a Wonderful Life* plays on television during the Christmas season. Over fifteen years ago, a very popular television show entitled "Touched by an Angel" involved angels disguised in human bodies who interacted with average people in trouble or in morally compromised situations. They used their advanced angelic knowledge and insights to help steer the troubled individual to make the right moral choices in his or her life.

The fact remains that a belief in angels has fired the imagination of artists, musicians, authors, and theologians for millenniums in a way that cuts across all boundaries of race, nationality, or religion. While this, in and of itself, does not offer proof of their existence, it implies that angels are an archetype of the universal collective unconscious. Therefore, they should not be dismissed.

So Who Really Believes in Angels?

Linda has found that the vast majority of her clients profess a belief in the existence of their own personal "guardian angel." Time and again, they have regaled Linda with stories of a force that not only watches over them, but has actually rescued them from either serious injury or even death. Her clients cut across all ethnic and religious groups. In fact, most of Linda's clients are well-heeled professionals, including a significant number of doctors, business owners, lawyers, and teachers, as well as prominent rabbis and religious clergy of other faiths. When push comes to shove, even skeptical progressive secularists have admitted to Linda they believe in some personal force that protects them from or during dangerous situations. It is oddly amusing that people whose primary belief system is science are still willing to "couch their bets" by being open to the idea that angels are real.

Against a backdrop of increased secularization and atheism in our society, the personal experiences of Linda's clients testify to the intrinsic feeling so many of us have that a force larger than us is watching over and guiding us. This illogical feeling in one's bones is that spark from our divine soul speaking to us, letting us know there is a God and there are rules as to how His game is played. God's realm has an inherent moral order with laws of karma that ultimately manifest as reward and punishment.

SCIENTISTS WHO ARE OPEN TO A BELIEF IN ANGELS

Albert Einstein always remained open to divine possibilities. Although he said, "Science without religion is lame, [and] religion without science is blind,"[4] he ultimately professed a belief that the final knowledge would somehow be centered around God, declaring, "I want to know God's thoughts . . . the rest are details."[5] His desire to maintain an openness to that which is deemed "mystical" stems from his conviction to pursue the truth wherever it may lead. "There remains something subtle, intangible and inexplicable. Veneration for this force beyond anything that we can comprehend is my religion."[6]

Proof of the existence of angels has never been accepted by the scientific community, and yet a new cadre of scientific thinkers, including Amit Goswami, Rupert Sheldrake, Fred Alan Wolf, Stanislav Grof, Michio Kaku, Deepak Chopra, Bruce Lipton, and Gregg Barden, profess a belief in their existence.

An example of this new breed of scientist is Amit Goswami, Ph.D., a theoretical nuclear physicist and a professor at the University of Oregon Institute in theoretical physics since 1968, who has taught physics for thirty-two years. His research interests also range from quantum cosmology, quantum measurement theory, and applications of quantum mechanics to the body/mind/spirit connection. He became best known as one of the scientific experts featured in the 2004 film *What the Bleep Do We Know!?* Goswami is also a prolific author of a well-regarded university textbook on quantum mechanics as well as a series of popular books relating to physics and spirituality, including *The Self-Aware Universe, Physics of the Soul, The Quantum Doctor,* and *God Is Not Dead.* These books call the materialist paradigm into question and offer in its place a new paradigm based on the idea that "quantum physics demands that science be based on the primacy of consciousness."[7] Goswami posits that the universe requires a sentient being to be aware of it; without an observer it only exists as a possibility. His work covers recent developments in physics that demonstrate how science is capable of validating mysticism that previously required a leap of faith.

Astrophysicists have been unable to produce any scientific evidence to support the idea of *a universe that is predisposed to sustain life.* On the contrary, the evidence is so overwhelmingly against it that it led physicist and author Paul Davies to remark "the universe seems unreasonably suited to the existence of life—almost contrived—you might say a 'put-up job.' "[8] This is why a concept called the anthropic principle, first posited by Australian cosmologist Brandon Carter in 1974, has gained traction in recent years among leading astrophysicists and astronomers.

The Anthropic Principle

The anthropic principle contends that the universe was brought into existence intentionally for the sake of producing humanity. The sheer degree of fine tuning and precision required for the confluence of physical, chemical, and biological laws and values to create and sustain carbon-based life on earth or elsewhere is extraordinary and mathematically remote. So much so that Michael Turner, an astrophysicist at the University of Chicago and Fermilab (a theoretical physics laboratory), likened it to "[throwing] a dart across the entire universe and [hitting] a bull's eye one millimeter in diameter on the other side."[9] Given the utterly inhospitable nature of outer space, the existence of carbon-based life in the universe must be either an incredibly fortuitous coincidence or the result of intelligent design of a Creator. This Creator intentionally planned purposeful adjustments to the laws of physics so that humanity could both discover and observe His universe.

The controversy within the scientific community arises from the insinuation that an intelligently designed universe actually verifies the existence of God. What is fascinating is that many leading astrophysicists and astronomers, including Sir Fred Hoyle, Paul Davies, John Wheeler, David Deutsch, Roger Penrose, Michael Turner, Steven Weinberg, and Stephen Hawking, subscribe to at least some aspect of this theory.[10]

How the universe evolved from the inception of the big bang to such complex structures as galaxies and planetary systems cannot be explained by any scientific model of a turbulence-driven structure. In his best-selling book, *A Brief History of Time*, astrophysicist Stephen Hawking states, "The remarkable fact is that the value of these numbers [the constants of physics] seem to have been very finely adjusted to make possible the development of life . . . For example, if the electric charge of the electron had been only slightly different, stars would have been unable to burn hydrogen and helium, or else they would have not exploded . . . " Hawking maintains this is potential evidence of "a divine purpose in Creation and the choice of the laws of science [by God]."[11]

Scientists who agree with the anthropic principle should also be open to efforts to seek direct communication with celestial beings that a majority of human beings believe in. Without even a shred of evidence to support their hypothesis, scientists involved in the search for extraterrestrial intelligence (SETI) speak glowingly of the possibilities that carbon-based intelligent beings from other planets or galaxies might transmit radio signals to us that will confirm the existence of intelligent life elsewhere in the universe. The assumption that another "lonely" civilization will reach out to broadcast radio signals of a mathematical nature in hopes of finding another like-minded civilization strikes us as a bit arrogant. It begs the question: Why would a truly evolved civilization communicate through radio waves when mind telepathy is much more advanced? Furthermore, in *The Physics of Angels*, biologist Rupert Sheldrake and theologian Matthew Fox offer a scientific reality check. Since the Andromeda Galaxy, which is nearest to ours, is approximately 1,800,000 light years away, a successful two-way communication via radio waves would take 3,600,000 years to complete.[12]

Thus far, the SETI experiment, which began in 1960, has been a total failure. Granted since the axiom "absence of evidence is not evidence of absence" still applies, we must therefore persist in playing out the scientific hand behind it. The same is true for UFO research and the crop circle phenomenon in England. However, given the improbable odds against the success of such investigations, coupled with the divine repercussions of the anthropic principle, it is looking more and more like scientists have painted themselves into a corner by also not exploring the scientifically virgin territory of angels—a non-carbon-based life form.

A Proposal to Include Angels in the Search for Intelligent Life in the Universe

In previous eras, there was always an association between heaven and what actually existed in the sky above. The sky or cosmos teemed with intelligent, conscious beings. There were, for example, celestial choirs of angels whose daily function was to sing praises to God. Praising God with awe and wonder for His creation was a centerpiece of angelic existence. This sense of awe and wonder also affected that which is most noble in the human spirit. The ceiling of the Sistine Chapel in the Vatican, considered Michelangelo's crowning achievement (along with frescoes painted by Raphael, Botticelli, Perugino, and Ghirlandaio), is replete with visions of angels in the depiction of important events in the Old and New Testaments.

This aspect of human consciousness began to be filtered out of the spiritual imagination in the 17th century when Newtonian laws dictated a clock-like, mechanized universe, leaving us largely bereft of the awe and wonder of a glorious cosmos borne of intelligent design by a supernal Creator. For far too many, the phrase "Our father who art in heaven" is now a quaint metaphor, having nothing to do with modern astronomy and its focus on galaxies, super novas, black holes, and the like. Although contemporary physics readily acknowledges the presence of time-space dimensions and even parallel universes, the idea that these may also be *spiritual* time-space dimensions, including angelic realms that transcend the physical world, was lost in the Newtonian equation. Science fiction and UFOs have replaced and trivialized angels and Godliness as the way most people now view the cosmos.[13]

Linda has channeled that the timeline of human consciousness has progressed to the point where we must look past conventional scientific thinking. We propose that scientists and theologians unite to call upon a higher power to reveal the physical and spiritual secrets of the universe. To begin with, *the search should not be limited to carbon-based life forms—our preconceived notion of what extraterrestrial life must be like.* Instead, why not attempt to scientifically validate the possibility of a cosmic intelligence that can communicate telepathically in a manner that has already been recognized and accepted by all major religions and a significant majority of their adherents on earth? The reason is that many scientists have an irrational fear of discovering what Einstein yearned for—"knowing God's thoughts." The idea of intelligent life on other planets is not nearly as threatening to science as is the idea of God. The existence of an extraterrestrial life form with far superior intelligence to our own does not necessarily imply a reality where we are beholden to that entity. The existence of God or His messengers does.

Kabbalah: Using the Tree of Life as a Basis for Scientific Exploration

At the same time as the scientific envelope of discovery of the physical universe is being pushed, there is a general lack of awareness that a spiritual cosmology could exist, even though *modern physics consistently raises questions that can only be answered by this domain.* Linda has channeled that without such a spiritual framework, the envelope of scientific knowledge can only be pushed incrementally. Our angelic guides tell us that the requisite framework is the Tree of Life contained within Kabbalah. Figure 19-1 is a simple overview of the Tree of Life, which is explained briefly here and more extensively at www.thehealinggift.com.

Kabbalah, which in Hebrew means "to receive," is the oldest known metaphysical system that, among other things, describes the cosmological evolution of creation. Predating the existence of humanity, *it is what God taught His angels.* This system is based on the Tree of Life, which is the divine template for the entire universe and a divine mini-template for the human body. It includes ten time-space dimensions called *sefirot* that function as a spiritual step-down transformer for the attenuation of light energy. So complex is this subject that

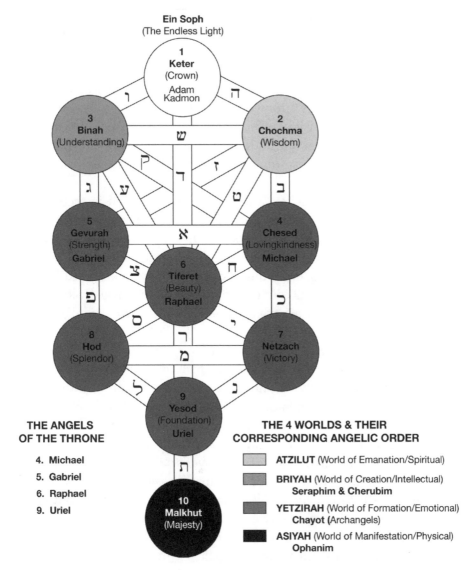

Figure 19-1. The Tree of Life and the Ten Sefirot of Creation.

I plan to write a book in the future describing the core principles of Kabbalah. The book will include a glossary of spiritual terminology needed to understand the architecture of the upper worlds and the vast communication network used by angels to receive prayers and dispense blessings.

In his book *The Way of God*, Kabbalist Rabbi Chaim Luzzatto (1707–1747) describes the mechanism that the angelic realms provide for putting the judgments and decrees of God into action. "When we speak of God's Influence, we are speaking of the system and order [called the Tree of Life] that He desired to make use of in translating His Will into action. God arranged all created things in [this tiered] system of steps and sequences . . . Through this system, all details of existence are sustained and influenced by God as He desires. God thus first influences an angel, who in turn influences another angel on a lower level. This continues step by step until the final angel acts upon a physical thing. This can either sustain this thing, or bring about something new, all according to the decree ultimately emanating from God."[14]

The concept of an angelic parallel universe is verified in the spiritual axiom "as above, so below." The principal text of Kabbalah, the Zohar, states: "Everything below, no matter how small, has a counterpart on high."[15] According to Rabbi Luzzatto, "Because of the linkage between the physical world and the [angels] . . . every time a physical thing is influenced [below], it also has an effect upon its counterpart among these [angels]. Since man's deeds in the world below are what influences these forces on high, man's influence is said to be directed upward."[16]

The world of astronomy pertains only to the various sublevels of the tenth and lowest sefirot named *Malkhut*, which includes the earth plane as well as the rest of the physical universe. Although modern astronomy is obsessed with an ever-expanding universe that includes galaxies, super novas, black holes, quarks, and gravitational fields, the physical universe constitutes only a part of *Asiyah*, which in Kabbalah is the lowest of "the four worlds." (Note that Malkhut and Asiyah overlap.) Included within several of the higher sefirot are three worlds named *Briyah, Yetzirah*, and Asiyah inhabited by a complex hierarchy of angelic orders that carry out God's Divine Will of assisting humanity in a variety of ways. These are the worlds that Linda has access to when she channels angels. The world of astronomy does not recognize the existence of the higher spiritual realms: *Atzilut*, Briyah, and Yetzirah.

We are fast approaching a time when science will truly be knocking on heaven's door. Linda has channeled that a new spiritual cosmology involving quantum physics and the Tree of Life will emerge. While this book is not a forum for speculation on quantum physics, it's fascinating to ponder the implications of an important new theory on that. Superstring theory and M-theory, its latest derivative, require ten space-time dimensions that emanate from a separate and distinct eleventh dimension. This is the same core concept described in the spiritual world of Kabbalah!

GOD'S ANGELIC UNIVERSE

This section and much of the next chapter contain information on angels and the angelic realms that is derived from Jewish and Kabbalistic sources. They include the Torah (the five books of Moses); the Talmud, a collection of rabbinic teachings pertaining to Jewish law, customs, and ethics from the 2nd to the 5th centuries A.D.; the Zohar, the principal books of Kabbalah (23 volumes) from the 1st century A.D. that were communicated from the angel/ prophet Elijah to Rabbi Shimon bar Yochai; and the writings of several prominent rabbis and scholars who are acknowledged authorities on the subject.

Angels Are God's Messengers

The word for angel in Hebrew is *malach*, which means messenger. An angel is a divine emissary and servant specifically created to carry out the Will of God. This may be directed toward the earth and all its inhabitants or to other worlds below Yetzirah. Angels transmit prayers from our physical world to the upper worlds of Yetzirah, Briyah, and Atzilut. When angels descend to the earth to fulfill a specific mission, they take on a human or animal form or appear within the elements of air or fire. Once the mission is complete, they divest themselves of bodies and return to the world from whence they came. An example of an angel appearing in the element of fire is in the famous biblical encounter between Moses and the burning bush (see Chapter 20).

An angel is an intelligent vibrational energy, a metaphysical "thought form" expressing a particular emotion or attribute created for a specific function. This explains why there are angels of love and healing as well as angels of death and destruction. According to Rabbi Shneur Zalman of Liadi (1745–1812), "Angels are called 'stationary,' while human souls are referred to as 'goers' or [walkers]. Since the angels, like everything else, were created 'by the breath of [God's] mouth' . . . referred to as God's 'speech,' they cannot change their character or develop spiritually. Angels like Archangel Michael, which God created for the sole purpose of serving Him with love, possess a fixed degree of love for God; angels like the Archangel Gabriel, whose function is to serve God with fear, possess a fixed level of fear. Each has their particular role to play, and they play it with eternal constancy. They are thus called 'stationary.' "[17] (For more about archangels, see Chapter 20.)

Angels are closer to God than humans because they can see Godliness. This is an important distinction. God's ultimate purpose for angels is for them to act as agents for the Divine Will, using love, mercy, healing, judgment, and tough love so that humanity can see Godliness as clearly as they do. The key difference bears repeating: Most of humanity is overly preoccupied with the material world, with little or no concern about *the spiritual preparation for what lies ahead. In short, angels see divinity in almost everything, while humanity sees divinity in almost nothing.*

In spite of this, humans also differ from angels in that we are capable of spiritual growth and development. A person who starts out with a low level of love and fear of God is not necessarily destined to stay on that level. On the contrary, God desires humanity to be more like angels as people undergo a refinement of emotions and attitudes to expand consciousness. Because humanity is largely blinded to the pervasive reality of God, the Creator gives humanity the illusion of free will. If we succeed, we pass our own unique test of tikkun, which was what we were reincarnated to perfect. If we fail, it is a failure of our character. There is no one to blame. There is no place to hide. There are repercussions.

Guardian Angels in the Jewish Faith

The first mention in the Torah of guardian angels watching over a person occurred when the patriarch Jacob was leaving Canaan (the future land of Israel). As he rested for the night, he saw a transfer of angels—those assigned to the Holy Land went back up to heaven, while those assigned to other lands came down to meet him. Upon his return to Canaan, he was greeted by angels assigned to the Holy Land.

Unbeknownst to many Jewish people, the concept of the guardian angel is profoundly Jewish. This was a common understanding mentioned in multiple places in the Talmud and the Zohar. One passage in the Talmud states, "Two ministering angels escort a person and testify for and against him."[18] That means every person has at least two guardian angels: a yetzer tov angel (good inclination) and a yetzer hara angel (evil inclination) who are with him or her at all times. A good way to think of them would be as human friends. By treating your friends well, they remain loyal to you. However, they will desert you if you abuse the trust behind their friendship. You now attract the type of low-consciousness individuals (human or angel) who put out the same energy as well—a case of water seeking its own level. However, if you are fortunate enough to regain your moral footing, a better class of friend (human or angel) will soon follow. If people become truly virtuous and kind, a special angel guides them on a more enlightened path where they are given inner strength that allows them to endure any pain or hardship.[19]

Several Kabbalist rabbis wrote extensively about guardian angels. For example, Rabbi Chaim Vital (1543–1620) wrote in *Etz Chaim (Tree of Life*, Gate 39, Chapter 4) that every person is born with two guardian angels who are appointed from birth to help us navigate through life to fulfill our soul's destiny. We may reach certain goals and milestones in any aspect of our lives or get sidetracked, ignoring the guidance from our good guardian angel. However, when our inevitable spiritual wake-up call arrives—punishment or an unplanned reduction in ego in the form of either divine or human tough love—our good guardian angel is always there to pick up the pieces, ready to guide us back to our true pathway in life. Our ability to at least sense or preferably communicate with this angelic force depends on spiritual refinement. This process awakens within us an inner knowingness that there is far more to life than what meets the physical eye. By seeing the good in people, and carefully choosing your words to avoid slanderous speech, good angels will surround you.

How Angels Are Created

According to Kabbalah, when God wishes to send an angel on a mission, He merely thinks the thought and an angel is dispatched. Such is the power of Divine Thought. Though angels have existed since the beginning of time, countless more have been created on an as-needed basis by God during the course of cosmological and human history.

The highest level of angels are those that were created during the "six days of creation," which to the Kabbalistically uninitiated, were *never* meant to imply six 24-hour days.[20] Although there are differing opinions about which angels were created on each of the six days and which time-space dimension they are associated with, they are an integral part of a fixed order of God's universe and perform vital roles essential to its functioning.

God created other hierarchies of angels to perform specific tasks. In *The Wisdom of the Zohar*, Isaiah Tishby states that the lower hierarchies of angels "survive only for a limited amount of time and then perish after they have fulfilled their function."[21] Tishby explains that this is the meaning of Lamentations 3:23 in the Bible: "Every day ministering angels are created from a river of fire, and they utter a song and die, as it is said, 'They are new every morning. Great is your faithfulness.' " He also cites a legend that certain angels referred to as angels of destruction are thought to undergo a continuous cycle of death and rebirth. "Some of [the angels] are stricken with terror (because of the seraphim), and they burn them in fire, and then they are renewed as in the beginning."[22]

Humanity has the unique ability to create these lower hierarchies of angels as a result of prayer or by the performance of good deeds, called *mitzvah* in Hebrew. In *The Thirteen Petalled Rose,* author Rabbi Adin Steinsaltz states: "Angels . . . are continuously being created anew, in all the worlds, and especially in the world of Asiyah, where thoughts, deeds, and experiences give rise to angels of different kinds." In this angelic communications network, he explains, the spiritual holiness contained within a mitzvah or prayer ascends to become the chief component of what becomes a new angel in the world of Yetzirah.[23] The act of creating an angel in an angelic realm is an integral part of human existence. Although, by design, we cannot comprehend what is occurring, the action is part of a cosmic gestalt that results in blessings coming back to us.

Communicating with Angels

With the exception of those few individuals who have been granted a gift of prophecy, an angel cannot reveal its true form to the rest of humanity whose perception belongs only to the world of Asiyah. This limitation prevents us from grasping the presence of an angel that belongs to the time-space dimensions of the angels—the worlds of Briyah and Yetzirah. According to the great sage Maimonides, "[divine insight is bestowed upon] all the prophets [other than Moses] through the medium of an angel."[24]

According to Kabbalah, one's ability to communicate with angels is determined by the level at which the "root" of the person's soul originates on the Tree of Life. It is just a fact of life that certain individuals are born with certain God-given gifts, while others are not. It is also true that this ability is determined by whom that person has been in their past lives. However, Linda tells her clients that as they physically detox it is possible for them to deepen their consciousness and awareness to an extent where they may achieve a level of communication with their guardian angels or spirit guides.

Angelic Hierarchies

Besides sensing a particular weight of the pendulum that determines which archangel she is talking to, Linda can see angels in one or more colors hovering in midair. Of this much she is sure: with the exception of cherubs, angels are not cute, baby-faced children with pretty wings. The hierarchies of angels all look different. To the more advanced Hebrew prophets such as Ezekiel or Isaiah, it was clear that angels take on a phantasmagorical, even psychedelic, appearance of creatures. Most importantly, they describe the *chayot* or archangels that speak to Linda—Michael, Gabriel, Raphael, and Uriel. They are also referred to as the living creatures or angels of the throne that carry the King's chariot and the throne of glory.[25] Although several additional orders exist, we will briefly discuss four hierarchies of angels and the worlds they inhabit. As described in Figure 19-1, these include *seraphim*, *cherubim*, chayot, and *ophanim*.

• **Seraphim.** The four chayot, located in Yetzirah, contain the seraphim, located in Briyah, within them. This means they control the seraphim and mitigate the judgment and fire in them.[26] The prophet Isaiah (6:1–3) describes the seraphim, which in Hebrew means "burning ones," as follows: ". . . I saw the Lord sitting upon a throne, high and lifted up; and His train filled the *Hekhal* (sanctuary). Above Him stood the Seraphim; each had six wings: with two he covered his face, and with two he covered his feet, and with two he flew." In his vision, the seraphim cry continually to each other, "Holy, holy, holy is the Lord of hosts: the whole earth is filled with His glory."[27]

• **Cherubim.** The Zohar states that the cherubim are from Briyah. The prophet Ezekiel describes them as having four faces and four wings. After Adam and Eve were expelled from the Garden of Eden in the world of Yetzirah down to the physical world of Asiyah, they were prevented from returning there by cherubim, who guarded the entrance to Garden of Eden with "flaming rotating swords." In Exodus (25:22) God spoke to Moses between two cherubs that stood facing one another on the Ark in the Holy of Holies in the Tabernacle in Jerusalem. The cherubs were made out of gold in the form of two young children with wings.

• **Chayot (archangels).** A biblical prophecy called Ezekiel's Vision of the Chariot [*merkavah*] gives an amazing description of what the lower two angelic hierarchies, chayot and ophanim, look like and how they communicate with each other. [Note: I have taken slight liberties in editing the following excerpt from Ezekiel's Vision of the Chariot (1:5–1:18). Without such editing, the description is somewhat incoherent. I've also included some material provided by scholar Howard Schwartz, author of the excellent book *Tree of Souls*, to clarify some of the language which otherwise is awkward and confusing.]

> I saw, and behold a stormy wind came sweeping out of the north—a huge cloud and flashing fire, surrounded by a radiance; and from its midst was the likes of a Speaking Silence in the center of the fire.

From its midst was the form of four Chayot [Archangels Michael, Gabriel, Raphael, and Uriel]. This was their appearance: They had human form. Each had four faces, and each of them had four wings. The legs of each were fused into a single rigid leg; and the feet of each were round like those of a single calf's hoof; and they shined like a vision of polished copper. Human hands were under their wings on all four sides. Their wings were separated on top: two of them touching those of the others, while the other two wings covered their bodies. Their wings were joined [to lift up the throne of glory], and they did not turn when they went. The form of their faces was the face of a man to the front, with the face of a lion to the right of the four, the face of an ox to the left of the four, and the face of an eagle to the back. Each one moved in the direction of their faces as they went, going wherever the spirit impelled them to go, without turning when they moved. The form of [these angels] had the appearance of burning coals of fire. This fire, suggestive of torches, had a radiance, and the Chayot angels ran and returned, like a vision of lightning.[28]

Here is spiritual insight into angelic anatomy. As mentioned earlier, an angel is the personification of a particular divine attribute. Angels are fixed and do not grow or develop in any way. This is why they are depicted as having the physical characteristic of "a single rigid leg." Since walking is synonymous with growth and development, an angel has no need for two legs; their one "leg serves only as a pedestal to stand on."[29] In contrast, humans are "goers" or "walkers," requiring two legs, free to choose a path of enlightenment or one of spiritual decline.

• **Ophanim.** The chayot control the four ophanim (wheels of the chariot angels), which are from the world of Asiyah. According to the Zohar, these four rule over thirteen million other ophanim.[30] The description from Ezekiel's Vision continues:

Then I gazed at the Chayot angels and behold, I saw four Ophan angels on the earth near the Chayot angels. There was one Ophan angel on each wheel. Their appearance and actions were like a vision of topaz. Each had four faces that moved in tandem with the Chayot angels. The rims of all four wheels were tall and frightening for they were all covered over with eyes. The structure of each wheel was like an Ophan angel within an Ophan angel—two wheels cutting through each other. And when they moved, each could move in the direction of any of its four quarters. When the Chayot angels moved, the Ophan angels went near them. When the Chayot angels rose up from the earth, the Ophan angels were also lifted.

Wherever the spirit of the Chayot angels had to go, the Ophan angels were taken because the spirit of the Chayot angels was in the Ophan angels.[31]

Further research in the Zohar and a book entitled *Innerspace* by Rabbi Aryeh Kaplan reveals that the chayot receive a primal life force from the highest spiritual dimensions and then transmit it to their progeny, the ophan angels.[32]

With a clear visual image of what angels look like in mind, we see in the daily Jewish prayer book a specific description of how these angels interact with each other as they pray to God. It states:

Holy, holy, holy is the Lord, Master of Legions, the whole world is filled with his glory. Then the *Ophanim* and the holy *Chayot*, with great noise raise themselves towards the Seraphim. Facing them they give praise saying: Blessed is the glory of the Lord from his place.

THE NATURE OF ANGELS

God created different hierarchies of angels to perform their own specific functions in service to Him. Although descriptions of them vary widely, we can draw specific conclusions about their personalities and innate "fixed" nature. In researching this, I was struck by the fact that this aspect of understanding angels was similar in the Jewish and Christian faiths.

• **A loving and compassionate nature.** With the exception of Satan, angels of destruction, fallen angels, demons and harmful spirits, described later in this chapter, the very existence of angels is predicated on their understanding that they were literally created to serve God in love, with a healthy fear and awe. As a result, their innate nature is loving. Although certain hierarchies of angels (archangels and seraphim) have a more intellectual approach than other angelic orders, they do not dabble in abstractions. Their core essence is that of a loving, understanding being. Their knowledge is heart knowledge[33], borne of deep supernal wisdom, not superficial understanding. Cherubim approach their devotion of service to God from a perspective that is skewed toward the emotions.

• **A powerful, strong-willed nature.** Angels are driven by blind faith to serve the Creator as it is their very reason for being. Some angels such as Archangel Michael serve God from the right side of the Tree of Life and show mercy, compassion, or tough love, as needed. Some angels such as Archangel

Gabriel serve God from the left side of the Tree of Life and execute from mild to strict judgment in carrying out the Divine Will. There is also a militaristic side to angels who go forth and serve the Lord in battle. They move in formations called camps. (See www.thehealinggift.com.)

• **A high level of intuition.** According to Catholic theologian St. Thomas Aquinas, angels are highly intuitive beings.[34] They do not require a left-brain, analytical, deductive reasoning process or the outcome of a hypothetical experiment to get an answer. Nor do they require an advanced degree to learn the essence of things.[35] They get it all intuitively, right away. Communicating with one's guardian angel helps people develop their intuitive nature in accordance with a focus on spiritual development and meditation.

The Functions of Angels

Just as no two people are exactly the same, no two angels are either. Each serves the Creator in its own way, performing that function for which it was expressly created. This may include a wide variety of activities:

• **Guarding us.** Jewish and Christian prayer books are replete with such examples. Psalm 91 is used to ward off forces of evil and invoke supernatural protective qualities. "For He orders his angels to protect you wherever you go. They will hold you with their hands to keep you from striking your foot on a stone." Another example from the Jewish daily prayer book (*siddur*) is the Wayfarer's Prayer for one embarking on a journey, which states: "Jacob went on his way and angels of God encountered him. Jacob said when he saw them, 'This is a Godly camp.' So he named the place *Machanayim* . . . Behold I send an angel before you to protect you on the way and to bring you to the place that I have prepared." Two other dramatic examples of this in Hebrew scripture are:

o The story of the Akeida where Archangel Michael prevents Abraham from carrying out the execution of his son Isaac when tested by God (see Chapter 20).

o During the captivity of the Jews in Babylon in the 6th century B.C., the prophet Daniel continues to pray to the Hebrew God *Yahweh* (YHVH) against the expressed orders of the king. As a result, Daniel is thrown into a lions' den to be devoured. However, God sends an angel to protect him, and he emerges miraculously unharmed the next day.

• **Defending us.** The greatest example of this is the splitting of the Red Sea, where Moses utilized Kabbalistic technology to activate seventy-two angels to part the Red Sea so the Jewish people could cross safely and avoid certain death at the hands of the Egyptian soldiers. (See www.thehealinggift.com.)

• **Healing us.** Archangel Raphael assists in healing Abraham after he circumcised himself at God's command. The principal book of healing used by the patriarchs was the Book of the Angel Raziel.

• **Instructing and inspiring us.** Here are some examples of archangels instructing biblical leaders: Archangel Raziel taught Adam the mysteries of the cosmos that were unknown even to other angels. Archangel Gabriel taught Joseph seventy languages needed to earn the respect of the pharaoh and be appointed viceroy of Egypt. Moses learned the secrets of God from Archangel Michael.

• **Accusing us.** Angels sit in judgment of humanity at different times during our lives, including the day of our death. An astonishing testimonial that involves accusing angels at the end of this chapter is a frightening reminder of this. The chief prosecutor in these matters may be Satan himself, called Samael, or one of his underlings, described later in this chapter.

• **Heralding major announcements.** Archangel Michael disguised as a wayfarer tells Abraham about the upcoming birth of his son Isaac. Abraham was also told by Archangel Gabriel disguised as a wayfarer about the upcoming destruction of Sodom. In the Book of Judges (13:21), an angel comes to the wife of Manoach to inform her that she will bear a son named Samson who will save the Israelites from the Philistines.

• **Facilitating prophecy.** According to Rabbi Luzzatto, with the exception of Moses, "the experience of prophecy must come about through [angelic] intermediaries" who act as a lens through which one who is prophesizing receives a vision. Luzzatto explains that during the act of prophecy "a prophet is greatly overwhelmed. His body and all his limbs immediately begin to tremble and he feels as if he is being turned inside out."[36]

• **Mediating between God and humanity.** Angels transmit the prayers of humanity to God. Regarding the Archangel Metatron, the Zohar says, "He carries the prayers of Israel up to the firmament and deposits them there in order to arouse the compassion of the Holy One, blessed be He."[37]

• **Overseeing the laws of nature.** To explain this phenomenon, we must understand the difference between two of the several names that God is called in the Jewish faith: Elohim and Yahweh. If you look in the Torah, you find that Elohim is the God who spoke to Abraham, Isaac, and Jacob. However, when Moses spoke to God, he spoke to Yahweh. Why would God change his name? Isn't that the point of monotheism—that He is One? It seems a bit confusing at first, but it isn't if you apply the following analogy:

Think of the names of God (and there are many) as different facets of a diamond. The facets are all different, but ultimately they are all different aspects of the same diamond. The various names of God represent various aspects of His ultimately complex and incomprehensible nature. Elohim is the facet of the diamond that refers to God at the level of nature. Even Ramses, the pharaoh who tried to prevent Moses and the Jews from leaving Egypt, understood God at this level. Only Moses dealt with God at the higher level or a bigger facet of the diamond that represents God at a level that is beyond nature. These involve phantasmagorical events of multidimensional complexity such as the burning bush episode, the ten plagues, or the crossing of the Red Sea (see Chapter 20) that required angelic interaction. Ramses could not comprehend God at this level. Nor can science—although in the early 21st century, quantum physics is finally beginning to knock on heaven's door.

Just as invisible vibrating strings of energy control all matter from various time-space dimensions according to superstring theory, God's agents and messengers operate from the upper worlds. Angels act as an invisible force, triggering, like the first falling domino, a scientific chain reaction that initiates all extraordinary geological and weather events on earth—from Hurricane Katrina to the 2005 tsunami in the Philippines and the 2010 earthquake in Haiti, albeit based on incomprehensible upper world logic. It is a logic similar to the reasons why a past life personality attribute or event can affect one's current life—or the real reasons why cancer suddenly appears in the body.

It is no coincidence that every major religion has prayers specifically designed to modify nature. When this construct eventually becomes accepted by science, it will necessitate new scientific and spiritual understandings of our natural world.

• **Presiding over the guardian angels of the seventy nations.** The metaphysical construct "as above, so below" is of vital importance regarding the political strife that exists in the world today. It is mentioned in Daniel (10:20-21) that each of the seventy nations that descended from Adam are collectively ruled over by each nation's own guardian angel. The Book of Enoch (89:59) states that Archangel Michael, as Israel's angel-prince, presides over the "seventy shepherds" who are the guardian angels of the 70 nations. With these 71 angel-princes of the world, God sits in council when holding judgment over the world; each angel-prince is able to plead the cause of its nation before God.[38]

As astonishing as Isaiah (24:21) may sound, "The fate of a particular nation below depends on the status of its guardian angel. When the angel prospers, so does his nation; when he fails; so does his nation. Thus it is written that YHVH will punish the host of heaven [guardian angels], and the kings of the earth [government leaders] on earth."[39]

What is of greatest relevance in our current age is the spiritual understanding that there are angels who preside over nations in conflict with one another. When Jacob had his dream about the ladder, among the angels he saw ascending and descending were the angel-princes of the nations of Babel, Media, Greece, Syria, and Rome.[40] Linda receives hints of information when she channels about world affairs that "angelic wars" are raging in the upper realms among these presiding angels. When Israel is oppressed by other nations because of its own transgressions, it is in a state of exile and under the dominion of the guardian angels of the other nations. However, it can never be destroyed because of God's ultimate relationship to Israel.[41] Since no human logic can possibly explain events as they are unfolding in the Middle East, perhaps it is time to consider a metaphysical/spiritual solution.

• **Ushering certain righteous individuals into the angelic realms.** See the story of Moses ascending into the angelic realms later in this chapter.

• **Assisting at the time of death.** The role of the angels of death begins in earnest thirty days before a person is ordained to die and continues through a remarkable process that occurs right after burial called the "beating of the grave" (*chibut hakever*), in which the yetzer hara (the dark angelic force) is forcefully separated from the soul by four angels whose job it is to "take him by the 'corners' and shake and beat him with fire." The process is far more painful for evil-doers who are more attached to their yetzer hara than for righteous individuals.[42] Although there may be differences in how various angels of death appear, the Zohar describes one particularly macabre vision of a dying man on his sickbed meeting Dumah, the angel of death: "The King's guard [an executioner angel] descends and stands before him at his feet with a sharpened sword in his hand. The man raises his eyes and sees the walls of the room burning with the fire that emanates from [the angel of death]. And then he sees himself in front of [the angel of death], covered with eyes, clothed in fire, burning in the man's presence."[43]

Negative Angels

Several years ago Bob Dylan wrote a simple but insightful song called "Serve Somebody" with the lyrics: "It may be the devil, or it may be the lord, but you gotta serve somebody."[44] Here are the various types of negative angels that exist:

• **Satan.** Both the Jewish and the Christian faiths agree that Satan, also known as *Samael* or Lucifer, respectively, was thrown out of heaven by God for transgressions against the Creator. However, to suggest that this is merely a question of God versus Satan in the battle for souls is, from a Kabbalistic perspective, an overly simplistic notion. It is important to remember that *God created Satan and the other dark forces* for a reason. Satan has a specific job to do, and that is to make us believe he doesn't exist. He nurtures this illusion by boosting our egos to the extent that we forget about our relationship with God. This causes us to put a premium on the physical world at the expense of our own spiritual growth. God does not interfere with our free will and our moral and spiritual decision-making processes. He tests us to see if we possess the consciousness required to exercise the proper free will in accordance with the divine plan. Satan *cooperates* with God by providing a litany of negative temptations. Satan or one of his operatives then presides as our accuser before God when we falter and succumb to the illusion he has so artfully woven—that he and negative repercussions of evildoing do not exist. In fact, Satan or his operatives can also function in the role of the angel of death or the evil inclination. In Chapter 20 we describe his ongoing battle and complex relationship with Archangel Michael.

In Judaism, *Gehennom* is the equivalent of hell, a place of punishment. It has much in common with the Christian concept of hell, except for one significant difference: In the Jewish view, punishment in Gehennom never lasts more than a year, while in the Christian view it is eternal.[45]

• **Angels of destruction.** There are other types of negative angels as well. According to Rabbi Luzzatto, "Everything in the world, whether good or bad, is done through them . . . [and they] are divided into two groups . . . one appointed to do good, whether it be physical or spiritual, and the others appointed for evil, both physical and spiritual. Those appointed for evil are called angels of destruction (*malachei chavalah*), harmful spirits (*mazzikim*), and demons (*shedim*)."[46] These subversive angels are actually created by the evil behaviors of humanity. They exist as permanent parasites, growing in power as they feed off a person's sins. The sinner is punished by being brought into contact with the level and domain of evil he creates.[47] According to the Zohar, the task of the *malachei chavalah* is one of punishment: "to crush the souls who dwell in Gehennom."[48] Legend has it that shedim were conceived through a union between Adam and Lilith, his first wife. Shedim can wreak havoc in various ways that include affecting one's dreams. A demon stands next to a person while he sleeps a light sleep and whispers frightening things in his or her ear, troubling the person's mind and making them afraid. These demons remain standing at a person's side, rejoicing and laughing that they were able to cause such fear.[49]

- **Fallen angels.** Not all angels fulfill their God-given destiny and are subject to similar metaphysical scrutiny and judgment as humanity is before the Creator. There is a Jewish legend about two angels in heaven, Uzza and Azael, who originally rebelled against their Master by objecting to the creation of humanity and the sin of Adam and Eve. According to the Zohar, God replied: If you had been with them, you would have sinned as well. As punishment for their rebellion, God cast them down from heaven and sent them to earth. They became the fallen angels (*nefilim*)[50] who ran after women and caused humankind to err. Genesis (6:2–4) describes the fallen angels: "The sons of God saw that the daughters of man were good, and they took themselves wives from whomever they chose . . . [and fathered the titans]. The titans were on the earth in those days and also later . . . The titans were the mightiest ones who ever existed, men of renown."[51]

Testimonial: How the heavenly angelic court dispenses divine judgments and decrees

---

As we continue to expand our knowledge of the angelic realms, we have been amazed to discover a complex legal system that in many ways parallels our own system of jurisprudence. Although we were familiar with the Talmudic axiom "as above, so below," we were nonetheless astonished to find major similarities between the ways in which divine justice and decrees are meted out by various hierarchies of angels and the ways that justice is meted out by our court system. These discoveries only served to confirm our suspicions of the degree to which the upper realms are a parallel universe to our own.

The story of how we became aware of this phenomenon happened quite by accident. However, as we know, there really are no accidents. The information gleaned from the following story was not only meant for the individual doing a health reading with Linda on behalf of his dying uncle. It was meant for our own edification as well.

A friend of ours, whom we will call Nathan, came to us concerning his dying uncle, a man in his late 50s whom we will call Sam. Nathan told us that Sam, who had been diagnosed with stage 4 lung cancer that had metastasized in the liver, had just been discharged from a local hospital in Los Angeles. His oncologists told him to "go home and get his affairs in order" as they had exhausted all attempts to aggressively treat his cancer with both chemotherapy and radiation without success. After describing the urgency of the situation, Nathan told us the family was wealthy, and they were prepared to spend whatever was required to save Sam by alternative means.

At the reading the next day, Nathan gave Linda a detailed summary of what his uncle had recently endured. Although Nathan knew that Linda did not diagnose or treat cancer unless it was to deal with negative emotions and past-life issues associated with the disease, the family wanted to know if any alternative cancer clinics might be effective in providing the miraculous cure they all deeply desired. They were prepared to take Sam anywhere in the world, if need be.

Nathan described Sam as a driven businessman who consumed large quantities of coffee and smoked one to two packs of cigarettes a day. As his health began to fade, his family pleaded with him to either cut back or eliminate both of these habits. He ignored all their requests and possessed an almost cavalier attitude that these habits had no negative effect on his health. He was driven to succeed in his business ventures to the exclusion of everything else.

Linda did a detailed reading on Sam's health. She rattled off a litany of toxins that were the physical cofactors behind the cancer. These included heavy metal toxicity, fungi, parasites, and acidosis, among other things. There were also negative emotions and unresolved past-life issues, but there was certainly no time for any of that. The fire first had to be put out—and fast.

Linda then channeled from an extensive list of alternative clinics/physicians outside the United States. The only one that came up for her to recommend was Dr. Hans Dorfmann, a brilliant German doctor whom we had worked with in 1991. He had successfully treated both of us and had taught us many aspects of German Biological Medicine, which we hold in high esteem. Among his protocols were injections of a specially prepared and purified thymus gland fraction obtained from a one-week-old lamb, which can literally jump-start the immune system to start fighting back against the cancer. Other protocols he used were similar to the brilliant pioneering work of Dr. Hans Nieper, M.D.[52], who had been his associate.

Linda stressed that there was literally no time to waste and that if everything went down like a military operation, the angelic guides told her there was only a 20 percent chance of survival. Still, 20 percent was 20 percent. The family understood the risks and, deciding to leave no stone unturned, immediately contacted Dr. Dorfmann. Linda's work was finished, and Nathan was soon engaged in direct talks with Dr. Dorfmann to sort out the details of how to proceed.

They devised the following plan. Dr. Dorfmann would take the train from Germany to a remote arctic area of a certain Scandinavian country where the sheep farm/laboratory that processed the thymus extract fraction was located. He would call Sam's family from there to tell them when he had the extract, packed in dry ice, in hand and was ready to take the train back to Cologne. Sam's family members would immediately fly with him to Germany to check into the medical clinic where Dr. Dorfmann worked. This had to go down like clockwork as the fresh thymus extract only has a potent shelf life of four to six weeks. It must be injected several times a week within this time period before it loses potency.

After Sam's family agreed to a price for these services, the money was immediately bank-wired to Germany and arrangements were made with the clinic. The doctor then wired funds to the laboratory to have them make the thymus extract. Then the waiting period started. After about a week, Dr. Dorfmann called to tell Nathan there had been a breakdown of lab equipment and it would take another ten days to get the thymus extract made. The doctor was rather embarrassed and commented to Nathan that in all the years he had known this lab, nothing like this had ever happened before. Finally, the doctor got word that the thymus extract was ready. Just as Dr. Dorfmann was getting ready to go to the train station, he tripped and fell down a flight of stairs, badly bruising his hip and leg. Since he was now in no condition to walk, much less travel, the trip had to be delayed for at least another week.

During this protracted period of waiting, Sam's condition continued to deteriorate. The family was getting frustrated and despondent. After the initial elation of real hope, the process had bogged down into a waiting game for the most bizarre and illogical of reasons. As Nathan described the whole frustrating ordeal, Linda immediately sensed that something was very wrong and told Nathan he should come to her office later that day. The information revealed in that session was a bombshell that has increased our awe and respect for the power of angels as a mechanism for facilitating divine judgment and executing divine decree.

After Linda went into trance and astral-traveled to Yetzirah, she received information that clarified the utter illogic of the situation. Although the information she initially received regarding the 20 percent possibility of saving Sam's life was technically correct, she had failed to ask the right question. That question, as surreal as it may seem, was this: "Is there any blockage from the angelic realms that will prevent a healing from occurring?"

The answer, unfortunately, was an unwavering "yes." The angels revealed that Sam's preoccupation with his material life, his reckless disregard for the sanctity of his physical temple—his body—and other personal issues they would not reveal had influenced the presiding angelic court to render a verdict whereby *no attempt, no matter how heroic or medically correct, would be allowed to succeed!* Getting lung cancer should have been a spiritual wake-up call to force Sam to deal with his own mortality. However, even this had not resulted in any meaningful level of soul searching that would transform his negative behaviors so he could reconnect to the lightforce of God. His insistence on rationalizing all aspects of his life and ignoring all the physical, emotional, and spiritual warning signals around him had been his undoing. An accusing angel had persuaded the angelic court to pass judgment so that the lab equipment had to break and the unsuspecting doctor had to bruise his hip and knee so the life-saving remedies would never reach Sam. The best-laid plans of mice and men had been rendered powerless by the angelic court.

Upon witnessing this communication, we were all rendered speechless—indeed awestruck by not only the finality of the judgment, but how powerless we are before the Creator. We bore witness to the futility that humanity faces, believing we can ultimately outsmart, outthink, or even fudge the laws of karma. It was a lesson of extreme humbleness and contrition before God that was necessary for our spiritual development. (See "Lessons Learned Through Angelic Communication.")

Lessons Learned Through Angelic Communication

We are constantly modifying the databases as new medical, emotional, or spiritual information becomes available. In the unfortunate case of Sam, Linda had simply not thought of the right question to ask. From this episode, we amended the Metaphysical Database to include the following categories: "accusing angels," "defending angels," and "angelic court verdict."

To verify our experience with accusing angels and angelic courts, we turned to Rabbi Chaim Luzzatto, who described such matters in detail in his book *The Way of God*. We urge those of you who have an interest in understanding divine intervention in human affairs to read the relevant sections of this book. The angels have confirmed to Linda that what Rabbi Luzzatto wrote is absolutely true. (Details of this phenomenon are also discussed in various writings of the Hebrew prophets.) Here are the key points Rabbi Luzzatto makes in describing how the heavenly court works as well as how it compares to our legal systems on earth.[53] Again, as above, so below:

- The spiritual realm contains courts of justice and deliberating bodies, with appropriate rules and procedures consisting of spiritual beings in particular systems and levels that resemble an earthly government. All earthly events are brought to courts in the spiritual realm, which decide heaven's response and issues decrees.

- God may appoint a special prosecutor, Satan, who seeks judgment before the tribunals where he indicts and arraigns the defendant.

- Angels that oversee earthly matters provide testimony at the heavenly tribunal.

- Each court member presents his argument, revealing insights into the case.

- The head judge must listen to all sides and issue the final decree.

ANGELS AND HUMANITY: AN UNEASY BUT HOLY ALLIANCE

As stated earlier, angels are messengers of God who live to do his Will. Though angels remain firmly committed to helping humanity, the relationship between them has not always been on such great footing. There exists, to this day, a sort of angelic consternation bordering on jealousy due to God's devotion to humanity in spite of its deeply flawed, intrinsic proclivity for the evil inclination. The angels' grievance stems from the fact that they were created long before humanity and were imbued with the ability to see Godliness more clearly than we can.

In 3 Enoch, an Old Testament apocryphal book written by high priest Rabbi Ishmael around 90–135 A.D., the angels object to the elevation of Enoch into heaven to become transformed into the angel Metatron, in much the same way as they objected to the creation of humanity and of giving the Torah to the Israelites.[54] It is important to understand that God created the Torah, the owner's manual of creation, before He actually created the universe. The Talmud states: He "looked into the Torah," meaning He consulted His blueprint of Creation before creating the universe. However, the Torah He gave the angels was actually a rearrangement of the Hebrew letters, making it substantially different from the Torah he gave to humanity. The Angelic Torah containing secrets of Kabbalah is the most beloved possession of the angels. If angels are not singing songs of praise to the Almighty or performing an assigned task, they obsess with studying secrets of the Creation and the cosmos contained within *their* Torah. It was therefore with shock and dismay that they observed Moses climbing up Mount Sinai to receive the variation of their Torah that was God's gift to humanity![55]

When Moses left the Jewish people to climb Mt. Sinai to receive the Torah, he metaphorically left the earth and ascended into the angelic realms. Moses was then transported to the archangelic court, where it was time for him to defend the Jewish people from the accusing angels, the metaphysical prosecutors of the court. What sort of leader would he be? Moses was functioning in a new role—that of metaphysical defense attorney for the downtrodden Jewish people. Here is a summary of this courtroom drama as described in the Talmud (Shabbos 88B): Why, the angels pleaded before God, would he want to give the Torah—the owner's manual of all Creation—to a people whom Moses had admittedly called "a stiff-necked people" and who, as a formerly enslaved people, still exhibited an unappreciative slave mentality, even after they had been liberated? God chose to overrule His angels, and the essence of His argument was: The angels had never endured the hardships that the Israelites had and could not therefore "walk a mile in their sandals."

In the 21st Century, Humanity Comes Full Circle with the Sin of Adam and Eve

According to Kabbalah, the future of humanity is integrally connected to its origins with Adam and Eve. When God first created the Adamic race, Adam, the first "modern" man, did not possess a mortal body. He was created like angels as a body of light. The "brightness" of his light was far beyond that of other angels. Quoting from various Torah commentaries, biblical scholar Howard Schwartz writes in *Tree of Souls:* "So astonishing was the sight of Adam that the ministering angels became confused, and mistook him for a divine being, and wished to proclaim him as God. So God caused Adam to fall into a deep sleep, and then all the angels knew he was but a man."[56] However, in many ways Adam had abilities far beyond that of other angels. Of enormous stature as well as being immortal, Adam possessed the ability to see all the way until the end of time. In fact, God intended to set Adam up as king over the angels. All this changed, however, after he and Eve sinned and were expelled from the Garden of Eden, which resides in the world of Yetzirah. They then took on human bodies and became mortal instead of immortal. Adam's perception of the divine and the other amazing gifts that he had been given were lowered to the level of Asiyah, below the attributes and abilities of the angels.

To discuss the metaphysical implications for humankind during this most difficult 6000-year cycle we are now nearing the end of is beyond the scope of this book. Kabbalah contains detailed information on this subject. What we can say in generalized terms is that when Adam and Eve sinned, that caused a cataclysmic rearrangement of the worlds. Much of the evil that exists in the world today had it origins in the aftereffects of this cosmic shock.

Linda has channeled that humanity must return to the consciousness that Adam experienced in the Garden of Eden. According to Kabbalah, humanity must fix that which it has broken (*tikkun olam* = heal the world). Linda has channeled that humanity, in its current state, is at a crossroads facing one of two options. Either ascend spiritually and become "fully human" as was Adam, in order to view the universe from a *Yetziric* perspective as the angels do, or devolve into our lower animal nature and become "fully animal." If the latter scenario happens, it is because humanity has collectively allowed its evil inclination to triumph over its good inclination. If we exercise our free will in such a manner, we will certainly face a dangerous and horrific future. The main question both now and in the future will then be: How much patience will God have with a fallen humankind? We can remember Noah and the flood or, for that matter, the tsunami in Asia in 2005 and the earthquake in Haiti in 2010. Or ignore them at our own risk.

CHAPTER 20

Meet the Archangels: A Guide to Those Angels That Speak to Linda

Holy, Holy, Holy is the Lord, Master of Legions,
the whole world is filled with His glory.
—THE PROPHET ISAIAH

SINCE 1993 WHEN HER CHANNELING GIFTS began to manifest, Linda has communicated with various archangels on an almost daily basis. Linda has revealed that she can distinguish which particular archangel she is communicating with by the "weighting" of the pendulum in her hand (weighting is Linda's term for the degree of weight she feels in the pendulum). Indeed, I have held the pendulum in my hand right after Linda has told me which archangel she is speaking with, and I can verify that the actual weight of the pendulum varies in accordance with the archangel she is speaking to. Although she has the ability to call on many different archangels, the ones with whom she communicates on the most regular basis are the four chariot angels of the throne—Michael, Gabriel, Raphael, and Uriel—and Metatron, the "king of the angels." The angel that is primarily involved with medical issues is Raphael.

Our understanding of archangels is through the lens of the Old Testament (Torah). Although the archangels are not mentioned by name there, they are found in the writings of the Hebrew prophets and in Talmudic, Chassidic, and Kabbalistic texts. In fact, even the daily Jewish prayer book (siddur) has an important prayer called the Bedtime Shema which states: "In the name of Hashem, God of Israel: may Michael be at my right, Gabriel at my left, Uriel before me, Raphael behind me; and above my head the presence of God." Our spiritual life revolves around the study of these sacred texts, coupled with ongoing personal refinement within that perspective.

Linda and I are not authorities on the New Testament or the Koran. We therefore do not delve into the subtle energetics of angelology from the Christian and Islamic perspectives. When the archangels communicate with Linda, they speak to us only from the perspective that we know and understand. We therefore do not represent that this information is the only valid approach to the subject of angels. It is just our approach.

With that in mind, here are brief biographical portraits of Metatron, Michael, Gabriel, Raphael, and Uriel, the most important archangels that have conversed with Linda since 1993.

THE CURRICULUM VITAE OF METATRON

Unlike Michael or Gabriel, Metatron is not directly mentioned by name in the writings of the prophets. However, due to his level of holiness, his name, unlike that of Michael or Gabriel, cannot be spoken directly out loud but is said silently to oneself. For this reason, when his name is spoken, it is phonetically pronounced "Ma-tat." In the Zohar, he is also identified as being the twin brother of Archangel Sandalphon, who has the ability to transform himself into the angelic prophet Elijah. It is Elijah who transmitted the information contained in the Zohar to Rabbi Shimon bar Yochai, who authored it in the 2nd century A.D.

In the Book of Enoch, an important but obscure piece of Jewish mystical literature, Metatron is revealed to have been a biblical figure named Enoch, who was the son of Jared and father of Methuselah, the man with the longest recorded lifespan in the Bible. Enoch was a descendant of Adam's third son, Seth, as well as an ancestor of Noah. He lived for 365 years, and at the end of his life he was taken away by God, ascending up to the heavens to become the angel Metatron. "And Enoch walked with God, and he was no more, because God had taken him" (Genesis 5:18–24).[1]

In the Book of Enoch, Metatron describes his journey to the upper worlds and transformation into an angel: "As soon as the Holy One, blessed be He, took me in [His] service to attend the Throne of Glory and the wheels of the *Merkavah* [chariot] and the needs of [the] *Shekhinah* [the female aspect of God], forthwith my flesh was changed into flames, my sinews into flaming fire, my bones into coals of burning juniper, the light of my eyelids into splendor of lightnings, my eyeballs into firebrands, the hair of my head into hot flames, all of my limbs into wings of burning fire, and the whole of my body into glowing fire."[2]

Why had Enoch been accorded such a glorious sendoff? In his own life on earth, Enoch had been the embodiment of supernal perfection that was originally destined for Adam prior to his fall from grace. The Creator had designed the Adamic race, with Adam as its prototype, to be imbued with a radiance that embodied this supernal perfection. However, when Adam's sin was brought about by the deception of the snake, coupled with his own lapse in judgment, this supernal radiance was removed from his soul and transferred to the soul of Enoch so it could "perfect itself in this world. Once it had achieved its full perfection in mortal existence, it ascended and took up its position at the head of the angelic throngs."[3] Since human and angelic perfection are combined in Metatron, he achieved the loftiest of positions in the celestial realms where he acts as an intermediary between man and God and [nourishes] the [righteous] souls with light from above."[4] He is referred to as the "lesser Yahweh" (the anglicized spelling of the holy name of God, YHVH) or "the king of the angels."

Linda has revealed that Metatron has the heaviest or densest weighting on the pendulum of any angel she communicates with. When he communicates with her, it is usually on very serious topics. Sometimes they are of a personal nature, and sometimes they are of global significance. Linda's most dramatic encounter with Metatron to date occurred in the summer of 2006 while our family was on vacation in Switzerland.

Revelations from Grindelwald

We drove to a mountain village named Grindelwald to take our seven-year-old son Aryeh on a ride called the Rodelbahn, which is basically a bobsled on wheels for children. After that we went to an outdoor roof garden restaurant for some coffee and ice cream. The restaurant offered a truly spectacular open-air view of three glorious mountains in the Swiss Alps—the Eiger, Jungfrau, and Monch.

As we gazed out across the valley at the incredible mountain view while waiting for our food to arrive, we suddenly heard a massive rumble and saw a large billowing cloud of smoke and ash coming from the side of the Eiger. At first we thought that either a bomb had gone off or that we were experiencing an earthquake, but we quickly realized that neither was the case. We stared in rapt astonishment as a bulbous plume of smoke and ash began to expand rapidly and started wafting over the city center of Grindelwald in the most dramatic fashion. Figures 20-1 and 20-2 are two photographs from the entire sequence that I took as the explosion unfolded.

After approximately thirty minutes the smoke and ash on the Eiger began to clear away, and we saw that a rather sizable chunk of a lower portion of the mountain had simply fallen off and crashed to the ground below (Figure

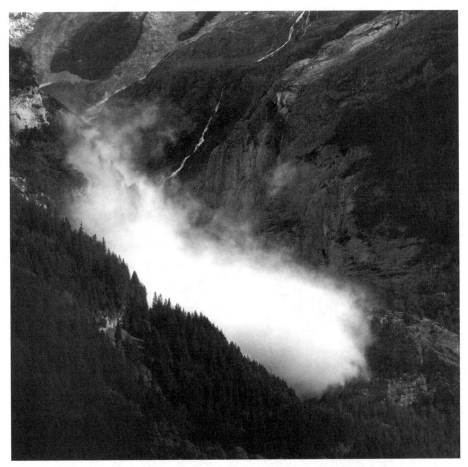

Figure 20-1. During explosion in Grindelwald, Switzerland, in 2006.

20-2). We asked two of the waitresses if they had ever seen anything like this before, and they both said that as far as they could remember, nothing of this magnitude had ever occurred. After the shock of realizing that we had just witnessed a historic geological event, it dawned on Linda and me that we had experienced this event just seconds after sitting down to look at the Eiger out of harm's way. What amazed us was that it did not happen when we were on the bobsled ride quite close to the Eiger or walking through Grindelwald earlier in the day. It happened precisely at the moment that we were given a ringside view of this natural disaster!

Suddenly Linda started shaking uncontrollably, and we immediately knew that an angel wanted to give her a message regarding what we had just witnessed. Linda got out her pendulum and soon found that Metatron had

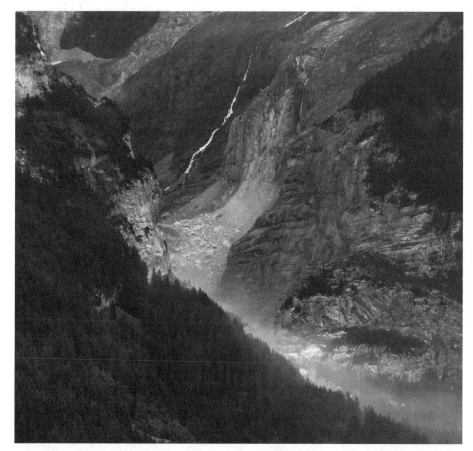

Figure 20-2. Thirty minutes after the explosion.

come to talk to her. He revealed to us that we had been maneuvered into position at just that precise moment to witness this extraordinary geological event. At that point, I decided to take Aryeh for a walk so that Linda could concentrate and get into her zone to find out what the metaphysical reasons were behind this astonishing display of nature's fury. After going into trance, Linda wrote the following exact word-by-word transmission from Metatron on the back of a napkin:

"Metatron speaking at 5:50 p.m. The Shekhinah manifestation is asserting divine displeasure regarding humanity. So we ask what are we able to do to change or gain pleasure of our God, our King, to change this judgment. He will not destroy the world, but there may be substantial damage and loss of life. [Linda got a shake when she heard this.] The physical manifestation to allow this to occur is significant climate and earth changes. There is still time."

Linda has interpreted this to be a warning as well as a message of hope. While upcoming planned disasters exist *in potentia*, there is still a window of time for a spiritual shift in consciousness that can prevent this from happening. What that window is we do not know. Suffice it to say, Linda and I were profoundly shaken by what we had witnessed. Even in an Alpine paradise we are never on vacation from God and his angels.

THE CURRICULUM VITAE OF MICHAEL

The archangel that exhibits the second densest weighting of the pendulum is Michael. In Hebrew, the name Michael means "Who is like God" or "Who is as God." Along with Gabriel, he is the only angel mentioned by name in the writings of the Hebrew prophets. Like Metatron, he is unique and powerful among angels in a multitude of ways. Linda interacts with him on a regular basis, and he gives us information on a wide range of topics, ranging from the international political landscape to more personal information that guides us in many aspects of our lives. He is the primary angel that Linda consults on the Metaphysical Database and the angel she invokes to help clear dybbuks (earthbound spirits). Since he is my guardian angel, he is heard from often. He has, on occasion, revealed himself in health readings for clients for whom he functions as guardian angel.

One of the seven archangels that God first created (Enoch, xc:21–22), Michael is said to have been created on the second day of creation.[5] He is from the time-space dimension called *Chesed* (lovingkindness) and is the "king over the holy living creatures [angels] that are in [the world of] *Yetzirah*."[6] (See Figure 19–1.) He has the highest rank of the four chariot angels of the throne, the forerunner of the Shekhinah, and the angel of forbearance and mercy (Enoch, xl:3). It is said that he taught Enoch the mysteries of clemency and justice (lxxi:2). Michael is also the guardian angel of Jacob and teacher of Moses. In the Zohar, Michael is revealed as the angel who appeared in the fire of the burning bush; he headed a group of angels who split the Red Sea; and he guided the Jews through the desert for forty years. From an astrological perspective, he rules over the planet Mercury. One of his more unusual job descriptions is that Michael leads the angels in song in the daily morning prayer service in his role as conductor of the angelic choir![7,8]

Linda characterizes Michael as being a very busy, hard-working angel. He works in multitasking mode, tirelessly performing many varied functions in both the upper and lower worlds as part of his never-ending love, service, and devotion to God. It is his very nature and essence. God created Michael for the sole purpose of serving Him with love.[9] His two most important functions in the Jewish faith are protecting the Israelites and being the high priest in the Holy Temple in the angelic parallel universe.

The Guardian Angel of Israel

In the Zohar, Michael is designated as "the guardian of Israel."[10] He was appointed by God to be the guardian angel of Israel on the day he visited Abraham, along with Gabriel and Raphael disguised as wayfarers, to announce to Abraham that Sarah, his ninety-nine-year-old wife, was pregnant with his son, Isaac. As the principal advocate of Israel, Michael has had to fight with the angelic princes of other nations. The Book of Daniel (10:13–14) speaks of Michael's assistance in helping Daniel in his struggles with the angel of Persia.[11] His principal enemy in the upper worlds, however, is Samael, the chief accuser of Israel. Michael may deal with Samael in the archangelic court, defending Israel and the Jewish people before God, or on the battlefield, defending Israel against its enemies.

However, the real origin of Michael's ongoing metaphysical battle with Samael predates the existence of the patriarchs and the Jewish people. According to legend, Michael, who represents the good inclination (yetzer tov), was already in an adversarial role with Samael, who is Satan. Samael represents the evil inclination (yetzer hara), dating from a time when he was thrown out of heaven. Samael took hold of the wings of Michael, whom he wished to bring down with him in his fall. God intervened, however, choosing to save Michael.[12]

The holiday of Rosh Hashanah is actually a universal holiday, as it is the birthday of Adam. The battle for the soul of not just Jewish people but for that of all humanity, on both an individual and collective level, is fought between Michael and Samael on this day. Rosh Hashanah falls on the first day of the astrological sign of Libra (*Tishrei*), beginning the Month of Scales, and is known as the Day of Judgment. On this auspicious day, Samael is given free reign to present all our negative actions before the Almighty and demand retribution for our deeds.

Michael as High Priest

In the Talmud, Michael is the ruler of the fourth heaven called *Zevul*, where lies the heavenly Jerusalem—the parallel universe equivalent of the Holy Temple[13], also referred to as Metatron's Tabernacle.[14] In keeping with the metaphysical concept of "as above, so below," Michael in the Holy Temple in the upper worlds is the equivalent of the High Priest (*Kohen Gadol*) who makes sacrifices in the Holy Temple in Jerusalem. The Zohar says that "if a soul deserves to pass through the gates of the terrestrial Jerusalem, the great angel Michael hastens to greet and walk with it."[15]

Genesis (28:12–17) states, "[Jacob] had a vision in a dream. 'God's angels were going up and down on it [a celestial ladder reaching to heaven] . . . How awe-inspiring this place is!' Jacob exclaimed. 'It must be God's temple. It is the gate to heaven!' " On the earth plane, the *precise place* where Jacob slept when he had this dream is none other than Mount Moriah, the very same spot where Michael prevented Abraham from slaughtering his son Isaac. This "awe-inspiring" place was to be the future home of the Holy Temple Mount in Jerusalem. This particular location, the mother of all vortexes on earth, is the most direct link to the angelic realms, and the future home of the Third Temple.

Peak Moments in the Torah Involving Michael

More than any other archangel, Michael is the unnamed angel in the Old Testament that carries out the Will of God in a most dramatic fashion for the leaders of Israel and the Jewish people. Four of the most important passages are discussed here.

1. The Binding of Isaac, Genesis (22:11–19)
In one of the most dramatic events in the Old Testament called the Binding of Isaac (Akeida), Abraham magnificently passes his test by demonstrating total allegiance to God. He shows this by his willingness to sacrifice his only son, Issac, based solely on his direct communication with God. At the last possible moment, Michael intercedes and stays the hand of Abraham, who was on the verge of slaughtering his son with a knife. Afterward, speaking on behalf of God, Michael issues a blessing for Abraham and his descendants:

> God's angel called to him from heaven and said, "Abraham, Abraham!" "Yes." "Do not harm the boy. Do not do anything to him. For now I know that you fear God. You have not withheld your only son from Him." Abraham then looked up and saw a ram caught by its horns in a thicket. He went and got the ram, sacrificing it as a burnt offering in his son's place. Abraham named the place, "God will see." Today, it is therefore said, "On God's mountain He will be seen." God's angel called to Abraham from heaven a second time and said, "God declares, I have sworn by my own

essence, that because you performed this act, and did not hold back your only son, I will bless you greatly and increase your offspring like the stars of the sky and the sand on the seashore. Your offspring shall inherit their enemies' gate. All the nations of the world shall be blessed through your descendants—all because you obeyed my voice."

2. Jacob Wrestles with an Angel, Genesis (32:25–33)

It is night and Jacob is exhausted after escaping from his father-in-law, Laban. He and his men are facing the very real possibility of an imminent attack from his brother, Esau, and his brood. Separated from his family at the banks of the river Yabbok, Jacob wrestles with "a stranger" that all rabbinic sources agree was an angel.

> Jacob remained alone. A stranger appeared and wrestled with him just before daybreak. When the stranger saw that he could not defeat him, he touched the upper joint of Jacob's thigh. Jacob's hip joint became dislocated as he wrestled with the stranger. "Let me leave!" said the stranger. "Dawn is breaking." "I will not let you leave until you bless me." "What is your name?" "Jacob." "Your name will no longer be said to be Jacob, but Israel. You have become great before God and man. You have won." Jacob returned the question. "If you would," he said, "tell me what your name is." "Why do you ask my name?" replied the stranger. He then blessed Jacob. Jacob named the place Divine Face (*Peniel*). He said, "I have seen the Divine face to face, and my soul has withstood it." The sun rose and was shining on him as he left Peniel. He was limping because of his thigh.

There is a highly regarded *Midrashic* interpretation[16] (a corpus of religious commentary written from the 2nd to the 8th century) of this passage named the "Midrash Avkir" that provides a fascinating glimpse into the various roles of Michael. "At the break of day a band of ministering angels came saying, "Michael, the hour of singing in praise of the Lord has arrived" (Song of Songs 2:12 by King Solomon). These angels were members of the angelic choir whose expressed purpose for being was their daily morning glorification of God in song. They were anxiously awaiting the presence of Michael to begin their performance as he led the angels in song in his role as conductor of the angelic choir. The seriousness of this position was such that Michael was quite anxious to quickly return to his conducting podium, as he was concerned that he would be "incinerated" by the other angels if he were late for the appointed performance to begin. This is the inner meaning of the passage "Let me leave!" said the stranger. "Dawn is breaking."

Jacob then demands that he receive a blessing from the angel before he releases him. Michael replies, changing his name to Israel. By surviving the fight with the angel, Jacob's spiritual tenacity allowed him to be transformed into Israel. Michael is now understood to be not only the guardian angel of Israel, but also the guardian angel of Jacob, the patriarchal prototype of Israel. However, this passage remains a mysterious episode in the Torah. As is often the case with rabbinic commentary, there are several differing opinions as to which angel actually wrestled with Jacob, let alone opinions about the underlying motivations. (See "Linda's Role as an Arbitrator in Biblical Research.")

Linda's Role as an Arbitrator in Biblical Research

The old adage, "Two Jews, three opinions," still applies, particularly in the realm of rabbinic commentary. The Zohar identifies the angel that wrestled with Jacob as Samael while the Midrash Avkir claims it was Michael. Still other commentaries suggest it was Metatron, Gabriel, or Uriel. It certainly seems unlikely that all of them could have been wrestling Jacob. Linda's objective was to positively identify which angel wrestled with Jacob.

Among those involved with Torah scholarship, it is generally agreed that certain sources are generally more accurate for esoteric information than other sources. Because the Zohar was channeled from Elijah the Prophet, who was an angel, to Rabbi Shimon bar Yochai, the Zohar provides a higher level of metaphysical knowledge since it is the angelic "take" of what the Torah really means. It would certainly seem to be the final word on such matters. Who better to ask than an angel, which is what you do when you read the slightly incoherent Zohar.

Linda called upon Michael and asked: "Is the information contained in the Midrash Avkir correct regarding its contention that it was Michael who wrestled with Jacob?" The pendulum spun to the right, indicating "yes" but with "qualified reservations." The next question was: "Is the information contained in the Zohar correct in alleging that it was Samael who wrestled with Jacob?" Again, the pendulum spun to the right but again with "qualified reservations." Linda proceeded to ask Michael if Gabriel, Uriel, or Metatron were also "contenders" in this wrestling match. In each case, the pendulum spun to the left, indicating a clear "no." At least we were able to narrow the playing field from five down to two. Obviously, some abstract level of higher thinking was at work here. So I left the room and let Linda get into a trance state so she could sort out what Michael was trying to tell her.

When I returned a few minutes later, Linda reported that Michael had provided a new, deeper understanding that for a certain scholarly crowd would be considered mind-boggling. Michael reported that what was lacking in all these commentaries was an integration of understanding of the parallel worlds that were simultaneously at play here—yet another reaffirmation of "as above, so below." Although Michael and Samael represent diametrically different viewpoints of consciousness, they are, on a primordial level, connected at the metaphysical hip. This is because they are allegorical warriors, representing the ongoing battle between the yetzer hara (evil) on earth and the yetzer tov (good) in the angelic realms.

When I called our rabbinic consultants to report what Linda had gotten—after pausing a moment to ponder the weightiness of what had just occurred—they all agreed that this integration of Michael representing the yetzer tov and Samael representing the yetzer hara was an elegant solution that really solved this age-old mystery. Jacob had, in fact, wrestled with both angels simultaneously, albeit in different worlds. Linda had resolved this rabbinic conflict that had existed for thousands of years. We researched to see if any reliable Jewish source had drawn the same conclusion and were surprised to find that one did not exist. Clearly, our rabbinical consultants concurred that this was an example of Linda channeling Torah research on a whole new level. The authenticity of Linda's contribution to Torah research, we wish to remind the reader, is based on the validity of her medical credibility established in Chapters 2–13 and 15–16. This is why all the metaphysical information revealed in the second half of this book should be taken just as seriously—because it all comes from the same spigot.

3. The Burning Bush, Exodus (3:1–5)

Michael is the guardian angel and teacher of Moses. Michael's intervention carries on during the life of Moses after he is introduced to Yahweh. On his last day as a member of the royal family in good standing, Moses killed an Egyptian taskmaster after watching him beat a Hebrew slave to death. After this, he was forced to escape the wrath of Pharaoh by fleeing to Midian where he meets and marries his future wife, Zipporah. While tending the flock of sheep of his father-in-law, Jethro, Moses experiences a most extraordinary mystical vision. In his role as a forerunner to the Shekhinah, Michael appears to Moses in the heart of a bush ablaze with fire that was not being consumed by the fire. After this peak mystical experience, Moses undergoes a complete transformation from a reluctant prophet into the champion of the Jewish people, the counterpart of Michael on earth.

> Moshe [Moses] tended the sheep of his father-in-law Yisro [Jethro], priest of Midian. He led the sheep to the edge of the wilderness and he came to God's mountain, in the Horeb area. God's angel appeared to [Moshe] in the heart of a fire in the middle of a thornbush. He looked and behold the

bush was on fire, but was not being consumed. Moshe said, "I must go over there and investigate this great sight. Why does the bush burn and is not being consumed?" When God saw that [Moshe] was going to investigate, God called to him from the middle of the bush, and said, "Moshe, Moshe."' "Yes," replied Moshe. "Do not come any closer," said [God]. "Take your shoes off your feet. The place upon which you are standing is holy ground."

4. The Parting of the Red Sea, Exodus (14:15–22)

The most miraculous interaction between Michael and Moses involved Michael's role as the guardian angel of Israel that traveled with Moses and the Jewish people in the pillar of cloud formation to the Red Sea. In one of the most astonishing displays of angelic power ever unleashed on earth, Michael was the leader of a group of seventy-two angels that assisted Moses to do "the heavy lifting" in parting the Red Sea.

> God said to Moses, "Why are you crying out to Me? Speak to the Israelites and let them start moving. Raise your staff and extend your hand over the sea. You will split the sea and the Israelites will be able to cross over on dry land. I will harden the heart of the Egyptians and they will follow you. Then I will triumph over Pharaoh and his entire army, his chariot corps and his cavalry. When I have this triumph over Pharaoh, his chariot corps and cavalry, Egypt will know that I am God." God's angel had been traveling in front of the Israelite camp, but now it moved and went behind them. The pillar of cloud thus moved from in front of them and stood at their rear. It came between the Egyptian and Israelite camps. There was cloud and darkness that night, blocking out all visibility. All that night the Egyptians and Israelites could not approach one another. Moshe extended his hand over the sea. During the entire night, God drove back the sea with a powerful east wind, transforming the seabed into dry land. The waters were divided. The Israelites entered the seabed on dry land. The water was on their left and right like two walls."[17,18]

What is most unusual is the opening line of this section. God asks Moses why he would cry out to Him just as the Egyptian troops were about to annihilate the Israelites who were trapped at the Red Sea. What God was really saying to Moses was: "Look, I taught you how to access the angelic energies, now do it by invoking Michael and the accompanying band of angels who will split the Red Sea for you!" Of course, it took a soul of the grade of Moses to unleash the full power of these angelic forces to part the Red Sea.

This same spiritual technology that Moses used to split the Red Sea can be used to access the same seventy-two angels for assistance in overcoming our own personal Red Sea—our limitations. Each of these angels is also a specific attribute of God. They are invoked through three-letter Hebrew codes that can be used to overcome a physical, emotional, or spiritual blockage to achieve a specific goal through Kabbalistic meditations. (For more information visit www.the healinggift.com.)

THE CURRICULUM VITAE OF GABRIEL

The archangel who exhibits the third heaviest weighting of the pendulum is Gabriel. His name means "God is my strength." He is from the time-space dimension of *Gevurah* (strength) and is the angel assigned by God to perform many tasks involving the divine enforcement of strict judgment and restraint. In a word, he is the angelic bad news bear for evildoers. He is also associated with mercy, vengeance, death, revelation, language, and dream interpretation. Gabriel rules over the cherubim. As one of the four angels of the throne, Gabriel sits on the left side of God. In the same way that Michael is analogous to the High Priest (*Kohen Gadol*), Gabriel is analogous to the Priest (*Levi*).

Gabriel can also function as an angel of destruction to implement divine displeasure against any group of people, including the Jewish people or their leaders. For example, Talmudic scholars claim that God was so incensed by the marriage of the daughter of the pharaoh to King Solomon that Gabriel was sent to drive a reed into the sea around which slime would gather to form what would become the city of Rome, the destroyer of Jerusalem in 68 A.D. God was critical of the fact that Solomon allowed his wife to continue to worship idols and did not ask her to worship Yahweh. God punished Solomon's legacy by having Israel split in two, northern (Ephraim) and southern (Judah), following the death of King Solomon.[19]

In the Book of Enoch, God implores Gabriel to destroy the offspring of traitorous angels who bred with the "daughters of man" (Genesis 6:2), resulting in the evil generation that was destroyed by the flood, with the exception of Noah and his family.[22] Gabriel was the angel who warned Lot of the impending doom that would come to the sinful inhabitants of Sodom and Gomorrah. It was Gabriel who implemented the death and destruction of these cities that was clearly the Will of God.

First mentioned in the Book of Daniel, Gabriel is the heavenly messenger who appears in order to reveal God's will. Gabriel interprets the prophet's vision of the ram and the he-goat (8:15–26)[21] and explains the prediction of the seventy weeks of years (or 490 years) for the duration of the exile from Jerusalem (9:21–27).[22] In fact, the Zohar explains that a dream is a lower grade of vision than prophecy because it contains both truth and lies and thus requires interpretation. Gabriel acts as a conduit for prophetic dreams as well as their interpretations for the patriarchs, prophets, and even ordinary people.[23]

The Guardian Angel of Joseph and Beyond

When Jacob's son Joseph is a newly captured slave in servitude to Potipar, an officer in Pharaoh's military, Gabriel plays a major role as Joseph's guardian angel by helping him resist the sexual advances of Potipar's wife.[24] Gabriel was responsible for assisting Joseph in interpreting two dreams of Pharaoh. This so impressed Pharaoh that it led to Joseph's improbable elevation from slave to viceroy of Egypt, the second most important position in Egypt after Pharaoh.[25]

Prior to Joseph's ascent as the viceroy of Egypt, his astrologers asked Pharaoh: " 'What! Shall a slave who was bought for twenty pieces of silver rule over us?' Pharaoh replied: 'I find him endowed with kingly attributes!' 'If that is the case,' they answered, 'he must know the seventy languages.' Then Gabriel taught Joseph all the seventy languages spoken at Babel."[26] Gabriel was not only uniquely brilliant in his command of Hebrew, the holy mother tongue, but of all other languages including Aramaic. (The Zohar states that the angels know all the languages except Aramaic.)

Gabriel and Moses

Gabriel played a major role in the early life of Moses, saving the child's life when Pharaoh gives him a test of loyalty. When Pharaoh sets before the child coals of fire and jewels, Gabriel pushes Moses's hands to touch the coals, which burned his tongue. Touching the jewels would be interpreted as an ominous sign of events in the future when Moses would attempt to usurp the throne of Pharaoh.

However, even Moses temporarily incurred the wrath of the Almighty when he didn't circumcise his son, Gershom, at the proper time. The Zohar states: "God confronted Moses and wanted to kill him." The text continues, "Gabriel came down in a flame of fire, having the appearance of a burning serpent," with the purpose of destroying Moses "because of his sin."[27] It was the quick thinking of his wife Zipporah who saved Moses when she took matters into her own hands and circumcised her son herself.

THE CURRICULUM VITAE OF RAPHAEL

The archangel who exhibits the fourth densest weighting of the pendulum is Raphael who possesses an extraordinary gift of healing. It is he who principally influences the direction that the pendulum turns as Linda scans the medical databases. His name in Hebrew means "God has healed," and he is associated with the time-space dimension of *Tiferet* (beauty and glory).[28] In The Book of Enoch, he is described as "one of the four presences, set over all the diseases and all of the wounds of the children of men." In the Zohar it states that "Raphael is in charge of healing the earth, and through him . . . the earth furnishes an abode for man, whom also he heals of his maladies."[29] There is also a Jewish tradition of a critically ill person adding another name to his first name, the most common of which is Raphael.

Raphael was involved in returning a sacred book that describes hidden angelic wisdom involving the healing of humanity that was originally given by Archangel Raziel to Adam. This amazing book is known as *Sefer Raziel* (Book of the Angel Raziel). "When Adam transgressed, the book flew away from him. But Adam begged God for its return, and beat his breast, and entered the river Gihon up to his neck, until his body became wrinkled and his face haggard. Then God made a sign for the angel Raphael, the angel of healing, to heal Adam and bring the book back to him."[30] The book was subsequently handed down through the generations and was used as the main book of healing by Noah, Abraham, Isaac, Jacob, Joseph, Moses, and Solomon.

When Michael, Gabriel, and Raphael were disguised as travelers, they were treated to gracious hospitality by Abraham. Raphael repaid the kindness by healing Abraham, eradicating his excruciating pain on the third day after his circumcision.[31] In another account, Raphael was sent by God to heal the patriarch Jacob of an injury to his sciatic nerve after he wrestled with the angel Michael.[32] In the Testament of Solomon it is reported that after King Solomon prayed to God for help in building the Holy Temple, God responded by having Raphael deliver a gift of a sapphire ring with magical powers. The ring was engraved with a five-pointed star called a *pentalpha* that had the power to subdue all demons. It is with the slave labor of demons that King Solomon was able to complete the building of the Holy Temple.[33]

THE CURRICULUM VITAE OF URIEL

The name Uriel means "fire of God." The last of the four throne angels, Uriel is associated with the time-space dimension of *Yesod* (foundation).[34] In the

Book of Enoch (x:1–2), Uriel is the divine messenger sent by God to warn Noah of the impending deluge.[35] It is Uriel who showed a copy of the Angelic Torah to Enoch before he was transformed into Metatron. For reasons we do not understand, Linda has had less communication with Uriel than with the other three archangels over the years. He is the guardian angel of a close friend of ours, so when he periodically has a session with Linda, Uriel appears to help oversee his reading.

ANGELIC TEAMWORK

In Linda's sessions with clients, there are times when angelic teamwork is required to do the specialized function of a particular angel. It is not uncommon, for example, for Raphael to work with Michael, Gabriel, or the client's guardian angel during the course of a session. This teamwork approach is described in the Old Testament. For example, Michael and Gabriel accompanied Moses when he came down from Mount Sinai with the Ten Commandments.[36] As mentioned above, Michael, Gabriel, and Raphael visited Abraham after his circumcision. Michael's task was to announce the astonishing news that Sarah, Abraham's ninety-nine-year-old wife, would be giving birth to their son Isaac. Gabriel's job was to execute divine judgment regarding the destruction of Sodom. Raphael's job was to heal the painful circumcision that Abraham had given to himself. Each angel performed a function uniquely suited to it. Michael heralded a major announcement for the Jewish people, Gabriel carried out the Divine Will of strict judgment, and Raphael utilized his unique gifts of healing.

We were able to find further corroborating evidence proving that the angelic team approach Linda works with has historical precedent. In describing Michael and Gabriel's work together as anonymous divine messengers jointly fulfilling a divine mission, the Zohar states, "Michael declares the glory of God while Gabriel embodies the power of God."[37] In his book called *Jewish Magic and Superstition*, Rabbi Joshua Trachtenberg states, "The names that appear most frequently are those of the three archangels, Michael, Gabriel, and Raphael, often mentioned in Talmudic literature. They are called upon to perform every sort of function imaginable, usually in conjunction with lesser assistants."[38] Our experience has confirmed exactly the same thing.

CHAPTER 21

Metaphysical Patterns in Time: Soul Connections Revealed

Learn to get in touch with the silence within yourself,
and know that everything in life has purpose. There are no mistakes,
no coincidences; all events are blessings given to us to learn from.
—Elisabeth Kubler-Ross

AN IMPORTANT QUESTION RAISED in Chapter 1 was: Why Linda? Who is Linda that she should possess such a staggering and verifiable gift of healing based on the ability to communicate with angels and spirits? I alluded to the fact that the reason has only to do with who her soul is on a reincarnated level, but I remained mum on the subject of just who that might be—until now. The full extent of Linda's metaphysical lineage is a private matter. However, through the following testimonial from one of Linda's most special clients, we are prepared to reveal a piece of it now.

As mentioned earlier, an outpouring of people responded to an article about Linda written by medical researcher and author Burton Goldberg for the July–August 2004 issue of *Alternative Medicine* magazine (reprinted on www.thehealinggift.com). While the vast majority of those who have seen Linda have no past-life relationship with her, a few of them did. Thus, the impetus for them to send an email to Linda in response to the article was not merely physical. They were, metaphysically speaking, being moved around like chess pieces by a higher force so that their soul connection would be reestablished for a higher good.

AN ASTONISHING METAPHYSICAL STORY

One of Linda's most astonishing metaphysical past-life case histories involves a woman named Marilyn, a fifty-six-year-old businesswomen and entrepreneur. She and her husband Ken own a successful corporate communications and software development company. Marilyn had been clinically diagnosed with angioedema, a severe form of hives that she had suffered with for several years. When an outbreak occurred, it started on her legs and hands and quickly spread to her chest. Finally it went to her face, which became quite swollen and disfigured. Doctor after doctor was completely baffled by her case, unable to pinpoint the cause of the outbreaks. Except for the temporary relief Marilyn got from anti-inflammatory drugs, the doctors utterly failed to make a dent in her condition.

Upon reading Goldberg's magazine article, Marilyn emailed Linda describing her condition, and an appointment was set. (Amazingly, Marilyn later told me that just prior to reading the article about Linda, she had prayed to God asking Him to dispatch Archangel Raphael to find her a healer who could cure her.) As a result of her work with Linda, Marilyn was completely healed of the debilitating condition that had stymied a bevy of high-priced dermatologists. Indeed, the miraculous cure she experienced was worthy of being included in the testimonials in this book.

However, what neither of them knew at the time, and what would turn out to be far more fascinating than the healing aspect of their relationship, was the real reason why Marilyn responded to the magazine article: to reestablish a bond of friendship that had existed in two previous lifetimes. During the course of Marilyn's healing, Linda discovered that they had been close friends and associates who had worked together in at least two other lifetimes spanning thousands of years. That's when it became quite clear why it was karmically correct for Linda to be the one to heal Marilyn.

As if that weren't enough, Marilyn also went through an extraordinary metaphysical and emotional crisis as part of her healing journey, which can only be described as being "poltergeistian" in nature. Thus, her story has three intertwined parts: a health story, a poltergeist story, and two past-life relationships with Linda.

Poltergeist in German means a noisy ghost (from German *polter*, "noise" or "racket"; *geist*, "spirit"). According to *Encyclopedia Britannica*, in occultism, poltergeist is a disembodied spirit or supernatural force credited with certain malicious or disturbing phenomena, such as inexplicable noises, sudden wild movements, or breakage of household items. Poltergeists are also blamed for violent actions—throwing stones or setting fire to clothing and furniture. Such events are said to be sporadic, unpredictable, and often repetitive. In 1982, Steven Spielberg co-wrote and co-produced a fascinating supernatural horror film called *Poltergeist*, where a group of seemingly benign ghosts begin communicating with a five-year-old girl in her parents' suburban California home via static on the family television. Eventually, they use the TV as their dimensional doorway to gain entrance into the home itself. That is all fine and well, but when one walks out of the movie theater, it is reassuring to know that wasn't real. It was just the sort of phantasmagorical escapist entertainment created with special effects wizardry that Hollywood excels at.

Yet the ability to traverse multiple universes and realities is an intrinsic part of Linda's healing gift. Even for Linda, the following true story was very special for her, as the information revealed was a karmic reconnection of a very complex relationship between her and Marilyn. It was hardly just another day at the office, which Linda sometimes jokingly refers to as the "Freudland Wax Museum."

The following edited testimonial is from an interview I had with Marilyn on the physical, metaphysical, and spiritual aspects of her work with Linda:

A few weeks after returning from our summer vacation to Ireland in 2006, my husband and I began to experience what can only be described as a significant number of paranormal phenomena in our house. It started with the breakdown of our fairly new washing machine, closely followed by the dishwasher's untimely demise. However, this was not the worst of it. We suddenly started experiencing the constant breaking of glasses, particularly in the kitchen and dining areas of the house. When either my husband or I held glasses or dishes in our hands, they suddenly either broke or mysteriously fell out of our hands, smashing to the floor. Dishes also fell from their place settings on the table. Over the next couple of weeks, there were over twenty separate such incidences. We are not normally clumsy people and knew that something was dreadfully wrong, but whom could we tell this to without people thinking we were crazy?

One day we were having a family gathering to celebrate my uncle's birthday. As we were washing dishes, one of them literally flew out of my hands, went up in the air, and crashed down on the ceramic tile floor. Two pieces from the broken dish shot into my leg, which began to bleed profusely. My husband and I were both startled, but kept this ensuing madness from our family. Things then went from bad to worse.

The following week our piano tuner came over for a semi-annual tuning of our Steinway grand piano. As he started working, he was stunned to find a major structural crack running the length of the bronze metal frame inside the piano. He remarked that he had never seen anything like it before. What made the situation even more peculiar is that there were no objects within range that could have fallen on the piano. It was not even possible that this kind of damage could have occurred from the sun or the elements.

One evening a short while later, we returned home after being out all day. We opened the front door to our house, which has a two-story foyer with polished marble floors and a very large and exquisite chandelier. As I walked into my darkened house, I felt a strange grinding feeling as my shoes stepped on something that felt like shards of glass. As we turned on the light, we gazed upwards and recoiled in horror at the sight of our beautiful showcase chandelier. It had been smashed sideways into the ceiling and essentially destroyed, with most of the glass crystals shattered all over our marble floor. My husband and I were completely spooked by this incident, and I remember hurrying to our bedroom to say a complete rosary before going to bed.

We came down in the morning to survey the wreckage. To adequately describe the level of destruction that we witnessed first requires a brief explanation about the chandelier, which has a special motorized relay system with four cords that lower the chandelier down to eye level for cleaning and then raise it up to its original position. The control panel, which normally remains shut, is located in a closet near the front of the foyer. A special key in the control panel needs to be turned to lower or raise the chandelier. It appeared to us that one of the cords had actually wrapped around the chandelier, and as the cords were rising to put the chandelier back in place, it had twisted, turning the chandelier sideways, crashing it with great force against the ceiling.

A few days later a manufacturer's representative came to assess the damage. We asked him how this could have happened, and he was momentarily at a loss for words. He then admitted that the device had never malfunctioned in such a manner before. It was, he remarked, as if a great, almost vindictive force had hurled it into the ceiling for this level of damage to occur. We stood there speculating on how this could have happened. Someone would have had to have gotten into the closet and physically turned the key to raise or lower the chandelier. However, no one had been in the house that day. There was simply no rational explanation for it.

The very next day, a man who has been a trusted employee of ours for several years declared that the house was haunted. We were dumbfounded, scared, and fearful, as we had no point of reference for such things. It was if we had entered into some sort of "Twilight Zone" episode with no end in sight. Fortunately, I was scheduled to see Linda the following day for a health reading. When I spoke to her, I was still quite upset, so I asked her if we could focus on the extraordinarily bizarre circumstances that my husband and I had been experiencing.

Linda went into trance for a few minutes. As she came back into her body, she told me that she had identified a ghost in our house. It was a female spirit who had come back through a "dimensional doorway" from Ashford Castle in Ireland, an ancient Irish castle that in recent years had been converted into a hotel.[1] That is one of the places where we stayed on vacation.

Her name was Mary and prior to her death she had been a chambermaid at Ashford Castle, where she later resided as a ghost. She was very angry with me because I had expressed an intense dislike for the castle when I was there. She traveled back to my house through a dimensional doorway, which Linda said was in my living room. She described it as a portal through which spirits can enter or leave the earth plane. The spirit was not "attached" to me, but instead roamed freely around my house causing intermittent destruction. I also remember that while Linda was in trance she uttered that she could hear Mary say she was "jealous of Marilyn's castle." Linda later indicated this was a typical reaction of a younger, more immature soul that appeared to be permanently stuck in her spiritual development.

Linda understood the urgency of the situation and promptly went into her metaphysical "Ghostbusters" mode. I was raised a Roman Catholic and am still active in my faith. Linda called upon Archangel Michael, who instructed her to have me invoke the name of a female saint. I tried invoking "Mary, Blessed Mother," and Linda channeled "no." I then called out for St. Teresa, and Linda channeled "no." I invoked St. Rita and Linda got "yes!" [In the Catholic tradition, St. Rita of Cascia (1381–1457) was an Italian nun who, according to legend, had her forehead pierced by a thorn from the crown of thorns from Jesus's crucifixion. She considered her wound a great gift from God and gladly bore it for the last fifteen years of her life. She is revered as a helper of the helpless, an advocate of the afflicted, and a guiding star in the firmament of the church.]

What was unusual about this ghost clearing, Linda told me later, was that she asked Archangel Michael if Mary, the Irish chambermaid spirit, was supposed to go back to the light. He told her that it was her soul's destiny and punishment to return to Ashford Castle for a long, long time.

Linda called on Archangel Michael and St. Rita to usher the errant and destructive chambermaid back through the dimensional doorway to Ashford Castle. Linda spoke to Mary directly and told her it was not proper for her to be in the house and that she must stop all hostile actions at once. Linda proceeded to chant several psalms of King David, which allowed Archangel Michael and St. Rita to facilitate Mary's return to Ireland.

After Mary was "vacuumed out," as Linda termed it, she did a ritual to seal the dimensional doorway in my living room. This involved astrally drawing a protective Star of David in all six directions–east, south, west, north, above, and below—while reciting different Hebrew names of God associated with each direction as she mentally affixed the star shape in the six directions to seal up the dimensional doorway. I was overwhelmed by the removal of this angry ghost and felt an intense relief that this nightmare was finally over. Linda also recommended that I get the Buddha Maitreya Solar Cross sculpture from the Shambhala Etheric Healing Tools Collection (www.tibetan foundation.org) to lessen the likelihood of a reoccurrence.

A Bit O' Metaphysical Blarney Revealed

Linda knew we had gone to Ireland on vacation earlier in the summer, but she had not yet heard of my terrible ordeal there. During my next reading, I relayed the entire story to her. After renting a car at the airport, we drove to Ashford Castle. As we approached it, I was suddenly overcome with a feeling of dread that I could not explain. In addition to being a famous historical attraction, it was a remarkably beautiful hotel with stunning grounds. I told Ken that I no longer wanted to stay at the castle even though it was I who had made the reservations at the hotel as a birthday present for him. But now we were tired after a long plane flight and drive, so I suppressed my illogical feelings as best I could.

After checking into our room, we noticed that the hotel had entertainment in a basement bar called "The Dungeon." Ken decided he wanted to go there to sing traditional Irish songs. A feeling of dread was beginning to wash over me, but wanting to be a good sport, I went down there with him because I knew he wanted to serenade me. I also wanted to hear my husband sing the Irish songs he knew and loved. We found a table and ordered some drinks. A female singer was entertaining the patrons at the bar with traditional Irish songs. Soon she called Ken up to the stage to sing. I avidly watched as my husband, who has a very good voice, broke into song.

Suddenly, I started getting an excruciating pain in my left side that felt like a knife had gone into me. I felt like I had to go to the hospital. When my husband finished singing, I told him that I was in tremendous pain and had to go up to the room to lie down. He could stay longer at the bar if he wanted, but I just had to get out of there. That night I tossed and turned in bed, unable to sleep. It felt like my very soul had been spooked, and I was desperate to leave. Finally, in the middle of the night, I brought the telephone into the bathroom, so I would not wake my husband. I called the Four Seasons Hotel where we were supposed to stay later in the trip and asked if it was possible to stay there the following night. I was willing to cancel our reservations at Ashford Castle even if it meant losing the money (which we did) just to get out of there.

After hearing this story, Linda went into trance and revealed this astonishing information: I had a past life in Ireland at this very castle where I had been forced, as a twenty-year-old woman, to witness rape, torture, and murder in the basement *in the same location* as The Dungeon! Linda explained that the excruciating knife-like pain I felt was a temporary paralysis due to the past-life recollection of what I had witnessed in the very same location! Linda also channeled that the trauma I had experienced in the bar had been stored in my bladder from that lifetime and was another negative cofactor in my overall health issues.

A DEEPER REVELATION

After recovering from the shock of the explanation, Marilyn regained her composure. Highly intuitive herself, Marilyn understood that there had to be some metaphysical purpose behind what she had endured in Ireland and at home. Why, she wanted to know, did she have to experience such misery and reconnect to an energy from a past life that dredged up such horrific memories in her soul? Because, Linda channeled, her current health issues were not only physical but also metaphysical in origin. Depending on a soul's journey, spiritual growth can occur in many ways, some more intense than others. In order to complete this aspect of her healing, Marilyn's soul needed to revisit the scene of the crime in order to reexperience it before it could be released.

Even for Linda, this moment of revelation was traumatic. What, she wanted to know, was so different about Marilyn that she had to endure this deeply personal and cathartic level of soul cleansing to regain her health, while the vast majority of her other clients did not? Suddenly she began to shake violently, and it was clear that the time had come for something important to be revealed: the true nature of Linda and Marilyn's past-life relationship to each other!

After going in and out of another trance, Linda revealed that the angels were guiding her to research an organization called the Hermetic Order of the Golden Dawn, a secret society of magicians and mystics formed in London in 1888. They performed mystical rituals designed to move energy and effectuate healing based on secret magical doctrines that were surgically lifted out of Kabbalistic knowledge from the Jewish faith and combined or hybridized with an impure "left column system" of Egyptian magic and idol worship.

There were also aspects of astrology, geomancy, and alchemy that were derived from Kabbalah. The society was headed by the occult mystic MacGregor Mathers and later involved Aleister Crowley, who had studied Kabbalah as well as Egyptian magic.

The Golden Dawn was nothing less than the original new age movement. Its members had a working knowledge of magical Kabbalah, Egyptian magic, and the angelic realms. It also attracted some of the leading literary figures of Victorian England, including writer and playwright George Bernard Shaw and the poet and playwright William Butler Yeats. There is no doubt in our minds that they were dealing with powerful energies. However, Linda has channeled that the admixture of a pure and an impure system ultimately contributed to the demise of the founding group.

The Golden Dawn was also noted for the equality it offered women in a leadership role as well as in its mystical ceremonies. Four principal women were involved in the upper political hierarchy of the group. These included an actress named Florence Farr, who later became one of the leaders of the Golden Dawn; a wealthy patron of the arts named Annie Horniman; an aristocratic revolutionary named Maud Gonne; and the wife of one of the cofounders, artist Moina Bergson Mathers. A wonderful account of the lives of these strong, independent women who refused to succumb to the restrictive morays of Victorian society can be read in *Women of the Golden Dawn* by Mary K. Greer.

It can now be revealed that Linda is the reincarnation of the actress Florence Farr (1860–1917) and that Marilyn is the reincarnation of Annie Horniman (1860–1937), repertory theater producer and principal financier of the Golden Dawn (see Figures 21-1 and 21-2). Florence and Annie participated in magical and healing ceremonies together, which further cemented their bond of friendship. Annie was an heiress to a tea fortune and due to her philanthropy is remembered as the "founder of modern English theater." She is also responsible for building and subsidizing the Abbey Theater in Dublin and the Gaiety Theatre in Manchester, England. Her father, wealthy tea importer Frederick John Horniman, founded the Horniman Museum, which exists to this very day in London. To find out more about Ms. Horniman read *Annie Horniman: A Pioneer in the Theater* by Shelia Gooddie.

In researching the life of Annie Horniman a little further, I stumbled upon the following excerpt from *The Annie Horniman Papers,* which are in the permanent collection of the John Rylands University of Manchester Library. It briefly describes the nature of the relationship between the two women as well as the company they kept.

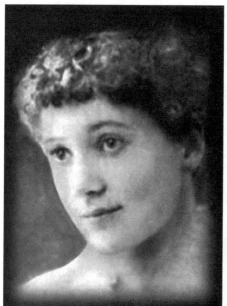

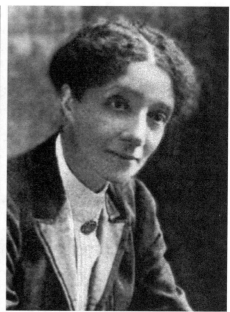

Figure 21-1. Florence Farr.

Figure 21-2. Annie Horniman.
*Used with permission of Manchester Archives
and Local Studies Central Library, St Peter's
Square, Manchester, England.*

During the 1880s and '90s, [Miss Horniman] also pursued another of her enduring interests and became deeply involved in the Order of the Golden Dawn, a secret occult society founded by Samuel Liddell "MacGregor" Mathers in 1888, where she first made the acquaintance of the Irish poet, W. B. Yeats, and the actress, Florence Farr. With the exception of the years 1897–1900, following a disagreement with Mathers, she remained a member of the Order until 1903, although during the final years there was growing acrimony amongst leading figures within the movement, leading to the resignation of both Yeats and ultimately Miss Horniman. A legacy from her grandfather gave Miss Horniman the opportunity to undertake her first theatrical venture: in 1894 she funded a season of experimental drama at the Avenue Theatre in London organized by her friend Florence Farr. She insisted on remaining an anonymous backer as she wanted to avoid provoking the displeasure of her family. The season was a financial disaster but was critically acclaimed; Miss Horniman subsequently referred to it as a "fruitful failure."[2]

A FINAL REVELATION

At the beginning of Marilyn's next session, Linda was instructed to continue the line of metaphysical thought from the last reading. They invited me to sit in on this session as they knew of my intense interest in past-life research. We all assumed more information would be forthcoming about Florence and Annie. Suddenly, without warning, Linda began to shake and convulse in a manner I have only witnessed a few times in the past. A far more shocking revelation about Linda and Marilyn was revealed: *Linda is the reincarnation of Queen Nefertiti (1370 BC–1330 B.C.: see Figure 21-3) and Marilyn is the reincarnation of Queen Nefertiti's aunt on her mother's side, a powerful high priestess who worked with her!*

The message from the angels was clear: The current lifetime between Linda and Marilyn is just a continuation of the same sort of

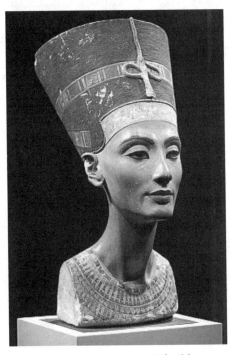

Figure 21-3. Queen Nefertiti.

work that Florence Farr and Annie Horniman and Nefertiti and her aunt had done together. This also explains why Florence and Annie were drawn to the rituals of the Golden Dawn. These things were very familiar to them. The ritual that Linda did to clear out the two dybbuks bears a resemblance to the type of rituals the two of them did when they were Florence and Annie or Nefertiti and the high priestess. Those past lives also explain, for example, why Marilyn is drawn to hypnotherapy and healing with crystals. Most importantly, it established the karmic necessity of why Linda had to be the one to heal Marilyn—to reestablish their ancient metaphysical lineage.

In summing up her feelings about Linda, Marilyn states: "After all I have been through, I am in a space where I follow my heart and soul rather than my head in these matters. Really, it all started with Linda. I am unbelievably grateful for the miraculous physical, emotional, and spiritual healing that I have experienced through her work. I believe her to be unique in the world."

OUR FINAL THOUGHTS

We have now come full circle from deep physical suffering to an awareness of our unique spiritual journey. The suffering we endured was for a purpose. There were no accidents. Linda's gift has allowed us to explore realms that bring us closer to God. It is a gift that welcomes receptive people of all faiths to join us on a journey to optimal wellness and expanded consciousness. With all the spiritual confusion in the world today, Linda's gift is a beacon of measurable clarity and light. Her gift is an olive branch from the angelic realms designed not only to heal, but also to validate the existence of a Divine Presence.

The Cardiovascular Database

HEART DISEASE

Angina pectoris

Stable
Unstable
Variant

Aortic valve stenosis

Aortic valve calcification
Bicuspid aortic valve
Congenital unicuspid
  aortic valve
Rheumatic valve disease

Arrhythmia

Atrial fibrillation
Bradycardia
Long QT syndrome
Supraventricular
  tachycardia
Ventricular fibrillation

Atherosclerosis

See Coronary heart disease

Atrial fibrillation

Chest pain
Edema
Heart failure
Heart palpitations
Irregular heartbeat
Shortness of breath
Stroke

Cardiomyopathy

Alcoholic
Dilated
Hypertrophic
Idiopathic
Ischemic
Peripartum
Restrictive

Chest pain

Angina
Aortic dissection
Blocked arteries
Pericarditis
Pneumothorax
Pulmonary embolism

Congenital heart disease

Cyanotic:
  Ebstein's anomaly
  Hypoplastic left heart
    syndrome
  Hypoplastic right
    heart syndrome
  Tetralogy of Fallot
  Total anomalous
    pulmonary venous
    return
  Transposition of the
    great vessels
  Tricuspid atresia

Truncus arteriosus
Non-cyanotic:
  Aortic valve stenosis
  Atrial septal defect
  Atrioventricular canal
    defect
  Coarctation of the
    aorta
  Patent ductus
    arteriosus
  Pulmonic stenosis
  Ventricular septal
    defect

Congestive heart failure

Cardiomyopathy
Congenital heart disease
Coronary artery disease
Endocarditis/myocarditis
Heart attack
Heart valve disease
Hypertension
Left-sided heart failure
Right-sided heart failure

Coronary heart disease

Symptoms:
  Angina
  Heart attack

Jaw, back, or arm pain
weakness
Shortness of breath
Palpitations
Recommended tests:
Coronary angiogram
Coronary
arteriography
Echocardiogram
Electrocardiogram
Electron beam
computed
tomography
Nuclear heart scan
Risk factors:
(See also Berkeley
HeartLab manual)
Alcohol
Bacteriological
infection
Calcification/plaque
Cellular waste
products
Cholesterol lipid panel
Cholesterol oxidation
LDL (elevate)
LDL/HDL ratio
Lipoprotein(a)
Low HDL
VLDL
C-reactive protein
Diabetic complications
Ferritin
Fibrogen (elevated)
Folate deficiency
Free Radicals
Fungal proliferation
Gum disease
Heavy metal toxicity
High blood pressure

Homocysteine
(elevated)
Hypercoagulation
Inflammation
Liver panel cofactors
Meridian imbalance
Metabolic syndrome
Mitochondrial
dysfunction
Nutrient deficiency
Obesity/overweight
Oxidative stress
Oxygen deficiency
Parasite infection
Sex hormone-binding
globulin
Smoking
Testosterone (low)
Thyroid-stimulating
hormone (TSH)
Thyroid-stimulating
hormone (low)
Triglyceride lipid panel
Viral infection

Cystic Hygroma
Birth defect
Knot in neck
Lymph filled sac in
head/neck

Endocarditis
See sections on bacteria
and fungi under
Pathogens

Heart Attack
Symptoms:
Cold sweat
Discoloration

Dizziness or fainting
Nausea
Pain or discomfort
that radiates to
arms, shoulders,
back, neck, jaw,
or abdomen
Persistent pressure,
fullness, squeezing,
or pain in the center
of the chest
Shortness of breath
Silent heart attack

Heart disease
Categories:
Coronary artery
disease
Congenital heart
disease
Hypertensive heart
disease
Inflammatory heart
disease
Ischemic heart disease
Pulmonary heart
disease
Valvular heart disease
Symptoms:
Angina
Congestion
Edema
Heart attack
High blood pressure
Jaw, back or arm pain
Low blood pressure
Palpitations
Shock (trauma or
surgery)
Shortness of breath

Skip beats
Slow beat
Spasms
Strain
Stroke
Tachycardia
Weakness

High cholesterol

Risk factors:
  Atherosclerosis
  Blood clots
  Coronary artery
    disease
  Heart attack
  Poor circulation
  Stroke

Hypertension

Risk factors:
  Arteriosclerosis
  Congestive heart
    failure
  Heart attack
  Kidney disease
  Stroke

Hypotension

Symptoms:
  Angina
  Chest pain
  Dizziness
  Dry skin
  Overactive bladder
Causes:
  Bleeding disorder
  Dehydration
  Heart disease
  Pregnancy
  Stroke

Myocarditis

See viruses, bacteria,
parasites, and fungi
under Pathogens; may
also be caused by
chemicals (arsenic,
hydrocarbons), drugs
(penicillin, sulfonamide,
cocaine, others), and
diseases like lupus,
connective tissue
disorders, inflammation
of blood vessels
(vasculitis), sarcoidosis,
and Wegener's
granulomatosis

Pericarditis (acute/chronic)

Causes:
  Kidney failure
  Lupus
  Medication
  Metastatic disease
  Radiation therapy
  Rheumatoid arthritis
  Trauma
  Viral infection

Pulmonary heart disease

Stroke

Ischemic stroke:
  Embolic infarct
  Lacunar infarct
  Thrombotic infarct
Hemorrhagic stroke:
  Epidural hematoma
  Intracerebral
    hemorrhage
Intracranial
  hemorrhage
Subarachnoid
  hemorrhage
Subdural hematoma

VALVULAR HEART DISEASE

Aneurysm

Abdominal aortic
Brain
Carotid
Cerebral
Mesenteric artery
Popliteal artery
Splenic artery
Thoracic aortic

Aortic regurgitation

Aortic valve stenosis
Carotid artery disease
Mitral regurgitation
Mitral valve stenosis
Mitral valve prolapse
Pulmonic regurgitation
Pulmonic stenosis
Raynaud's phenomenon
Causes:
  Connective tissue
    diseases
  Dermatomyositis
  Lupus
  Scleroderma
  Sjögren's syndrome

Tricuspid regurgitation

Tricuspid stenosis

HEART PATHOLOGY CAUSED BY PATHOGENS*

Acute myocarditis
Acute rheumatic fever
Arrhythmia
Cardiomyopathy
Deep vein thrombosis
Endocarditis
Heart inflammation
Hypercoagulation
Inflammation of heart
  muscle
Myocardial infarction
Myocarditis
Myocyte necrosis
Pericarditis
Systemic inflammatory
  disease

PATHOGENS*

Bacteria

Acinetobacter
Actinomyces
Botulinum toxin
Campylobacter jejuni
Chlamydia pneumoniae
  (pneumonia,
  atherosclerosis,
  Alzheimer's disease)
Clostridium
Clostridium tetani (tetanus)
Corynebacterium
Corynebacterium
  diphtheriae (diptheria)
Coxiella burnetii (Q fever)
Enterococcus
Francisella tularensis
  (tularemia)

Haemophilus influenzae
Helicobacter pylori
  (gastric ulcer)
Meningococci
Mycobacterium
  tuberculosis
  (tuberculosis pleurisy)
Neisseria gonorrhoea
  (gonorrhea)
Pertussinum
Pneumococcus
  (pneumonia, blood
  infections, meningitis)
Propionibacterium
Pseudomonas
Salmonella (all species)
Salmonella typhi (typhoid
  fever)
Staphylococcus aureus
Streptobacillus
Streptococcus
Streptococcus beta-
  haemolyticus, Group A
Streptococcus beta-
  haemolyticus, Group B
Streptococcus mutans
Streptococcus pneumoniae
  (meningitis,
  pneumococcal disease)
Streptococcus pyogenes
  (scarlet fever)
Streptococcus viridans

Fungi

Aspergillus niger
Candida albicans
Mucor racemosus
Coccidioides
Cryptococcus
Histoplasma

Parasites

Chlamydia psittaci
  (psittacosis)
Dirofilaria immitis
  (heartworm)
Plasmodium malariae
  (malaria)
Schistosoma
  (schistosomiasis)
Toxoplasma gondii
  (toxoplasmosis)
Trypanosoma cruzi
  (Chagas disease)

Rickettsia and Spirocytes

Bartonella species
Borrelia burgdorferi (Lyme
  disease)
Brucella spp. (brucellosis)
Leptospira
Lyssavirus (rabies)
Treponema pallidum
  (syphilis)

Viruses

Adenoviruses
Coxsackie A virus
Coxsackie B virus
Cytomegalovirus
Echovirus
Enteroviruses
  (Meningitis)
Epstein-Barr virus
Grippe
Haemophilus influenzae
  type b (viral
  meningititis)
Hepatitis C virus

Herpes simplex virus
type 1
Herpes simplex virus
type 2
Human
immunodeficiency
virus
Influenza virus (all
strains)
Morbillivirus (measles)
Oncogene (cancer)
Parovirus B$_1$9
Poliovirus
Rubella virus
Sepsis lenta
Varicella-zoster virus
Variola major (smallpox)
Variola minor (smallpox)

*Adapted from *Cell Wall Deficient Forms: Stealth Pathogens* by Lida H. Mattman. Boca Raton, FL: CRC Press, 2000

HEART STRUCTURE

Aorta

Atria

Atrium, left
Atrium, right
Auricles
Fossa ovalis
Interatrial septum

Cardiac arteries

Arterial blood supply

Coronary artery, left
Coronary artery, right
Cardiac arteries
Cardiac arteries, marginal

Cardiac nerves

Atrioventricular node
(AV node)
Deep cardiac nerves
Sinoatrial node
Sinoauricular node
Superficial cardiac
nerves

Cardiac veins

Anterior cardiac vein
Coronary sinus vein
Endothelium
Great cardiac vein
Middle cardiac vein
Oblique vein of left
atrium
Posterior vein of left
ventricle
Marginal vein, left
Marginal vein, right
Pulmonary veins, left
Pulmonary veins, right
Small cardiac vein
Vein tendons
Vein valves

Endocardium

Connective tissue
Elastic fibers
Connective fibers

Heart meridian

Heart valves

Aortic valve
Chordae tendinae (heart
valve tendons)
Mitral valve
Pulmonary valve
Tricuspid valve
Tubulus valve, left
Tubulus valve, right
Ventricular diastole
Ventricular systole

Myocardium

Cardiac muscle
Muscular longitudinal
tissue
Muscular transverse
tissue fiber
Connective tissue
Tendons
Purkinje fiber
Tendon of infundibulum

Pericardium

Fibrous pericardium
Lymphatic pericardial
fluid
Pericardium meridian
Serous pericardium

Ventricles

Ventricles, left
Ventricles, right
Ventricular septum

Phase II Liver Detoxification Pathways Used for Specific Compounds

Pathway	Xenobiotics		Drugs		Natural Compounds	
Glutathione conjugation	Styrene Acrolein Ethylene oxide Benzopyrenes Methyl parathion Chlorobenzene	Anthracene Toxic metals Petroleum distillates Naphthalene	Acetaminophen Penicillin Ethacrynic acid Tetracycline		Bacterial toxins Aflatoxin Lipid Peroxides Ethyl alcohol Quercitin	N-Acetylcysteine Prostaglandins Baterial toxins Bilirubin Leukotreine A4
Sulfation	Aniline Pentachbrophenol Terpenes Amines Hydroxylamines Phenols		Acetaminophen Methyl dopa Minoxidil Metaraminol Phenylephrine		DHEA Quercitin Bile acids Safrole Tyramine Thyroxine Estrogens Testosterone Cortisol	Catecholamines Melatonin 3-Hydroxy coumarin 25-Hydroxy vitamin D Ethyl alcohol CCK Cerebrosides
Gycine conjugation	Napthylacetic acid Alphatic amines		Salicylates Nicotinic Acid Chlorpheniramine Brompheniramine		Bile acids Cinnamic acids PABA	Plant Acids Benzoic acid Phenylacetic acid
Taurine conjugation	Propionic acid Caprylic acid				Bile acids Stearic acid Palmitic acid Myristic acid	Lauric acid Decanoic acid Butyric acid
Glucuronidation	Aniline Carbamates Phenols Thiophenol Butanol N-Hydroxy-2-napthylamine		Salicylates Acetaminophen Morphine Meprobamate Benzodiazepines Clofibric acid Naproxen Digoxin	Phenylbutazone Valproic acid Steroids Lorazepam Ciramadol Propranolol Oxazepa	Bilirubin Estrogens Melatonin Bile acids Vitamin E	Vitamin A Vitamin K Vitamin D Steroid hormones
Acetylation	2 Aminofluorene Analine		Clonazepam Dapsone Mescaline Isoniazid Hydralazine	Procainamide Benzidine Sulfonamides Promizole	Serotonin PABA Histamine Tryptamine	Caffeine Choline Tyramine Coenzyme A
Methylation	Paraquat Beta-carbolines Isoquinolines Mercury Lead	Arsenic Thallium Tin Pyridine	Thiouracil Isoetharine Rimiterol Dobutamine Butanephine	Elouphed Morphine Levaphanol Nalorphine	Histamine Epinephrine Dopamine Norepinephrine L-Dopa Apomorphine Hydroxyestradiols	

Reprinted by permission from Richard S. Lord and J. Alexander Bralley, eds. *Laboratory Evaluations for Integrative and Functional Medicine* (Duluth, GA: Metametrix Institute, 2008).

APPENDIX C

201 Chemicals Known to Be Neurotoxic in Humans

Metals and Inorganic Compounds

Aluminum compounds
Arsenic and arsenic compounds
Azide compounds
Barium compounds
Bismuth compounds
Carbon monoxide
Cyanide compounds
Decaborane
Diborane
Ethyl mercury
Fluoride compounds
Hydrogen sulphide
Lead and lead compounds
Lithium compounds
Manganese and manganese
    compounds
Mercury and mercury compounds
Methyl mercury
Nickel carbonyl
Pentaborane
Phosphine
Phosphorus
Selenium compounds
Tellurium compounds
Thallium compounds
Tin compounds

Organic Solvents

Acetone
Benzene
Benzyl alcohol
Carbon disulphide
Chloroform
Chloroprene
Cumene
Cyclohexane
Cyclohexanol
Cyclohexanone
Dibromochloropropane
Dichloroacetic acid
1,3-Dichloropropene
Diethylene glycol
Dimethylformamide
2-Ethoxyethyl acetate
Ethyl acetate
Ethylene dibromide
Ethylene glycol
n-Hexane
Isobutyronitrile
Isophorone
Isopropyl alcohol
Isopropylacetone
Methanol
Methyl butyl ketone
Methyl cellosolve

Methyl ethyl ketone
Methylcyclopentane
Methylene chloride
Nitrobenzene
2-Nitropropane
1-Pentanol
n-Propyl bromide
Pyridine
Styrene
Tetrachloroethane
Tetrachloroethylene
Toluene
1,1,1-Trichloroethane
Trichloroethylene
Vinyl chloride
Xylene

Other Organic Substances

Acetone cyanohydrin
Acrylamide
Acrylonitrile
Allyl chloride
Aniline
1,2-Benzenedicarbonitrile
Benzonitrile
Butylated triphenyl phosphate
Caprolactam
Cyclonite
Dibutyl phthalate
Diethylene glycol diacrylate
3-(Dimethylamino)-propanenitrile
Dimethyl sulphate
Dimethylhydrazine
Dinitrobenzene
Dinitrotoluene
Ethylbis(2-chloroethyl) amine
Ethylene
Ethylene oxide
Fluoroacetamide
Fluoroacetic acid

Hexachlorophene
Hydrazine
Hydroquinone
Methyl chloride
Methyl formate
Methyl iodide
Methyl methacrylate
p-Nitroaniline
Phenol
p-Phenylenediamine
Phenylhydrazine
Polybrominated biphenyls
Polybrominated diphenyl ethers
Polychlorinated biphenyls
Propylene oxide
2,3,7,8-Tetrachlorodibenzo-p-Dioxin
Tributyl phosphate
2,2`,2`-Trichlorotriethylamine
Trimethyl phosphate
Tri-o-tolyl phosphate
Triphenyl phosphate

Pesticides

Aldicarb
Aldrin
Bensulide
Bromophos
Carbaryl
Carbofuran
Carbophenothion
[alpha]-Chloralose
Chlordane
Chlordecone
Chlorfenvinphos
Chlormephos
Chlorpyrifos
Chlorthion
Coumaphos
Cyhalothrin
Cypermethrin

2,4-Dichlorophenoxyacetic acid
Dichlorodiphenyltrichloroethane
  (DDT)
Deltamethrin
Demeton
Dialifor
Diazinon
Dichlofenthion
Dichlorvos
Dieldrin
Dimefox
Dimethoate
Dinitrocresol
Dinoseb
Dioxathion
Disulphoton
Edifenphos
Endosulphan
Endothion
Endrin
EPN
Ethiofencarb
Ethion
Ethoprop
Fenitrothion
Fensulphothion
Fenthion
Fenvalerate
Fonofos
Formothion
Heptachlor
Heptenophos
Hexachlorobenzene
Isobenzan
Isolan
Isoxathion
Leptophos

Lindane
Merphos
Metaldehyde
Methamidophos
Methidathion
Methomyl
Methyl bromide
Methyl demeton
Methyl parathion
Mevinphos
Mexacarbate
Mipafox
Mirex
Monocrotophos
Naled
Nicotine
Oxydemeton-methyl
Parathion
Pentachlorophenol
Phorate
Phosphamidon
Phospholan
Propaphos
Propoxur
Pyriminil
Sarin
Schradan
Soman
Sulprofos
2,4,5-Trichlorophenoxyacetic acid
Tebupirimfos
Tefluthrin
Terbufos
Thiram
Toxaphene
Trichlorfon
Trichloronat

Reprinted by permission of the publisher from "Developmental neurotoxicity of industrial chemicals" by P Grandjean and PJ Landrigan. *The Lancet* 2006; 368: 2167–2178.

APPENDIX D

Negative Emotional Database

LIST OF NEGATIVE CHARACTERISTICS AND EMOTIONS

Abrasive
Abrupt
Absent-minded
Abusive
Afraid of people
Aggressive
Aimless
Alarming
Alcoholic
Aloof
Angry
Antagonistic
Argumentative
Attention-seeking
Avoiding
Awkward
Babyish
Barbaric
Base
Beating around bush
Belligerent
Bigoted
Bitter
Blame-passer
Blaming
Blocked
Blunt

Boastful
Boisterous
Boorish
Boring
Brazen
Brooding
Brutal
Bullying
Calculating
Callous
Careless
Caustic
Characterless
Charlatan
Chatter-box
Cheater
Cheerless
Childish
Closed
Clumsy
Coarse
Coercive
Cold
Cold-hearted
Colorless
Competitive
Complacent

Complaining
Compulsive
Concealing
Conceited
Confrontational
Confused
Contemptuous of others
Contradictory
Controlling
Covetous
Cranky
Critical
Crooked
Cross
Crude
Cruel
Cunning
Cynical
Dawdling
Decadent
Deceitful
Deceptive
Defensive
Defiant
Deficient in attention
Dejected
Demanding

Dependent
Depressed
Derisive
Deserting
Despairing
Destructive
Detached
Devious
Dishonest
Disloyal
Disobedient
Disorderly
Disrespectful
Distracted
Distrustful
Divisive
Domineering
Downcast
Dreamy
Drowsy
Dull
Egoistic
Egotistic
Elusive
Envious
Evasive
Evilly inclined
Excessive
Excitable
Exhibitionist
Exploitative
Extravagant
Faint-hearted
Faraway
Fearful
Ferocious
Fickle
Fierce
Finicky
Flaky

Flattering
Flighty
Flippant
Flustered
Foggy
Foolish
Forgetful
Frantic
Fraudulent
Frivolous
Frustrated
Histrionic
Headstrong
Hostile
Hyper
Hypercritical
Hypersensitive
Hypochondriac
Hypocritical
Hysterical
Idle
Ignorant
Illogical
Ill-tempered
Illusive
Immature
Immoderate
Immoral
Impatient
Impetuous
Impractical
Impudent
Impulsive
Inaccessible
Inactive
Incompetent
Inconsiderate
Inconsistent
Indecisive
Indifferent

Indiscreet
Ineffective
Inefficient
Infantile
Inferiority complex
Inflexible
Insecure
Intimidated
Intimidating
Intolerant
Intrusive
Irrational
Irresponsible
Irritable
Irritating
Isolated
Jealous
Judgmental
Jumping to conclusions
Juvenile
Loafing
Lonely
Loner
Loud
Lowly
Lustful
Malicious
Manipulative
Mean
Meddlesome
Mediocre
Mercenary
Merciless
Mischievous
Miserable
Misleading
Monotonous
Moody
Myopic
Nagging

Naïve
Narcissistic
Negative thinking
Neglectful
Negligent
Nervous
Neurotic
Nosy
Obnoxious
Obstinate
Odd
Offensive
Opportunistic
Oppressive Ostentatious
Overbearing
Overeater
Paranoid
Passive
Passive-aggressive
Patronizing
Pessimistic
Petty
Phobic
Phony
Pitiless
Pompous
Possessive
Prejudiced
Procrastinating
Punitive
Pushy
Quarrelsome
Quitter
Quixotic
Rebellious
Reckless
Reclusive
Regretful

Remorseful
Repulsive
Resentful
Restless
Revengeful
Rigid
Rough
Rude
Ruthless
Sad
Sadistic
Sarcastic
Scolding
Secretive
Self-blaming
Self-centered
Self-conscious
Self-contemptuous
Self-deceptive
Self-destructive
Self-hating
Self-important
Selfish
Self-pitying
Self-righteous
Self-serving
Self-tempting
Sensation-seeking
Servile
Shabby
Shallow
Shortsighted
Showing off
Shy
Sloppy
Slow

Smug
Snobbish
Spiteful
Squeamish
Stiff
Stingy
Stubborn
Submissive
Sulky
Superficial
Suspicious
Sycophant
Tactless
Tasteless
Tense
Thoughtless
Timid
Tyrannical
Uncertain of oneself
Uncompromising
Underhanded
Unethical
Unfair
Unforgiving
Unfriendly
Unhappy
Unproductive
Unrealistic
Unreliable
Unsociable
Unstable
Vain
Vengeful
Vindictive
Violent
Weak
Withdrawn
Worrying

Reprinted with permission from Rabbi Zelig Pliskin.

References and Notes

Chapter 1: Discovery of Linda's Gift

1. "EAV Discussions: The Basics." VeraDyne Corp.: www.veradyne.com/eav_basics.html.

2. Ulrich Arndt. "Diagnose & Medizin-Forschung." Horus Media (in German): www.horusmedia.de/ 1994-pilze/pilze.php.

3. Jost Dumrese and Bruno Haefeli. "Pleomorphismus: Blutsymbionten, Blutparasiten, Blutpilze." (In German): www.iape.de/html_ger/pub_pleobuch.htm and www.grayfieldoptical.com/papers.

4. Aryeh Kaplan. *Meditation and the Bible*. York Beach, ME: Samuel Weiser, 1978, p. 33.

5. Ibid., p. 31.

6. Ibid., pp. 32–33.

7. Ibid., pp. 31–32.

8. Carter Phipps. "John Haught: A Theologian of Renewal." *EnlightenNext*, Issue 42, (Dec. 2008–Feb 2009).

Chapter 2: Our Healing Philosophy

1. W. John Diamond and W. Lee Cowden with Burton Goldberg. *An Alternative Medicine Definitive Guide to Cancer*. Tiburon, CA: Future Medicine Publishing, 1997, p. 9.

2. Werner Heisenberg. *Physics and Philosophy: The Revolution in Modern Science*. London: Allen & Unwin, 1959, p. 161.

3. Richard Gerber. *Vibrational Medicine: The #1 Handbook of Subtle-Energy Therapies*. Rochester, VT: Bear & Co., 2001, p. 44.

Chapter 3: Introduction to Metaphysical Systems Engineering

1. Richard Gerber. *Vibrational Medicine: The #1 Handbook of Subtle-Energy Therapies*. Rochester, VT: Bear & Co., 2001, p. 39.

2. David M. Ojcius, Toni Darville, and Patrik M. Bavoil. "Can Chlamydia Be Stopped?" *Scientific American*. Vol. 292 (May 2005): 72–79.

Chapter 4: The Physical Databases

1. Anti-candida diet refers to a highly alkaline, vegetarian approach to diet that largely trumps Metabolic Typing and Glycemic Index for an individual suffering from mercury toxicity or a compromised immune system until such time that mercury detoxification is completed.

2. Metabolic Typing is a brilliant, customized nutritional approach to diet based on one's biochemical individuality as determined by lab analysis of the Krebs cycle and the autonomic nervous system. See Harold Kristal and James Haig. *The Nutrition Solution*. Berkeley, CA: North Atlantic Books, 2002.

3. "The Glycemic Index is simply a numerical means [scale from 1–100] of describing how much the carbohydrates in individual foods affect blood-glucose levels (*glycemia*). Foods with high GI values contain carbohydrates that cause a dramatic rise in blood-glucose levels while foods with low GI values contain carbohydrates that have much less impact." Jennie Brand-Miller et al., *The Low GI Diet Revolution*. New York: Marlowe & Co., 2005, p. 23.

4. P.H. Langsjoen and A.M. Langsjoen. "The Clinical Use of HMG CoA-reductase Inhibitors and the Associated Depletion of Coenzyme Q10. A Review of Animal and Human Publications." *Biofactors.* Vol. 18 (2003):110–111. "The depletion of the essential nutrient CoQ10 by the increasingly popular cholesterol lowering drugs, HMG CoA reductase inhibitors (statins), has grown from a level of concern to one of alarm." The Canadian government acknowledges the dangers of depleting the body's natural reservoir of CoQ10.

5. A de Corla-Souza and BA Cunha. "Streptococcal Viridans Subacute Bacterial Endocarditis Associated with Antineutrophil Cytoplasmic Autoantibodies (ANCA)." *Heart & Lung.* Vol. 32 (Mar–Apr 2003): 140–143.

6. David Schlossberg. *Clinical Infectious Disease.* New York: Cambridge University Press, 2008, pp. 1061–1062.

7. Robert Haas, M.S. "Lower Cholesterol Safely : Nutritional Interventions for Healthy Lipids." *Life Extension Magazine,* March 2010. The article states that the compound "Monacolin-K effectively lowers cholesterol by acting as an HMG-CoA reductase inhibitor." This is the same mode of action as in Lipitor. To support the claim of effectiveness, the article cites a meta-analysis of 93 randomized controlled trials involving almost 10,000 Chinese patients [Liu J., et al. "Chinese Red Yeast Rice (*Monascus purpureus*) for Primary Hyperlipidemia: A Meta-analysis of Randomized Controlled Trials." *Chinese Medicine.* Vol. 1 (2006):4]. Haas's article also cites an additional clinical study showing that red yeast rice along with healthy lifestyle practices lowers cholesterol as effectively as the prescription drug Simvastatin (Zocor) [D.J. Becker, et al. "Simvastatin vs Therapeutic Lifestyle Changes and Supplements: Randomized Primary Prevention Trial." *Mayo Clinical Proceedings.* Vol. 83, No. 7 (July 2008):758–764].

8. www.drweil.com/drw/u/QAA400513/Red-Rice-Yeast-for-Cholesterol-Control.html. 1/22/2009. Red yeast rice extract is known to contain several naturally occurring statins. It delivers a mix of these compounds instead of pharmaceutical statins, which deliver a single type of molecule. As a result, it is, according to Dr. Andrew Weil, M.D., "less likely to cause the side effects that sometimes occur with the pharmaceutical versions." It should be pointed out that many people experience no side effects from Lipitor. For these individuals, Lipitor may be the more economical choice. Your doctor is the final arbitrator in this decision.

Chapter 5: Fungal Disease

1. "Fungus, Yeast, Candida & Parasites." Fungus Focus: www.fungusfocus.com

2. Burton Goldberg. *Chronic Fatigue, Fibromyalgia, and Lyme Disease.* Berkeley, CA: Celestial Arts, 2004, p. 74.

3. Donna Gates and Linda Schatz. *The Body Ecology Diet: Recovering Your Health and Rebuilding Your Immunity.* Decatur, GA: B.E.D. Publishing, 2007, p. 15.

4. Carol Wilson. "Recurrent Vulvovaginitis Candidiasis; An Overview of Traditional and Alternative Therapies." *Advanced Nursing Practice.* Vol. 13 (May 2005): 24–29.

5. Thomas Rau. "The Value of Darkfield Microscopy." Hoya, Germany: Semmelweis-Institut GmbH.

Chapter 6: Pleomorphism

1. R. Monina Klevens, et al. "Invasive Methicillin-Resistant *Staphylococcus aureus* Infections in the United States." *Journal of the American Medical Association.* Vol. 298, No. 15 (Oct 2007): 1763–1771. According to CDC researchers, Methicillin-resistant *Staphylococcus aureus* (MRSA) was responsible for an estimated 94,000 life-threatening infections and 18,650 deaths in 2005. In that same year, approximately 16,000 people in the U.S. died from AIDS.

2. Cesar A. Arias, and Barbara E. Murray. "Antibiotic-Resistant Bugs in the 21st Century: A Clinical Super-Challenge." *New England Journal of Medicine.* Vol. 360 (Feb 2009): 439–443.

3. Personal correspondence with Dr. Kirk Slagel, N.M.D., Mar 2009.

4. Robert O. Young. *Sick and Tired? Reclaim Your Inner Terrain.* Pleasant Grove, UT: Woodland Pub., 2001, p. 19.

5. "There was a book published in 1932 that is still in print today: *Béchamp or Pasteur?* This book was written by E. Douglas Hume, whom it turns out was actually a woman who had to disguise her name as male to get the book published. Hume chronicles a contemporary of Pasteur, Antoine Béchamp, the most respected

researcher and teacher in France at the time, department head at the University at Lille." Quoted from an article by Tim O'Shea, DC, "The Post Antibiotic Age: Germ Theory," www.whale.to/vaccine/shea1.html.

6. E. Douglas Hume. *Béchamp or Pasteur? A Lost Chapter in the History of Biology*. New York: DLM, 2006. First published 1932 by C.W. Daniel Co. "Like Koch, Pasteur was very motivated by money. In the race for a vaccine for anthrax, for example, not only did Pasteur not test it on animals before using humans, but it was also established that Pasteur actually stole the formula from a colleague named Toussaint. Unable to prove his claim at the time, Toussaint died a few months later of a nervous breakdown. (Hume)." Quoted from an article by Tim O'Shea D.C., "The Post Antibiotic Age: Germ Theory," www.whale.to/vaccine/shea1.html.

7. Young, op. cit., p. 27.

8. Ibid., p. 26.

9. Christopher Bird. "To Be or Not To Be? The Mystery of Pleomorphic Organisms." *Raum & Zeit*. Vol. 2, No. 6 (1991). Quoting a translation of *The Blood* by Antoine Bechamp (1908).

10. Young, op. cit., p. 26.

11. Delhoume, Leon, De Claude Bernard d'Arsonval Lib. Bailliere et fils, Paris, 1939, p. 595 as quoted in "The Mystery of Pleomorphic Microbial Organisms" by Christopher Bird in *Raum & Zeit*, Vol. 2, No. 6 (1991).

12. Before he died, Pasteur instructed his family not to release some 10,000 pages of lab notes after his death. Not until 1975, after the death of his grandson, were these "secret" notes finally made public. A historian from Princeton, Professor Geison made a thorough study of the lab notes. He presented his findings in an address to the American Association for the Advancement of Science in Boston in 1993. Dr. Geison's conclusions: "Pasteur published much fraudulent data and was guilty of many counts of scientific misconduct,' violating rules of medicine, science, and ethics." Quoted from an article by Tim O'Shea, D.C., "The Post Antibiotic Age: Germ Theory," www.whale.to/vaccine/shea1.html.

13. In 1924, the German physiologist Otto Warburg showed that cancerous tumors contain up to ten times the level of lactic acid found in healthy human tissues. "Enderlein Therapy: A Cancer Therapy That Promotes Gentle Self-Healing" by Richard Walters. *Raum & Zeit* Vol. 3, No. 1 (1991): 24–27.

14. R Walters. "Enderlein Therapy: A Cancer Therapy That Promotes Gentle Self-Healing." *Raum & Zeit*. Vol. 3, No. 1 (1991): 24–27.

15. Peter Schneider. "The Sanukehl Preparations: Polysaccharides for Haptenic Therapy." Sanum-Kehlbeck (1998): www.sanum.com/sanukehl/index.htm.

Chapter 7: Parasites

1. Anne Louise Gittleman. "Are Parasites Making You Fat?" (Oct 20, 2006): www.annlouise.com/news-press/news-archives/are-parasites-making-you-fat.html.

2. Centers for Disease Control and Prevention. "About Parasites." (May 1, 2008): www.cdc.gov/ncidod/dpd/aboutparasites.htm.3. Ann Louise Gittleman. *Guess What Came to Dinner? Parasites and Your Health*. New York: Avery, 2001, p. viii.

4. Ibid., pp. 6–7.

5. Ibid., p. 33.

6. Anne Louise Gittleman. "Are Parasites Making You Fat?" (Oct 20, 2006): www.annlouise.com/news-press/news-archives/are-parasites-making-you-fat.html.

Chapter 8: Miasms

1. Ann Jerome Croce. "The Thought Behind the Action." *Homeopathy Today*, Sept 2000.

2. Ibid.

3. Brian Knight. "The Itch that Cannot Be Scratched: Understanding Eczema and Psoriasis for a Practitioner." The International Institute of Kinesiology in Australia, www.iikinesiology.com/news.htm

4. "Spenglersan Colloids: Biologically Immune Constitutional Means of Active and Passive Immunization." Literature from Meckel-Spenglersan Pharmazeutische Praparate. Compiled in English by the American Academy of Biological Medicine, p. 4.

5. Personal conversation with Helmut Schimmel, Oct 1992.

6. Konrad Werthmann. "Polysans: A New Way to Help Treat Chronic Disorders." *Explore Magazine* Vol. 10, No. 4 (2001): www.explorepub.com/articles/werthmann_10_4.html.

7. Spenglersan Colloids, op. cit., p. 5.

8. Ibid., p. 4.

9. Ibid., p. 4.

10. Ibid., p. 6.

11. Peter Schneider. "The Tubercular Constitution as a Common Cause of Chronic Diseases and Its Treatment with Naturopathic Regulation Therapy," Semmelweis-Institut GmbH, 2000, p. 2: www.poschneider.com/tubercular_constitution/index.htm.

12. D. Kimberly Slagel. "The History and Usage of the Polysan Remedies." *Pleo News*. Vol. 4, No. 5 (May 2005).

13. Julian Winston. "The Classical View on Miasms: Part III." American Homeopathic Collection. Tawa, New Zealand: Great Auk Publishing, 2004: www.julianwinston.com.

14. JWV Wait, et al. "Tuberculosis Meningitis and Attention Deficit Hyperactivity Disorder in Children." *Journal of Tropical Pediatrics*. Vol 48 (2002): 294–299.

15. Burton Goldberg. *Alternative Medicine: The Definitive Guide*. Berkeley, CA: Celestial Arts, 2002, pp. 584–585.

16. "According to renowned homeopath George Vithoulkas, miasms are broad-focused predisposing individuals to certain families of illness, whereas oncogenes are coded specifically not only for a certain type of illness (cancer), but actual varieties of that illness (breast, ovarian, lung, pancreatic cancers)." W. John Diamond, W. Lee Cowden, with Burton Goldberg. *Definitive Guide to Cancer*, Tiburon, CA: Future Medicine Publishing, 1997, p. 641.

Chapter 9: Mercury

1. RP Sharma, EJ Obersteiner. "Metals and Neurotoxic Effects: Cytotoxicity of Selected Metallic Compounds on Chick Ganglia Cultures." *Journal of Comparative Pathology*. Vol. 91, No. 2 (1981): 235–244.

2. World Health Organization (WHO). "Elemental Mercury and Inorganic Mercury Compounds: Human Health Aspects." (Jun 2004): www.who.int/pcs/cicad/full_text/cicad50.pdf.

3. Bernard Windham. "Facts about Mercury and Dental Amalgam." (Apr 2004): www.eatingalive.com/windham/windhamA.htm.

4. National Institute for Occupational Safety and Health (NIOSH). "A Recommended Standard for Occupational Exposure to Inorganic Mercury." NIOSH (1973): Publication No.73-11024.

5. L Friber, ed. *Environmental Health Criteria. 118: Inorganic Mercury*. Geneva: WHO, (1991): www.who.int/water_sanitation_health/medicalwaste/mercurypolpaper.pdf.

6. "Toxic Mercury: The Beautiful Poison." Toxic Mercury Amalgam: www.toxicmercuryamalgam.com

7. F Lorscheider, MJ Vimy. "Evaluation of the safety issue of mercury release from dental fillings." *FASEB Journal*. Vol. 7 (1993): 1432–1433.

8. MJ Vimy, F Lorscheider. "Intra-oral air mercury released from dental amalgam." *Journal Dental Research*. Vol. 64 (1985): 1069–1071; AM Aronsson, B Lind, M Nylander. "Dental Amalgam and Mercury." *Biological Metals*. Vol. 2 (1989): 25–30.

9. Dietrich Klinghardt, Joseph Mercola. "Mercury Toxicity and Systemic Elimination Agents." *Journal of Nutritional and Environmental Medicine*. Vol. 11 (2001): 53–62.

10. "Over 2,000 Flood FDA with Reports of Illnesses from Mercury Fillings but Agency Still Claims Secret Pandemic Is 'Rare." Consumers for Dental Choice. Press release (Nov 14, 2006): www.toxicteeth.org/ pressRoom_releases.cfm.

11. FN Kudsk. "Absorption of Mercury Vapour from the Respiratory Tract in Man." *Acta Pharmacologica. et Toxicool.* Vol. 23 (1965): 250–262.

12. Klinghardt and Mercola, op. cit., pp. 11, 53–62.

13. Hal A. Huggins and Thomas Levy. *Uninformed Consent: The Hidden Dangers in Dental Care.* Charlottesville, VA: Hampton Roads Pub. Co., 1999, p. 171.

14. Ibid., p.172.

15. L Friber, ed. *Environmental Health Criteria. 118: Inorganic Mercury.* Geneva: WHO (1991): www.who.int/ water_sanitation_health/medicalwaste/mercurypolpaper.pdf.

16. Russell L. Blaylock. *Health and Nutrition Secrets That Can Save Your Life.* Albuquerque, NM: Health Press, 2006, p. 45.

17. "Scientists and Consumer Advocates Charge FDA with 'Stacking the Deck' in Favor of Keeping Mercury in Tooth Fillings." Consumers for Dental Choice. Press release (Aug 21, 2006): www.toxicteeth.org/ pressRoom_releases.cfm.

18. Michael Bender. *Facing Up to the Hazards of Mercury Tooth Fillings.* Mercury Policy Project (2008): www.mercurypolicy.org.

19. This is why it comes as no surprise that in July 2009, the FDA defied all scientific reasoning by the manner in which they issued a regulation classifying dental amalgam as class II devices. On the one hand, this means that the FDA technically considers it to have more risk and that special controls may need to be put in place in specific situations. The official ruling does say "the developing neurological systems in fetuses and young children may be more sensitive to the neurotoxic effects of mercury vapor." However, the ruling provides no warning or contraindications for parents or pregnant women. According to Charlie Brown, director of Consumers for Dental Choice, "by omitting this critical information the FDA has created a legally gray area where it could give the appearance of contradicting itself. The ruling still could be interpreted as meaning that the FDA considers amalgam harmless for pregnant women and children under the age of six." For more information see "FDA's Mercury Ruling Defies All Scientific Reasoning" by Joseph Mercola at www. mercola.com/sites/articles/archive/2009/08/22/FDA-has-the-Audacity-to-Claim-Mercury-is-Completely-Harmless.aspx.

20. M Nylander, et al. "Mercury Accumulation in Tissues from Dental Staff and Controls in Relation to Exposure." *Journal of Swedish Dentistry.* Vol. 13 (1989): 235–243.

21. Huggins and Levy, op. cit., p. 111.

22. "Dental Products Manufacturer Update." Consumers for Dental Choice. (Oct 16, 2007): www.toxicteeth.org/RB__565608.pdf.

23. Citizen Petition to FDA from Consumers for Dental Choice. (Nov 10, 2005): 7–8: www.toxicteeth.org/ petition_withdraw_reg.pdf.

24. Blaylock, op.cit., p. 45.

25. Bernard Williams. "New Studies Find High Mercury and Adverse Effects of Dental Amalgam." Dental Amalgam Mercury Solutions: www.flcv.com/damspr1.html.

26. Consumers for Dental Choice. Press Release. www.toxicteeth.org/pressRoom_releases.cfm.

27. "Disadvantaged Kids Get a Mercury-Free Smile." Consumers for Dental Choice. Press Release (Jan–Feb 2005): www.toxicteeth.org/pressRoom_releases_gksd05.cfm.

28. Sierra Club, et al. "Dentist the Menace? The Uncontrolled Release of Dental Mercury." Mercury Policy Project, Health Care Without Harm (June 2002).

29. Bernard Windham. "Dental Amalgam Fillings and Chronic Health Conditions." DAMS International: www.flcv.com/indexa.html.

30. "Dental Mercury Use Banned in Norway, Sweden and Denmark Because Composites Are Adequate Replacements." Reuters (Jan 3, 2008): www.reuters.com/article/pressRelease/idUS108558+03-Jan-2008+PRN20080103.

31. LJ Hahn, et al. "Whole-body imaging of the Distribution of Mercury Released from Dental Fillings into Monkey Tissues." *FASEB Journal*. Vol. 4 (1990): 3256–3260.

32. Patrick Stortebecker. *Mercury Poisoning from Dental Amalgams*. Stockholm: Stortebecker Foundation for Research, 1985, p. 32.

33. Dietrich Klinghardt. "Art Laws." Klinghardt Academy for the Healing Arts: www.klinghardtacademy .com/Articles/ART-Laws.html.

34. BM Dooley. "Mercury Testing and Treatment." *Townsend Letter for Doctors & Patients*. (Nov 2008); phone conversation with Dr. Bruce M. Dooley.

35. Dietrich Klinghardt. Klinghardt Academy for the Healing Arts: www.klinghardtacademy.com.

Chapter 10: How the Monster Rears Its Head

1. Bernard Windham. "Mercury Exposure Levels from Amalgam Dental Fillings: Documentation of Mechanisms." DAMS International: www.flcv.com/amalg6.html.

2. Russell L. Blaylock. *Health and Nutrition Secrets That Can Save Your Life*. Albuquerque, NM: Health Press, 2006, pp. 50–51.

3. Maggie Spilner. "Over-the-Counter-Painkillers . . . Or Plain Killers." Stop Aging Now (Aug 7, 2009): www.stopagingnow.com/news/news_flashes/6232.

4. James B. LaValle. *Cracking the Metabolic Code: 9 Keys to Optimal Health*. Laguna Beach, CA: Basic Health Publications, 2004, p. 223.

5. Bernard Windham. "Mercury Exposure Levels from Amalgam Dental Fillings; Documentation of Mechanisms." DAMS International: www.flcv.com/amalg6.html.

6. LaValle, op. cit., p. 223.

7. Dietrich Klinghardt. "Amalgam/Mercury Detox as Treatment of Chronic Viral, Bacterial, and Fungal Disease." Mercury Exposure (Sept 1966): www.mercuryexposure.org/index.php?article_id=66.

8. AO Summers, et al. "Mercury Released from Dental Silver Fillings Provokes an Increase in Mercury and Antibiotic -Resistant Bacteria in Oral and Intestinal Flora of Primates." *Antimicrobial Agents and Chemotherapy*. Vol. 37 (1993): 825–834.

9. Mercola and Klinghardt, op. cit., pp. 11, 53–62.

10. Hal A. Huggins and Thomas E. Levy. *Uninformed Consent: The Hidden Dangers in Dental Care*. Charlottesville, VA: Hampton Roads Pub. Co., 1999, p. 175.

11. Ibid., pp. 29–30, 174.

12. Ibid., pp. 29–31.

13. Blaylock, op. cit., pp. 65–67.

14. Blaylock, ibid., p. 65.

15. Huggins and Levy, op.cit., p. 31.

16. CH Kirkpatrick. "Transfer Factors: Identification of Conserved Sequences in Transfer Factor Molecules." *Molecular Medicine*. Vol. 6, No. 4 (Apr 2000): 332–341.

17. M Nylander, et al. "Mercury Concentrations in the Human Brain and Kidneys and Exposure from Amalgam Fillings." *Swedish Dental Journal*. Vol. 11 (1987): 179–187.

18. LJ Hahn. "Dental 'Silver' Tooth Fillings: A Source of Mercury Exposure Revealed by Whole Body Scan and Tissue Analysis. *FASEB Journal*. Vol. 3 (1989): 2641–2646.

19. MJ Vimy, et al. "Mercury from Maternal Silver Fillings in Sheep and Human Breast Milk: A Source of Neonatal Exposure." *Biological Trace Element Research*. Vol. 56 (1997): 143–152.

20. In children, mercury inhibits the enzymatic process required to digest milk casein and wheat gluten. This is why the commonly prescribed casein-free, gluten-free diet (CFGF) is effective in reducing such effects. See Bernard Windham. "Developmental, Cognitive, and Behaviorial Effects of Toxic Metals." Dental Amalgam Mercury Solutions: www.flcv.com/indexk.html.

21. Bernard Windham. "Mercury Exposure Levels from Amalgam Dental Fillings: Documentation of Mechanisms." DAMS International: www.flcv.com/amalg6.html (338,3).

22. Crohn's & Colitis Foundation of America. www.ccfa.org.

23. Larry Clapp. "Lessons of 17 Years of Healing through Cleansing." Prostate Health Resources: www.prostate90.com/cleansing/heavymetals-nanochelation.htm.

24. Rita Ellithorpe, et. al. "Interim Report of Clinical Observations of the Effects with Detoxamin and Supportive Combination Therapy on Prostate Conditions." Online newsletter (Mar 28, 2007): www.detoxamin.com.

25. Rita Ellithorpe, et al. "Calcium Disodium EDTA Chelation Suppositories: A Novel Approach for Removing Heavy Metal Toxins in Clinical Practice." Online newsletter: www.detoxamin.com.

26. L Palkovicaova. "Maternal Dental Amalgam Fillings as the Source of Mercury Exposure in Developing Fetus and Newborn." *Journal of Exposure Science and Environmental Epidemiology*. Vol. 18 (2008): 326–331.

27. Huggins and Levy, op.cit., p.42.

28. W Karp, et al. "The Effect on Mercuric Acetate on Selected Enzymes of Maternal and Fetal Hamsters at Different Gestational Ages." *Environmental Research*. Vol. 36 (1985): 351–358.

29. Huggins and Levy, op.cit., p. 42.

30. Huggins and Levy, ibid., p. 42.

31. A Oskarsson, et al. "Total and Inorganic Mercury in Breast Milk and Blood in Relationship to Fish Consumption and Amalgam Fillings in Lactating Women." *Archives of Environmental Health*. Vol 51 (1996): 234–241.

32. Blaylock, op.cit., p. 64.

33. I Gerhard, et al. "Impact of Heavy Metals on Hormonal and Immunological Factors in Women with Repeated Miscarriages." *Human Reproduction Update*. Vol. 4 (1998): 301–309.

34. I Gerhard. "Amalgam aus Gynakologischer Sicht." *Der Frauenart*. Vol. 36 (1995): 627–628.

35. Bernard Windham. "Mercury Exposure Levels from Amalgam Dental Fillings: Documentation of Mechanisms." DAMS International: www.flcv.com/amalg6.html.

36. Huggins and Levy, op.cit., pp. 41–43.

37. According to Dr. T. Timothy Smith, PhD, HCLD, scientific director at North Hudson I.V.F., Englewood Cliffs, New Jersey. Online correspondence (February 27, 2006) http://sharedjourney.com/yabbse/Amorphous_heads_sperms_in_SA-6-1-2022-0.html).

38. Bernard Windham. "Mercury Caused Endocrine Conditions Causing Widespread Adverse Health Effects, Cognitive Effects, and Fertility Effects." DAMS International: www.flcv.com/endohg.html.

39. Bernard Windham. "Documentation of Common Cardiovascular Health Effects from Mercury form Amalgam." Dental Amalgam Mercury Solutions: www.flcv.com/cardio.html.

40. MC Houston. "The Role of Mercury and Cadmium Heavy Metals in Vascular Disease, Hypertension, Coronary Artery Disease, and Myocardial Infarction." *Alternative Therapies in Health Medicine*. Vol. 13, No. 2 (Mar–Apr 2007): S128–133.

41. Stephen T. Sinatra. *Reverse Heart Disease Now: Stop Deadly Cardiovascular Plaque Before It's Too Late*. Hoboken, NJ: John Wiley & Sons, 2007, p. 49.

42. Rita Ellithorpe, et al. "Interim Report of Clinical Observations of the Effects with Detoxamin and Support- ive Combination Therapy on Prostate Conditions." (Mar 2007). In a 90-day study involving mercury detox- ification conducted on thirty men, ages forty-eight to seventy-four, blood chemistry panels done on the study participants showed that high-density lipids (HDL, the good cholesterol), increased significantly over pre- treatment levels. In fact, the cholesterol to HDL ratios, low-density lipids (LDL, bad cholesterol) and plaque 2 (LPPLA2, a marker that detects cardiovascular plaque), all significantly decreased in the majority of par- ticipants. Online newsletter. www.detoxamin.com

43. Dietrich Klinghardt and Joseph Mercola. "Mercury Toxicity and Systemic Elimination Agents." *Journal of Nutritional and Environmental Medicine.* Vol. 11 (2001), p. 3.

44. Richard S. Lord and Alexander Bralley, editors. "Conjugation Pathways Used for Specific Compounds." *Laboratory Evaluations for Integrative and Functional Medicine,* 2nd ed. Duluth, GA: Metametrix Institute, 2008, p. 496.

Chapter 11: Neurotoxicity and Mercury

1. Dietrich Klinghardt. "Mercury Detoxification: Perpetuating Factors, Problems and Obstacles." Klinghardt Academy for the Healing Arts: www.klinghardtacademy.com/Articles/Mercury-Detoxification-Perpetuat- ing-Factors-Problems-and-Obstacles.html.

2. Bernard Windham. "Mercury Exposure Levels from Amalgam Dental Fillings: Documentation of Mecha- nisms." DAMS International: www.flcv.com/amalg6.html.

3. Ibid., (studies referenced: 19, 27, 34, 36, 39,43, 69, 70, 147, 148, 175, 207, 211, 258, 262, 273, 274, 291, 295, 301, 303, 305, 327, 329, 395).

4. C Pritchard, et al. "Pollutants Appear to Be the Cause of the Huge Rise in Degenerative Neurological Con- ditions." *Public Health* (Aug 2004): www.flcv.com/alzgh.html.

5. Ibid. (www.flcv.com/parkins.html).

6. Mark Breiner. *Whole Body Dentistry: Discover the Missing Piece to Better Health.* Fairfield, CT: Quantum Health Press, 1999, pp. 70–71.

7. Hal A. Huggins and Thomas E. Levy. *Uninformed Consent: The Hidden Dangers in Dental Care.* Char- lottesville, VA: Hampton Roads Pub. Co., 1999, p. 126.

8. Bernard Windham. "Mercury from Amalgam Fillings: A Major Factor in Periodontal Disease and Oral Health Problem." DAMS International: www.flcv.com/periodon.html.

9. ES Lain, et al. "Electro Galvanic Phenomenon of the Oral Cavity Caused by Dissimilar Metallic Restora- tion." *Journal of the American Dental Association.* Vol. 23 (Sept 1936).

10. DW Eggleston and M Nylander. "Correlation of Dental Amalgam with Mercury in Brain Tissue." *Journal of Prosthetic Dentistry.* Vol. 58. (1987): 704–707.

11. LJ Hahn, et al. op.cit., pp. 2641–2646.

12. MJ Vimy, et al. op.cit., pp. 143–152.

13. LJ Hahn, et al. op.cit., pp. 3256–3260.

14. JC Pendergrass, et al. "Mercury Vapor Inhalation Inhibits Binding of GTP to Tubulin in Rat Brain: Simi- larity to a Molecular Lesion in Alzheimer Diseased Brain." *NeuroToxicology.* Vol. 18 (1997): 315–324.

15. CW Leong, NI Syed, et al. "Retrograde Degeneration of Neurite Membrane Structural Integrity of Nerve Growth Cones Following in Vitro Exposure to Mercury." *NeuroReport.* Vol.12, No.4 (Mar 26, 2001): 733–737.

16. Naweed Syed Neuroscience Research Laboratory: www.ucalgary.ca/~neuro/syed/syed.htm.

17. "The Scientific Case Against Amalgam," IAOMT (2002, 2005): 17: www.iaomt.org/articles/category_ view.asp?intReleaseID=193&catid=30.

18. Personal phone conversation with Naweed Syed, Aug 2009.

19. CW Leong, et al. op. cit.

20. Personal phone conversation with Naweed Syed, Aug 2009.

21. Personal meeting and personal conversation with Naweed Syed, UCLA, Aug 2009.

22. According to Dr. Syed, the initial evidence from his rat brain cell research is even more powerful than the time-lapse photography techniques used in his earlier snail neuron research. The technique that his lab is now using provides direct electrophysiological evidence. Dr. Syed and his colleagues made recordings directly from two identified neurons. These recordings were made using glass microelectrodes that were inserted into the cells to measure their electric potentials. They showed that stimulating the presynaptic cell produces one-for-one excitatory potentials in its postsynaptic partner under normal recording conditions. However, no connectivity was observed when cells were cultured in the presence of mercury. The data clearly show that mercury blocks the formation of synapses between the two cells.

23. Alzheimer's Association. Alzheimer's Disease Facts and Figures (2009): www.alz.org/national/documents/report_alzfactsfigures2009.pdf.

24. Boyd Haley. "The Relationship of the Toxic Effects of Mercury to Exacerbation of the Medical Condition Classified as Alzheimer's Disease." *Int J Geriatr Psychiatry*. Vol. 16 (May 2001): 513–517.

25. BW Health Wire. "IAOMT Researchers Connect Mercury to Alzheimer's Disease." (Mar 26, 2001): www.ariplex.com/ama/amaucal1.htm. (The seven characteristics of the diseased Alzheimer's brain that this and other studies have shown to be affected by low levels of mercury include elevated amyloid protein, neurofibrillar tangles, dysfunctional tubulin, creatine kinase and glutamine synthetase, hyperphosphorylated tau, and low levels of reduced glutathione.)

26. Bernard Windham. "Toxic Exposures and Parkinson: The Mercury Connections." DAMS International: www.flcv.com/parkins.html.

27. G DePalma, et al. "Case Controlled Study of Polymorphic Xenobiotic Metabolizing Enzymes in Parkinson's Disease." Abstract of 7th Annual meeting of International Neurotoxicological Association (Jul 4–9, 1999, Leicester, UK). *Neurotoxicology*. Vol. 21 (2000): 615–640, 632.

28. A Seidler, et al. "Possible Environmental, Occupational, and Other Etiological Factors for Parkinson's diseases: A Case Controlled Study in Germany." *Neurology*. Vol. 46 (1996): 1275–1284.

29. Bernard Windham. "Mercury from Amalgam Fillings Is a Common Cause of MS, ALS, PD, SLE, RA, MCS, AD, etc." DAMS International: www.flcv.com/ms.html.

30. Ibid. (studies referenced: 35, 139, 163, 291).

31. Ibid. (studies referenced: 271, 302).

32. Ibid. (studies referenced: 34, 158, 207).

33. Ibid. (studies referenced: 183, 184, 207, 212 222, 244, 271, 289, 291, 302, 324, 326, 406).

34. www.autismspeaks.org.

35. RF Kennedy. "Deadly Immunity." *Rolling Stone* (Jun 20, 2005): www.rollingstone.com/politics/story/7395411/deadly_immunity.

36. Bernard Windham. "Neurological and Immune Reactive Conditions Affecting Kids." DAMS International: www.flcv.com/kidshg.html.

37. www.autismhelpforyou.com.

Chapter 12: Chelating Mercury Out of the Darkness

1. Dietrich Klinghardt. "A Comprehensive Review of Heavy Metal Detoxification and Clinical Pearls from 30 Years of Medical Practice." Klinghardt Academy of Neurobiology: www.neuraltherapy.com/heavyMetalDetox.pdf.

2. Donna Gates and Linda Schatz. *The Body Ecology Diet: Recovering Your Health, Rebuilding Your Immunity.* Decatur, GA: B.E.D. Publishing, 2007, p. 92.

3. Anonymous. MercuryLife weblog: www.mercurylife.com.

4. Dietrich Klinghardt. "Mercury Detoxification Perpetuating Factors, Problems and Obstacles." Klinghardt Academy of Neurobiology: www.neuraltherapy.com/Mercury%20Detoxification%20Perpetuating%20Factors.htm.

Chapter 13: A World of Natural Supplements

1. Patrick Holford. *New Optimum Nutrition for the Mind*. Laguna Beach, CA: Basic Health Publications, 2009, pp. 96–97.

2. T Rundek, et al. "Atorvastatin Decreases the Coenzyme Q_{10} Level in the Blood of Patients at Risk for Cardiovascular Disease and Stroke." *Archives of Neurology*. Vol. 61, No. 6 (Jun 2004): 889–892. A Columbia University study in New York found that thirty days of statin therapy (80 mg/day) decreased CoQ_{10} levels by half. This is associated with increased risk for mitochondrial dysfunction that is behind much heart disease and may be a cofactor in increasing diabetic tendencies.

3. PH Langsjoen and AM Langsjoen. "The Clinical Use of HMG-Coa Reductase Inhibitors and the Associated Depletion of CoQ_{10}: A Review of Animal and Human Publications." *Biofactors*. Vol. 18, Nos. 1–4 (2003): 101–111."The depletion of the essential nutrient CoQ_{10} by the increasingly popular cholesterol lowering drugs, HMG-CoA reductase inhibitors (statins), has grown from a level of concern to one of alarm."

4. Mark Hyman. *The UltraMind Solution: Fix Your Broken Brain by Healing Your Body First:* New York: Scribner, 2008, p. 63.

5. JS Cohen. "Seniors, Side Effects, and Celebrex: Does This Strong, One-Size-Fits-All Drug Put Seniors, Women, And Others At Unnecessary Risk?" *MedicationSense* E-newsletter: www.medicationsense.com/articles/oct_dec_03/seniors_celebrex.html.

Chapter 14: Our Work with Sigmund Freud

1. Paul Roazen. *Freud and His Followers*. New York: Knopf, 1975, p. 225.

2. Peter Gay. "Sigmund Freud: Psychoanalyst," *Time* (Mar 29, 1999).

3. William W. Meissner. *Psychoanalysis and Religious Experience*. New Haven, CT: Yale University Press, 1984, p.74.

4. Heinrich Meng and Ernest Freud, eds. *Psychoanalysis and Faith: Dialogues with the Reverand Oskar Pfister*. New York: Basic Books, 1963, p. 8.

5. Meissner, op. cit., p. 74.

6. Meng and Freud, op. cit., p. 9.

7. American Psychiatric Association, www.psych.org. On a personal note, it is our greatest hope that Joseph will one day win this prestigious award.

8. Lucy Freeman. *Freud and Women*. New York: Ungar, 1981, p. 86.

9. Ernest Jones. *The Life and Work of Sigmund Freud*, Vol. III. New York: Basic Books, 1961, p. 227.

10. Celia Bertin. *Marie Bonaparte: A Life*. New York: Harcourt Brace Jovanovich, 1982.

11. Robert M. Chalfin. Review. "Marie Bonaparte. A Life." *The Psychoanalytic Quarterly*. Vol. 54 (1985): 115–120.

Chapter 15: The Emotional Database

1. Mark Hyman. *The UltraMind Solution: Fix Your Broken Brain by Healing Your Body First*. New York: Scribner, 2008, p. 13.

2. Melinda Wenner. "Infected with Insanity: Could Microbes Cause Mental Illness?" *Scientific American Mind*. (Apr 17, 2008). Mental illness, once thought to be the result of neurological or psychological defects may be caused by viral or microbial infections.

3. Joe Dispenza. *Evolve the Brain: The Science of Changing Your Mind.* Deerfield Beach, FL: Health Communications, 2009, p. 91.

4. A Dubini, et al. "Do noradrenaline and serotonin differentially affect social motivation and behavior?" *European Neuropsychopharmacology.* Vol. 7(Supp 1) (1997): S49–S55.

5. Melanie Segala (ed.). *Disease Prevention and Treatment.* Ft. Lauderdale, FL: Life Extension Foundation, 2003, p. 682.

6. Nora D. Volkow, et al. "Depressed Dopamine Activity in Caudate and Preliminary Evidence of Limbic Involvement in Adults with Attention-Deficit/Hyperactivity Disorder." *Archives of General Psychiatry.* Vol. 64(8) (2007): 932–940.

7. Almut G. Winterstein, et al. "Cardiac Safety of Central Nervous System Stimulants in Children and Adolescents with Attention-Deficit/Hyperactivity Disorder." *Pediatrics.* Vol. 120 (2007): e1494–e1501.

8. Hyla Cass. *Natural Highs: Supplements, Nutrition, and Mind-Body Techniques to Help You Feel Good All the Time.* New York: Avery, 2002, p. 120.

9. Metametrix, Genova Diagnostics, and Doctor's Data are examples of such laboratories.

10. Patrick Holford. *New Optimum Nutrition for the Mind.* Laguna Beach, CA: Basic Health Publications, 2009, pp. 70–73.

11. Ibid., p. 71.

12. Patrick Holford. *Optimum Nutrition for the Mind.* Laguna Beach, CA: Basic Health Publications, 2004, p. 182.

13.Teodoro Bottiglieri, et al. "Homocysteine, folate, methylation, and monoamine metabolism in depression." *Journal of Neurology, Neurosurgery, and Psychiatry.* Vol. 69 (Aug 2000): 228–232.

14. David Perlmutter. *The Better Brain Book: The Best Tools for Improving Memory, Sharpness, and Preventing Aging of the Brain.* New York: Penguin Books, 2004, p. 47.

15. Richard S. Lord and J. Alexander Bralley. *Laboratory Evaluations for Integrative and Functional Medicine.* Duluth, GA: Metametrix Institute, 2008, p. 635.

16. Elson Haas. *Staying Healthy with Nutrition: The Complete Guide to Diet and Nutritional Medicine.* Berkeley, CA: Celestial Arts, 2006, p. 110.

17. MS Morris, et al. "Plasma pyridoxal 5'-phosphate in the U.S. population." The National Health and Nutrition Examination Survey, 2003–2004. *American Journal of Clinical Nutrition.* Vol. 87 (May 2008): 1446–1454.

18. Craig Weatherby. "Top Psych Panel Says Omega-3s Deter Depression, Bipolar Disorder." *Vital Choice Newsletter* (Jan 2007).

19. Holford, *New Optimum Nutrition for the Mind,* p. 67.

20. G Nowak, et al. "Zinc and depression. An update." *Pharmacol Rep.* Vol. 57(6) (Nov–Dec 2005): 713–718. Review.

21. Hyman, op. cit., p. 142.

22. Ibid., p. 143.

23. MB Youdim, et al. "Is Parkinson's Disease a Progressive Siderosis of Substantia Nigra Resulting in Iron and Melanin Induced Neurodegeneration?" *Acta Neurologica Scandinavica.* Vol. 126 (1989): 47–54.

24. K Linde, et al. "St John's Wort for Major Depression." *Cochrane Database of Systematic Reviews* (2008), Issue 3.

25. Segala, op. cit., pp. 686–687.

26. Mechthild Scheffer. *Bach Flower Therapy: Theory and Practice.* Rochester, VT: Healing Arts Press, 1988, p. 14–17.

27. Ibid., p.13.

Chapter 16: The Connection Between Emotions and Women's Hormones

1. Geoffrey P. Redmond. *It's Your Hormones*. New York: HarperCollins, 2005, p. 32.

2. Patrick Holford. *Optimum Nutrition for the Mind*. Laguna Beach, CA: Basic Health Publications, 2004, p. 122.

3. Uzzi Reiss. *Natural Hormone Balance for Women: Look Younger, Feel Stronger, and Live Life with Exuberance*. New York: Pocket Books, 2001, pp. 9–10, 36–46.

4. Ibid., pp. 9–10, 36–46.

5. Uzzi Reiss. "Important Published Medical Information the Media Does Not Share with You." URx. (Jan 1, 2008): www.uzzireissmd.com/importantinfo.html.

6. Writing Group for the Women's Health Initiative Investigators. "Risks and Benefits of Estrogen Plus Progestin in Healthy Postmenopausal Women." *Journal of the American Medical Association*. Vol. 228, (2002): 321–333.

7. Greg Peterson. "Water Worries: Drugs Are Turning Up in Drinking Water and Causing Bizarre Mutations." *Emagazine.com*. (Jul–Aug 2007): www.emagazine.com/view/?3773&src=.

8. AE Thomsen, et al. "Increased Risk of Developing Affective Disorders in Patients with Hypothyroidism: A Register Based Study." *Thyroid*. Vol. 15(7): 700–707.

9. M Bauer, et al. "Thyroid Hormones, Serotonin and Mood: Of Synergy and Significance in the Adult Brain." *Molecular Psychiatry*. Vol. 7(2), (2002): 140–156.

10. HE Carlson, et al. "Adverse Effects of Antipsychotics and Mood Stabilizers." *Psychiatric Times*. Vol. 25(1), (Dec 2007).

11. Mark Hyman. *The UltraMind Solution: Fix Your Broken Brain by Healing Your Body First*. New York: Scribner, 2008, p. 105.

12. RS Wilson, et al. "Proneness to Psychological Distress Is Associated with Risk of Alzheimer's Disease." *Neurology*. Vol. 61(11), (Dec 2003): 1479–1485.

13. D Buljevac, et al. "Self Reported Stressful Life Events and Exacerbations in Multiple Sclerosis: Prospective Study." *BMJ*. Vol. 327(7416), (Sept 2003): 646.

14. LE Carlson, et al. "Relationships Among Cortisol (CRT), Dehydroepiandrosterone-Sulfate (DHEAS) and Memory in a Longitudinal Study of Healthy Elderly Men and Women." *Neurobiology of Aging*. Vol. 20(3), (May 1999): 315–324.

15. Hyman, op. cit., p. 181.

16. "Bioidentical Hormones: Why Are They Still Controversial?" *Life Extension* (Oct 2009), p. 65.

17. Ibid. In a study published in the journal *Breast Cancer Research and Treatment*, 80,000 post-menopausal women using various forms of HRT were followed for more than eight years. Women who used estrogen in combination with non-bioidentical progestins had a 69 percent increased risk of breast cancer; compared to women who had never used HRT. However, for women who used bioidentical progesterone in combination with estrogen, the increased risk of breast cancer was completely eliminated with a significant reduction in breast cancer risk compared with non-bioidentical progestin use. (Fournier A, et al. "Unequal Risks for Breast Cancer Associated with Different Hormone Replacement Therapies: Results from the E3N Cohort Study. *Breast Cancer Research and Treatment*. Vol 107[1], [Jan 2008]: 103–111.)

18. This would include organizations such as the American Academy of Anti-Aging Medicine, the Bioidentical Hormone Society, or the World Society of Anti-Aging Medicine.

19. S Abbas, et al. "Serum 25-hydroxyvitamin D and Risk of Post-Menopausal Breast Cancer—Results of a Large Case-Control Study." *Carcinogenesis*. Vol. 29(1), (Jan 2008): 93–99. Vitamin D has been shown to prevent and even repair gene mutations, which substantially reduce risk. One controlled study involving over 2,000 post-menopausal women divided into two essentially equal groups showed that women with the highest blood levels of vitamin D had a nearly 70 percent reduced risk of breast cancer as compared to the other group of women with the lowest vitamin D levels!

20. P Muti, et al. "Estrogen Metabolism and Risk of Breast Cancer: A Prospective Study of the Alpha-Hydrox-yestrone Ratio in Premenopausal and Postmenopausal Women." *Epidemiology.* Vol. 11(6), (Nov2000): 635–640.

21. HJ Yoo, et al. "Estrogen Metabolism as a Risk Factor for Head and Neck Cancer." *Archives of Otolaryngology Head Neck Surgergy.* Vol. 124(3), (Mar 2001): 241–247.

22. S Sharma, et al. "Screening of Potential Chemopreventive Agents Using Biochemical Markers of Carcinogenesis." *Cancer Research.* Vol. 54(22), (Nov 1994): 5848–5855.

23. K Kuriki, et al. "Breast Cancer Risk and Erythrocyte Compositions of n-3 Highly Unsaturated Fatty Acids in Japanese." *International Journal of Cancer.* Vol. 151(2), (Jul 2007): 377–385.

24. V Maillard, et al. "N-3 and n-6 Fatty Acids in Breast Adipose Tissue and Relative Risk of Breast Cancer in a Case-Control Study in Tours, France." *International Journal of Cancer.* Vol. 98(1), (Mar 2002): 78–83.

25. S Yamamoto, et al. "Soy, Isoflavones, and Breast Cancer Risk in Japan." *Journal of the National Cancer Institute.* Vol. 95(12), (Jun 2003): 906–913.

26. HP Lee, et al. "Dietary Effects on Breast-Cancer Risk in Singapore." *Lancet.* Vol. 337(8751), (May 1991): 1197–1200.

27. SE McCann, et al. "Dietary Lignan Intakes and Risk of Pre- and Postmenopausal Breast Cancer." *International Journal of Cancer.* Vol. 111(3), (Sept 2004): 440–443.

28. F Boccardo, et al. "Serum Enterolactone Levels and the Risk of Breast Cancer in Women with Palpable Cysts." *European Journal of Cancer.* Vol. 40(1), (Jan 2004): 84–89.

29. LU Thompson, et al. "Dietary Flaxseed Alters Tumor Biological Markers in Postmenopausal Breast Cancer." *Clinical Cancer Research.* Vol. 11(10), (May 2005): 3828–3835.

30. RL Thangapazham, et al. "Green Tea Polyphenol and Epigallocatechin Gallate Induce Apoptosis and Inhibit Invasion in Human Breast Cancer Cells." *Cancer Biological Therapy.* Vol. 6(12), (Dec 2007): 1938–1943.

31. RL Thangapazham, et al. "Green Tea Polyphenols and Its Constituent Epigallocatechin Gallate Inhibits Proliferation of Human Breast Cancer Cells In Vitro and In Vivo." *Cancer Letters.* Vol. 245(1–2), (Jan 2007): 232–241.

32. AH Wu, et al. "Green Tea and Risk of Breast Cancer in Asian Americans." *International Journal of Cancer.* Vol. 106(4), (Sept 2003): 574–579.

33. Z Walaszek, et al. "Antiproliferative Effect of Dietary Glucarate on the Sprague-Dawley Rat Mammary Gland." *Cancer Letters.* Vol. 49(1), (Jan 1990): 51–57.

34. AS Heerdt, et al. "Calcium Glucarate as a Chemopreventive Agent in Breast Cancer." *Israel Journal of Medical Science.* Vol. 31(2–3), (Feb 1995): 101–105.

35. Z Walaszek, et al. "Metabolism, Uptake, and Excretion of a D-Glucaric Acid Salt and Its Potential Use in Cancer Prevention." *Cancer Detection and Prevention.* Vol 21(2), (1997): 178–190.

Chapter 17: Sigmund Freud Speaks

1. There was one other letter (359J) in 1923 that concerns a patient whom Jung referred to Freud.

2. Sigmund made a point of telling Linda that he thinks highly of Peter Gay, director of the Center for Scholars and Writers at the New York Public Library and Sterling Professor Emeritus at Yale University.

3. William McGuire, ed. *The Freud/Jung Letters* (unabridged edition). Princeton, NJ: Princeton University Press, 1974, p. xvii.

4. Carl Jung. *Memories, Dreams, Reflections.* New York: Vintage Books, 1989, p. 148.

5. Anthony Storr and Anthony Stevens. *Freud & Jung: A Dual Introduction.* New York: Barnes & Noble Books, 1998, p. 13.

6. William McGuire. *The Freud/Jung Letters* (unabridged edition). Princeton, NJ: Princeton University Press, 1974, 139F, p. 218.

7. Fritz Wittels. *Sigmund Freud: His Personality, His Teaching, His School.* New York: Dodd, Mead & Co., 1924, p. 138.

8. Ernest Jones. *The Life and World of Sigmund Freud* (Vol. 2). New York: Basic Books, Inc., 1955. p.149.

9. Paul Roazen. *Freud and His Followers.* New York: De Capo Press, 1992, p. 227.

10. Ibid., p. 226.

11. Jones, op. cit., p. 50.

12. Ibid., p. 33 Cf. *The Freud/Jung Letters,* pp. 196–197.

13. Ibid., p. 33.

14. McGuire, op. cit., Letter 84F, p. 140.

15. Ibid., Letter 86J, p. 144.

16. Storr and Stevens, op. cit., p. 14.

17. Peter Gay. *Freud: A Life for Our Time.* New York: W.W. Norton & Co., 1998, p. 226. quoting from *The Freud/Jung Letters,* 170J, Dec 25/31, 1909, p. 280.

18. Roazen, op. cit., p. 229.

19. Jones, op. cit., p. 141.

20. McGuire, op. cit., Letter 318J, p. 509.

21. Ibid., Letter 319F, p. 510.

22. Ibid., Letter 323J, p. 515.

23. Sigmund Freud. *On the History of Psychoanalysis.* SE XIV, New York: W.W. Norton & Co., 1966, p. 58.

24. McGuire, op cit., Letter 323J, p.516.

25. Ibid., Letter 324F, p. 517.

26. Sigmund Freud. *On the History of the Psychoanalytical Movement* (orig. 1914) SE XIV, New York: W.W. Norton & Co., 1966, p. 58, later commenting on the meaning of paragraph 1 on letter 324F, *Freud/Jung Letters,* p. 517.

27. McGuire, op cit., Letter 324F, p. 517.

28. Ibid., Letter 324F, p. 517.

29. Ernest Jones. *The Life and Work of Sigmund Freud* (Vol. I). New York: Basic Books, Inc., 1955, p. 317.

30. Gay, op. cit., p. 233.

31. Sigmund has told Linda from the spirit world that he still stands by this assertion.

32. McGuire, op. cit., pp. 521–522, the Munich Conference, which references a quote from the book *Putnam and Psychoanalysis,* p. 150.

33. Ibid., Letter 328J, p. 522.

34. Ibid., Letter 329F, p. 524.

35. Ibid., Letter 329F, pp. 523–524.

36. Gay, op. cit., p. 233.

37. McGuire, op. cit., Letter 330J, pp. 525–526.

38. Jung, op. cit., p. 158.

39. Gay, op. cit., p. 225.

40. Elsewhere, in other writings, Jung concluded that "This experience with Freud . . . is the most important factor in my relationship with him." *Analytical Psychology: Notes of the Seminar* given in 1925, ed. William McGuire (Bollingen Series XCIX), Princeton, NJ: Princeton University Press, 1989, p. 22.

41. McGuire, op. cit., Letter 338J, pp. 534–535.

42. Ibid., Letter 342F, pp. 538–539.

43. Gay, op. cit., p. 239. Psychoanalyst Lou Andreas-Salomé, who was at the International Conference of Psychoanalysts in Sept 1913, following their breakup, wrote in her journal that "where with Jung a kind of robust gaiety, abundant vitality, spoke through his booming laughter two years ago, his seriousness now holds pure aggressiveness, ambition, mental brutality. Freud has never been so close to me as here: not only because of his break with his son Jung whom he loved, for whose sake he had, as it where, transferred his cause to Zurich, but precisely because of the manner of the break—as though Freud were carrying it through in narrow minded stubbornness," an appearance that Jung had fabricated in defiance of the reality.

44. Z'ev ben Shimon Halevi. *Psychology and Kabbalah*. York Beach, ME: Redwheel/Samuel Weiser, LLC, 1992, p. 165.

45. Sigmund Freud. *The Interpretation of Dreams* (Vol. 5). Standard Edition, London: Hogarth Press, 1963, p. 483.

46. Carl Jung and Violet De Laszlo. "Christ, A Symbol of the Self." In *Psyche and Symbol: A Selection from the Writings of C.G. Jung*. Princeton, NJ: Princeton University Press, 1991, p. 71.

47. Jung, op. cit., p. 388. Synchronicity is a term coined by Jung to designate the meaningful coincidence or equivalence (a) of a psychic and a physical state or event that have no causal relationship to one another. Such synchronistic phenomenon occur, for instance, when an inwardly perceived event (dream, vision, premonition, etc.) is seen to have a correspondence in external reality: the inner image of premonition has come true; (b) of similar or identical thoughts, dreams, etc., occurring at the same time in different places.

48. Storr and Stevens, op. cit., p. 2.

49. Jones, op. cit., p. 47.

50. McGuire, op. cit., Letter 87F, pp. 144–146. Freud then remarked, "Do you remember the lines from the *Philoctetes*: (These arrows alone will take Troy)? My self-confidence has so increased that I am thinking of taking this line as a motto for a new edition of the *Collective Papers on the Theory of the Neuroses*."

51. Sigmund Freud, *The Interpretation of Dreams* (Vol. 5), p. 608.

52. Jung, op. cit., p. 147.

53. Ibid., p.169.

54. Sigmund Freud, *The Interpretation of Dreams* (Vol. 5), p.350–351.

55. McGuire, op.cit., letter 170J, p. 280.

56. Ibid., Letter 163F, p. 265.

57. Michael Vannoy Adams. *The Mythological Unconscious*. New York: H. Karnac Books, 2001, p. 2., quoting from *Freud & Jung*, 1974: 483.

58. Ibid., pp. 11–12.

59. Gay, op. cit., p. 226, quoting from the *Freud/Jung Letters*, 168J, Dec 14, 1909, p. 274.

60. Barry Strauss. *The Trojan War*. New York: Simon & Schuster, 2006, pp. 1–5.

61. Ibid., p. 3.

62. Homer. *The Iliad*. Translated by Martin Hammond. New York: Penguin Classics, 1987, p. vii.

63. Aristotle. *Poetics*. Translated by Malcolm Heath. New York: Penguin Books, 1996, Chapter 8.1, p. 25.

64. Freud has mentioned that a holographic parallel to this reconciliation in their lives as Freud and Jung was the Conference in Munich in 1912.

65. Storr and Stevens, op. cit., p. 16.

66. Jones, op. cit., p. 33.

67. Storr and Stevens, op. cit., p.13–14.

68. McGuire, op. cit., Letter 330J, p. 525.

69. Storr and Stevens, op. cit., p. 16.

70. Roazen, op. cit., p. 228.

71. Sigmund Freud. *The History of Psychoanalytical Movement*. New York: W.W. Norton & Co., 1966, p. 43.

72. Roazen, op. cit., p. 279.

73. Homer. *The Iliad*. Translated by E.V. Rieu, New York: Penguin Books, 1950, p. 4.

74. Jung, op. cit., p. 158.

75. Ibid., p. 150.

76. Ibid., pp. 150–151.

77. Ibid., pp. 167–168.

78. Storr and Stevens, op. cit., p.16.

Chapter 18: The Metaphysical Database

1. Anodea Judith. *Wheels of Fire: A Users Guide to the Chakra System*. St. Paul, MN: Llewellyn Publications, 1990, p. 1.

2. Cyndi Dale. *The Subtle Body: An Encyclopedia of Your Energetic Anatomy*. Boulder, CO: Sounds True, Inc., 2009, p. 99.

3. Ibid., p. 147.

4. CW Leadbetter. *The Chakras*. Wheaton, IL: Theosophical Publishing House, 1977, p. 1.

Chapter 19: Belief in Angels

Note to scholars: In Chapters 19–20 where I reference the Zohar, other than *The Wisdom of the Zohar* by Isaiah Tishby (London: The Littman Library of Jewish Civilization, 1989), I am specifically referring to the Zohar (Vols. 1–23) that were translated into English by the Kabbalah Centre International (2003). This, in essence, is a translated copy that follows the sequence of paragraph numbers of Rabbi Ashlag's Hebrew version of the Zohar called the "Sulam."

1. Rodney Stark. *What Americans Really Believe: New Findings from the Baylor Surveys of Religion*. Waco, TX: Baylor University Press, 2008, pp. 56–57.

2. David Van Biema. "Guardian Angels Are Here, Say Most Americans." *Time Magazine*, Sept 18, 2008: www.time.com/time/nation/article/0,8599,1842179,00.html.

3. Stark, op.cit., pp. 55–56.

4. Albert Einstein. *Science, Philosophy and Religion: A Symposium*, 1941, later reprinted in *The World as I See It*. New York: Philosophical Library, 1949, pp. 24–28.

5. Alice Calaprice. *The Expanded Quotable Einstein*. Princeton, NJ: Princeton University Press, 2000, p. 202.

6. "Albert Einstein, response to atheist, Alfred Kerr," (1927) quoted in *The Diary of a Cosmopolitan* (1971).

7. Amit Goswami. *God Is Not Dead: What Quantum Physics Tells Us About Our Origins and How We Would Live*. Charlottesville, VA: Hampton Roads Pub., 2008, p. 7.

8. *The Anthropic Principle* (VHS & DVD). London: BBC, 1988.

9. "The 'Fine-Tuning' of the Universe." 2001 Principle: www.2001principle.net/2005.htm.

10. For specific quotes on the anthropic principle from each of these scientists, go to www.2001 principle.net/2005.htm.

11. Stephen Hawkings. *A Brief History of Time: From the Big Bang to Black Holes*. New York: Bantam Books, 1988, p. 125.

12. Matthew Fox and Rupert Sheldrake. *The Physics of Angels: Exploring the Realm Where Science and Spirit Meet*. San Francisco: Harper San Francisco, 1996, p. 17.

13. Ibid., p. 13.

14. Chaim Luzzatto. *The Way of God*. New York: Feldheim Publishers, 1997, pp. 147–149.

15. Zohar (Vol. 5), Vayatze #195, p. 119.

16. Luzzatto, op. cit., p. 81.

17. Rabbi Shneur Zalman of Liadi. "Walk with Me." An adaptation by Yitzchok Wagshul of a discourse Likutei Torah. www.kabbalaonline.com

18. Talmud, Tractate Tanith, p. 11a.

19. The Talmud even speaks about one's guardian angels functioning as inspectors of the psyche at the beginning of the Sabbath on Friday night. "There are two of God's ministering angels who accompany one home on Shabbat evening from the synagogue to his home—one is good and one is evil. If when entering the house, one finds a candle lit, a table set and a bed made—the good angel declares: 'May it be Your will, God, that next Shabbat be just like this one.' The evil angel is required, even against his will, to say 'Amen.' However, if the household is not prepared, the malicious angel declares: 'May it be Your will, that next Shabbat be just like this one.' Then the beneficent angel is required, even against his will, to say Amen" (Talmud Shabbat, p. 119b).

20. For a brilliant dissertation that reconciles scientific understanding with scripture, read the Kabbalistic interpretation of how the world was created in six twenty-four-hour days. Aryeh Kaplan. *Immortality, Resurrection, and the Age of the Universe: A Kabbalistic View*. Hoboken, NJ: Ktav Pub., 1993.

21. Isaiah Tishby. *The Wisdom of the Zohar: An Anthology of Texts* (Vol. 2). Oxford, New York: Oxford University Press, 1989, p. 601.

22. Ibid., p. 601.

23. Adin Steinsaltz. *The Thirteen Petalled Rose: A Discourse on the Essence of Jewish Existence and Belief*. New York: Basic Books, 2006, p. 7.

24. Rabbi Maimonides. "Becoming a Prophet." In *Mishneh Torah: Hilchot Yesodei HaTorah*, Chapter 7, adapted by Eliyahu Touger: www.kabbalaonline.org/kabbalah/article_cdo/aid/380357/jewish/Becoming-a-Prophet.htm

25. Tishby, op.cit., p. 616.

26. *Zohar Vol. 2 Beresheet* #78, p. 74.

27. Aryeh Kaplan. *Innerspace*, Brooklyn, NY: Moznaim Publishing Co., p. 28.

28. Ibid. Ezekiel's Vision 1:15–1:19, pp.140–141; and Howard Schwartz, *Tree of Souls*, p. 182.

29. Moshe Wisnefsky, *Apples from the Orchard: Gleanings from the Mystical Teachings of Rabbi Yitzchak Luria*. Malibu, CA: Thirty Seven Books, 2008, p. 852.

30. *Zohar Vol. 2 Beresheet* #67, p. 67.

31. Kaplan, op. cit., p. 141; Ezekiel's Vision 1:15–1:19; and Howard Schwartz, *Tree of Souls*, p. 182.

32. Ibid., p. 176.

33. Fox and Sheldrake, op. cit., p. 3.

34. St. Thomas Aquinas. *Summa Theologiae* (1a, Vol. 9), q. 58, "How an Angel's Mind Functions, a. 1–7. London: Blackfriars, 1968, pp. 145–168.

35. Fox and Sheldrake, op. cit., p. 2.

36. Luzzatto, op. cit., p. 217

37. Zohar Hadash, Beresheit, 10b, and Midrash ha-Ne'elam

38. Hebrew Enoch; Jellinek, "B.H." v. 181, Targ. Yer. Gen. xi. 7–8, Pirke R. El. xxiv.

39. Howard Schwartz. *Tree of Souls: The Mythology of Judaism*. Oxford, NY: Oxford University Press, 2004, p. 408.

40. Gen. R. lxviii., Pesi. xxiii. 151a.

41. Schwartz, op. cit., p.408.

42. Rabbi Yitzchak Luria. *Sha'ar HaGilgulim (The Gates of Reincarnation)*. Chapter 23. Malibu, CA: Thirty Seven Books Pub., 2003, p. 190–191. Regarding the concept of *Chibut HaKever*, after a person dies and is buried in the dust of the earth, immediately four angels arrive and deepen his grave to the height of the man, as it says in *Meseches Perek Chibut HaKever*. Then they return his soul to his body like during his lifetime since the k'lipah (a figurative "husk" of evil that surrounds and conceals the sparks of Divine light) remains attached to both necessitating that the soul be returned to the body. Then, these angels take him by the "corners" and they shake and beat him with fire, just like a garment is held from the ends and shaken to remove dust, until the k'lipah leaves him completely. This is called Chibut HaKever, which is like the beating and shaking of a garment. They deepen the grave in order to create an area within which to shake and beat him. However, the judgment is not the same for everyone. Righteous people distance themselves from the yetzer hara during their lifetimes, and humble themselves and use their suffering as self-affliction. As well, Torah and mitzvahs (good deeds) weaken them until the day comes for them to die. Such righteous people do not need much suffering, just a minor "beating" to separate the yetzer hara from them. It is just the opposite for evil people. Through indulging in the pleasures of this world they become even more strongly attached to the k'lipah of their bodies and souls. This is the *sod* (secret) of why a person is not saved from Chibut HaKever, as mentioned in *Meseches Perek Chibut HaKever*.

43. Tishby, op. cit., p. 847.

44. Reprinted with permission: "Gotta Serve Somebody" written by Bob Dylan. Copyright © 1979 by Special Rider Music. All rights reserved. International copyright secured.

45. Schwartz, op. cit., pp. 232–233.

46. Luzzatto, op. cit., p. 367.

47. Steinsaltz, op. cit., pp. 19–21.

48. *Zohar* (Vol. 2), *Beresheet* B 15, #44. The Third Compartment, p. 37.

49. Rabbi Ariel Bar Tzadok. *The Difference Between Dreams That Come from Angels* & [Those] *That Come from Demons* (Parashat Miqetz 47) from the Teachings of Rabbi Yehuda Fatiyah of Yerushalayim: www.kosher torah.com

50. Tishby, op. cit., pp. 650–651.

51. Aryeh Kaplan (trans.). *The Living Torah*. Brooklyn, NY: Moznaim Publishing Co. 1981, p. 25.

52. Dr. Nieper's patients included many world stars, royalty, and politicians: Anthony Quinn, John Wayne, Yul Brynner, William Holden, and Princess Caroline of Monaco. He advised the ailing ex-president Ronald Reagan . . . Nancy Sinatra lavished praise on this great German physician: "He is a fabulous person, a recognized scientist, a marvelous doctor." His patients both loved and respected him: www.explore pub.com/articles/neiper1.html.

53. Luzzatto, op. cit., p. 155–161.

54. Sources: B. Sanhedrin 38b; Genesis Rabbah: 4, 8:5, 8–6, 8:8; Midrash ha-Ne'elam, Zohar Hadash 16a–b; Midrash ha-Gadol on Genesis 1:26; Enoch 4:6–9

55. Schwartz, op. cit., pp. 261–262.

56. Ibid., p. 130.

Chapter 20: Meet the Archangels

Note to scholars: See note at top of References for Chapter 19.

1. The Book of Enoch is considered to be one of the most important pieces of Jewish mystical literature (Craig

A. Evans, *Noncanonical Writings and New Testament Interpretation*, 1992, p. 23). It is an ancient pseudepigraphical work (a work that claims to be by a biblical character, but is actually written under a pen name).

2. Hugo Odeberg. *3 Enoch or The Hebrew Book of Enoch*. Part 2, Chapter 15. London: Cambridge University Press, 1928, p. 39.

3. Isaiah Tishby. *The Wisdom of the Zohar: An Anthology of Texts*. Vol. 2. New York: Published for the Littman Library by Oxford University Press, 1989, p. 627, quoting from the Zohar Hadash, Terumah, 42d–43a, and Shir ha-Shirim, 69b.

4. Tishby, op. cit., p. 630.

5. Midrash Rabba, Bereshit Chapter 1, Paragraph 3.

6. Zohar, Vol. 17, Naso #10, p. 57.

7. Midrash Avkir from a text entitled *Yalkut Re'uveni 1:132*.

8. In an interesting footnote to this, I recall an incident several years ago that occurred when Linda and I were at home listening to a recording of the fourth movement of Gustav Mahler's "Symphony of a Thousand," (1906) a monumental tour de force for orchestra and choir, the libretto of which concerns an angelic choir singing praises to God. During one especially poignant passage, Linda suddenly started to shake. I immediately turned down the volume on the stereo to find out from her what was happening. She channeled that she had been visited by Michael who had revealed his particular fondness for this piece of music!

9. Rabbit Shneur Zalman. "Walk with Me." An adaptation by Yitzchok Wagshul of a discourse Likutei Torah: www.kabbalaonline.com

10. Zohar, Vol. 11, Parashat Trumah #233, p. 145.

11. Book of Daniel. Art Scroll History Series. Brooklyn, NY: Mesorah Publishing, 1998, p. 277.

12. Pirke R. El.xxvi.

13. Babylonian Talmud, Tractate Chagigah 12B.

14. Tishby, op. cit., p. 645.

15. Zohar, Vol. 4, Chayei Sarah #150, p. 89.

16. Midrash Avkir from a text entitled *Yalkut Re'uveni 1:132*.

17. As a footnote to this most dazzling display of angelic prowess, Michael, prior to the actually "parting," first exercised his function as an advocate of Israel in front of the Archangelic Court when Samael accused the Israelites of idolatry declaring that they were deserving to die by drowning in the Red Sea (Ex. Rabbah xviii. 5). Uzza, the tutelary angel of Egypt summoned Michael to plead the cause of the Hebrews before the court. However, Michael remained silent and it was God Himself who defended Israel.

18. Exodus 23: 20–23. God explains to Moses that he "will send an angel [Michael] before you to safeguard you on the way" through the desert for what will turn out to be the next forty years (Abravanel). God then tells Moses that neither he nor the Jewish people should rebel against Michael and that Michael must be related to with the utmost reverence as "my name is within him" (The Torah Commentary of Rebbeinu Bachya). Survival is conditional upon obeying the word of Michael as God says to Moses that "If you obey him [Michael] and do all that I say, then I will hate your enemies and attach your foes. My angel [Michael, will act as a guide and] will go before you and bring you among the Amorites, Hittites, Perizzites, Canaanites, Hivites, and Yebusites, and I will [then] annihilate them."

19. Babylonian Talmud, Tractate Shabbat, 56b.

20. Enoch, op. cit., p. 14.

21. Daniel, op. cit., pp. 228–236.

22. Ibid., 257–266.

23. Zohar (Vol. 6), Parashat Vayeshev, #82–87, pp. 44–47.

24. Babylonian Talmud Sotah 13b.

25. In a most fascinating metaphysical story, Gabriel's role as the guardian angel to Joseph extended long after the earthly death of Joseph. Gabriel is involved in the famous and gruesome story of the slaughter of the Ten Martyrs of Rome, which is retold on Yom Kipper. A section of the service called the "Avodah" retells the story of the horrific torture and execution of the ten most important Rabbis at the hands of the Romans. Although many Christians may be unaware of this, shortly after the slaying of Jesus, the Romans turned their wrath on the most righteous of rabbis whose only crime was their devotion to living and teaching a life of Torah and spirituality (Midrash Eleh Ezkerah). The real untold metaphysical story of the Avodah that involves Gabriel goes as follows: Rabbi Akiva, the spiritual leader of his generation and one of the ten martyrs, had the ability to astral travel to receive spiritual information from angels. After learning of their death sentence, Rabbi Akiva ascends to the upper realms to ask Gabriel why these righteous rabbis merited death after leading lives of holiness. Gabriel replies that these ten rabbis are in fact the reincarnated souls of the brothers of Joseph who sold their brother into slavery in Egypt. These biblically primordial souls must now get their metaphysical comeuppance by atoning for this sin even though these souls are now housed in the bodies of righteous rabbis, living a life that occurred many lifetimes after the actual crime was committed! Such are the ways of divine logic where the karma surrounding the reincarnated journey of the soul from lifetime to lifetime is of paramount importance to God and his angels.

26. Babylonian Talmud Sotah 36b; "Yalkut. Re'ubeni," section "Mikkez" p. 71b.

27. Zohar (Vol. 3), Lech Lecha, essays on circumcision #396, pp. 208–209.

28. Zohar (Vol. 12), Vayak'hel #296 acknowledges that there is also another opinion in the Ashlag commentary that Uriel is in the East. #297 states that Raphael is also referred to as Boel.

29. Gustav Davidson. *The Dictionary of Angels*. New York: Free Press, 1967, p. 240. The author has taken slight liberties with the translated original text (see Zohar [Vol. 2], Beresheit B #167, p. 117) to deduce a clearer meaning.

30. Howard Schwartz. *Tree of Souls: The Mythology of Judaism*. Oxford, NY: Oxford University Press, 2004, pp. 253–254.

31. Sources: Gen. Rabbah 48:9–50:2, BT Yoma 37a; Baba Metzia 86, Zohar 1, 98b–99a, Sitrei Torah.

32. Babylonian Talmud Tractate Chullin 92a.

33. Gustav Davidson. *The Dictionary of Angels*. New York: Free Press, 1967, p. 242.

34. Chaim Vital, *Etz Chiam*, Gate 43, Section 3 states that Uriel is associated with the direction of West, which is yesod. However, the Zohar, Vol. 12, Vayakhel suggests that it also an opinion that it may be east which is tiferet. Zohar, Vol. 12, Vayakhel # 298 also mentions an angel named Nuriel that appears to be another angel that is a related "aspect" of Uriel.

35. Book of Enoch 10:1–2.

36. Deut. Rabbah 2:34

37. Shabtai Teicher, ed. *Zohar—Sabba d'Mishpatim* #44. Jerusalem, Israel: self-published, p. 58.

38. Joshua Tractenberg. *Jewish Magic and Superstition*. Philadelphia, PA: University of Pennsylvania Press, 1939, 2004, p. 98.

Chapter 21: Metaphysical Patterns in Time

1. The website for the Ashford Castle is www.ashford.ie/index.php.

2. *The Anne Horniman Papers*, John Rylands University of Manchester Library. "The season stands as an important landmark in the modern theatre movement: included in the programme were productions of Arms and the Man, the first play by George Bernard Shaw to be seen in the commercial theatre, and The Land of Heart's Desire, the first play by W.B. Yeats produced in London. Anne Horniman had a great admiration for Yeats' work, and for some years she acted as his amanuensis in London."

Suggested Readings and Resources

Preface

Scott-Mumby, Keith. *Virtual Medicine*. La Quinta, CA: Polimedia Communications, 2008.

Chapters 2–3

Diamond, W. John, and W. Lee Cowden. *An Alternative Medicine Definitive Guide to Cancer*. Tiburon, CA: Future Medicine Publishing, Inc., 1997.

Gerber, Richard. *Vibrational Medicine: The #1 Handbook of Subtle-Energy Therapies*. Rochester, VT: Bear & Co., 2001.

Goldberg, Burton. *Alternative Medicine: The Definitive Guide*. Berkeley, CA: Celestial Arts, 2002.

Sinatra, Stephen T. *The Sinatra Solution*. Laguna Beach, CA: Basic Health Publications, 2005.

Chapter 4

Schlossberg, David. *Clinical Infectious Disease*. New York: Cambridge University Press, 2008.

Chapters 5–6

Goldberg, Burton. *Chronic Fatigue, Fibromyalgia, and Lyme Disease*. Berkeley, CA: Celestial Arts, 2004.

Hume, Ethel Douglas. 1932. *Béchamp or Pasteur? A Lost Chapter in the History of Biology*. New York: DLM, 2006.

Young, Robert O., with Shelley Redford Young. *Sick and Tired*. Pleasant Grove, UT: Woodland Publishing, 2001.

Chapter 7

Gittleman, Ann Louise. *Guess What Came To Dinner*. New York: Avery, 2001.

Chapter 8

Diamond, W. John, W. Lee Cowden, and Burton Goldberg. *Definitive Guide to Cancer*. Tiberon, CA: Future Medicine Publishing, 1997.

Chapters 9–12

Blaylock, Russell L. *Health and Nutrition Secrets*. Albuquerque, NM: Health Press, 2006.

Breiner, Mark A. *Whole Body Dentistry*. Fairfield, CT: Quantum Health Press, 1999.

Cousens, Gabriel. *Conscious Eating*. Berkeley, CA: North Atlantic Books, 2000.

Cutler, Andrew Hall. *Amalgam Illness: Diagnosis and Treatment*. Sammamish, WA: andycutler@aol.com, 1999.

Gates, Donna, and Linda Schatz. *The Body Ecology Diet: Recovering Your Health and Rebuilding Your Immunity*. 10th edition. Decatur, GA: B.E.D. Publishers, 2007.

Huggins, Hal A., and Thomas Levy. *Uninformed Consent*. Charlottesville, VA: Hampton Roads Publishing Company, 1999.

Kristal, Harold J., and James M. Haig. *Nutrition Solution*. Berkeley, CA: North Atlantic Books, 2002.

LaValle, James B., with Stacy Yale. *Cracking the Metabolic Code*. Laguna Beach, CA: Basic Health Publications, 2004.

Lord, Richard S., and Alexander Bralley, eds. *Laboratory Evaluations for Integrative and Functional Medicine*. 2nd edition. Duluth, GA: Metametrix Institute, 2008.

Queen, H.L. "Sam," and Betty Queen. *The IV-C Mercury Tox Program: A Guide for the Patient*. Colorado Springs, CO: Queen & Co., 1991.

Sinatra, Stephen T., and John Roberts. *Reverse Heart Disease Now: Stop Deadly Cardiovascular Plaque Before It's Too Late*. Hoboken, NJ: John Wiley & Sons, 2007.

Stortebecker, Patrick. *Mercury Poisoning from Dental Amalgam*. Stockholm: Stortebecker Foundation for Research, 1985.

Chapter 13

Cass, Hyla. *Supplement Your Prescription*. Laguna Beach, CA: Basic Health Publications, 2009.

Crayhon, Robert. *Robert Crayhon's Nutrition Made Simple*. New York: M. Evans & Co. 1994.

Chapter 14

Bertin, Celia. *Marie Bonaparte: A Life*. New Haven, CT: Yale University Press, 1987.

Chapters 15–16

Cass, Hyla, and Patrick Holford. *Natural Highs*. New York: Avery Books, 2002.

Dispenza, Joe. *Evolve the Brain: The Science of Changing Your Mind*. Deerfield Beach, FL: Health Communications Inc., 2007.

Haas, Elson. *Staying Healthy with Nutrition*. Berkeley, CA: Celestial Arts, 2006.

Holford, Patrick. *New Optimum Nutrition for the Mind*. Laguna Beach, CA: Basic Health Publications, 2009.

Hyman, Mark. *The UltraMind Solution: Fix Your Broken Brain by Healing Your Body First*. New York: Scribner, 2008.

Perlmutter, David, and Carol Colman. *The Better Brain Book: The Best Tools for Improving Memory, Sharpness, and Preventing Aging of the Brain*. New York: Penguin, 2004.

Redmond, Geoffrey. *It's Your Hormones*. Los Angeles: Regan, 2006.

Reiss, Uzzi. *Natural Hormone Balance for Women*. New York: Pocket Books, 2001.

Scheffer, Mechthild. *Bach Flower Therapy: Theory and Practice*. Rochester, VT: Healing Arts Press, 1988.

Segala, Melanie, ed. *Disease Prevention and Treatment*. 4th edition. Hollywood, FL: Life Extension Media, 2003.

Somers, Suzanne. *The Sexy Years: Discover the Hormone Connection.* New York: Crown Publishers, 2004.

_____. *Ageless: The Naked Truth about Bioidentical Hormones.* New York: Crown Publishers, 2006.

Chapter 17

Adams, Michael Vannoy. *The Mythological Unconscious.* London: H. Karnac Books, 2001.

Bertin, Celia. *Marie Bonaparte: A Life.* New Haven, CT: Yale University Press, 1987..

Freeman, Lucy, and Dr. Herbert S. Strean. *Freud and Women.* New York: Continuum Publishing Company, 1987.

Freud, Sigmund. *On the History of Psychoanalytical Movement.* New York: W.W. Norton, 1966.

_____. *The Interpretation of Dreams.* (Standard Edition) Vol. 5. London: Hogarth Press, 1975.

Gay, Peter. *Freud: A Life for Our Time.* New York: W.W. Norton, 2006.

Halevi, Z'ev ben Shimon. *Kabbalah and Psychology.* New York: Weiser Books, 1992.

Homer, trans. Martin Hammond. *The Iliad.* London: Penguin Books, 1987.

Jones, Ernest. *The Life and Work of Sigmund Freud.* Vol. 2. New York: Basic Books, 1955.

Jung, C.G., ed. Aniela Jaffe. *Memories, Dreams, Reflections,* New York: Pantheon Books, 1963.

McGuire, William, ed. *The Freud/Jung Letters.* Princeton, NJ: Princeton University Press, 1994.

Roazen, Paul. *Freud and His Followers.* New York: Da Capo Press, 1992.

Storr, Anthony, and Anthony Stevens. *Freud and Jung: A Dual Introduction.* New York: Barnes & Noble Books, 1998.

Strauss, Barry. *The Trojan War.* New York: Simon & Schuster, 2006.

Chapter 18

Dale, Cyndi. *The Subtle Body: An Encyclopedia of Your Energetic Anatomy.* Boulder, CO: Sounds True, Inc. 2009

Gerber, Richard. *Vibrational Medicine for the 21st Century.* New York: William Morrow, 2000.

Judith, Anodea. *Wheels of Fire: A Users Guide to the Chakra System.* St. Paul, MN: Llewellyn Publications, 1990.

Winkler, Gershon. *Dybbuk.* Brooklyn, NY: Judaica Press, 1982.

Chapters 19–20

Book of Daniel. Art Scroll ed. Brooklyn, NY: Mesorah Publishing, 1998.

Davidson, Gustav. *The Dictionary of Angels.* New York: The Free Press, 1971.

Fox, Matthew, and Robert Sheldrake. *The Physics of Angels: Exploring the Realm Where Science and Spirit Meet.* San Francisco: Harper-San Francisco, 1996.

Goswami, Amit. *God Is Not Dead: What Quantum Physics Tells Us About Our Origins and How We Would Live.* Charlottesville, VA: Hampton Roads Publisher, 2008.

Hawking, Stephen. *A Brief History of Time: From the Big Bang to Black Holes.* New York: Bantam Books, 1988.

Kaplan, Aryeh. *Immortality, Resurrection, and the Age of the Universe: A Kabbalistic View.* Hoboken, NJ: Ktav Publishing House, 1993.

Kaplan, Aryeh. *Innerspace.* Brooklyn, NY: Moznaim Publishing Company, 1990.

Luzzatto, Moshe Chaim. *The Way of God*. Natnuet, NY: Feldheim Publishers, 1997.

Schwartz, Howard. *Tree of Souls: The Mythology of Judaism*, New York: Oxford University Press, 2004.

Stark, Rodney. *What Americans Really Believe: New Findings from the Baylor Surveys of Religion*. Waco, TX: Baylor University Press, 2008.

Steinsaltz, Adin. *The Thirteen Petalled Rose: A Discourse on the Essence of Jewish Existence and Belief*. New York: Basic Books, 2006.

Tishby, Isaiah. *The Wisdom of the Zohar: An Anthology of Texts*. Vol. 2. London: Littman Library of Jewish Civilization, 1989.

Trachtenberg, Joshua. *Jewish Magic and Superstition*. Philadelphia: University of Pennsylvania Press, 2004.

Wisnefsky, Moshe. *Apples from the Orchard: Gleanings from the Mystical Teachings of Rabbi Yitzchak Luria*. Malibu, CA: Thirty Seven Books, 2008.

Yochai, Shimon Bar. *The Zohar*. Vols. 1–23. Los Angeles: Kabbalah Center International Inc., 2003.

Chapter 21

Gooddie, Shelia. *Annie Horniman: A Pioneer in the Theater*. Portsmouth, NH: Heinemann, 1991.

Greer, Mary K. *Women of the Golden Dawn*. Rochester, VT: Park Street Press, 1995.

RESOURCES ON MERCURY TOXICITY

In addition to the books listed in Suggested Readings, there are several amazing websites and books available on the scourge of mercury toxicity from dental amalgam and other sources. Much of the information contained in Chapters 9–12 was derived from the following sources.

Science

The most complete repositories of information on what mercury does to the body and brain are found at www.flcv.com/indexa.html and www.flcv.com/dams.html. These materials were compiled by Bernard Windham, president of the DAMS (Dental Amalgam Mercury Solutions) organization, and contain information derived from over 5,000 worldwide research or government agency studies. Windham, who formerly suffered from mercury toxicity, is a venerable research genius as well as a chemical engineer, mathematician, government planner, and university professor. This compilation of data is an extraordinary labor of love on his part, and I am most grateful to him for it. Medical researchers can reach him by email at berniew1@embarqmail.com. In addition, Leo Cashman, executive director of DAMS (www.dams.cc; 651-644-4572), provides valuable information and resources on holistic-oriented doctors and biological dentists for people suffering from mercury poisoning due to amalgam fillings and other sources.

In Chapter 11, I discuss the revolutionary work of several scientists who have made major contributions to understanding the dangers of mercury toxicity. Dr. Naweed Syed, Ph.D., at the University of Calgary in Alberta, who works with snail neurons, offers visual proof of what mercury can do to the brain. The website for his laboratory is www.ucalgary.ca/~neuro/syed/syed.htm. A video entitled "How Mercury Causes Brain Neuron Degeneration," produced by the University of Calgary, can be seen at www.thehealinggift.com.

Dr. Boyd Haley, Ph.D., former chair of the chemistry department at the University of Kentucky in Lexington, is a passionate spokesperson for the dangers of mercury toxicity and a leading authority on its relationship with Alzheimer's disease and autism. For an overview of his work, go to www.whale.to/v/haley.html. I urge you to watch "Mercury Toxicity & Autism, Parts 1–3" on video.google.com.

Biological Dentistry

The International Academy of Oral Medicine and Toxicology (IAOMT, www.iaomt. org) promotes biological dentistry and finances important research. The IAOMT provided funding for "How Mercury Causes Brain Neuron Degeneration" and "The Smoking Tooth," which can be viewed at www.thehealinggift.com. Another important source of information on biological dentistry and the damaging effects of mercury is Dr. Hal Huggins, D.D.S. (www.hugginsappliedhealing.com).

Medical

From a practitioner's perspective, Linda and I think very highly of Dr. Dietrich Klinghardt, M.D., whose clinics are located in Washington State, England, Germany, and Switzerland. Dr. Klinghardt uses Autonomic Response Testing (ART), his advanced hands-on examination technique, to evaluate the patient. His website is www.klinghardtneurobiology.com.

Legal

From a legal perspective, attorney Charlie Brown is waging a vigorous campaign to combat bureaucratic fraud, deception, and disinformation on the dental amalgam issue through his organization Consumers for Dental Choice. I urge you to support his organization and highly recommend its website (www.toxicteeth.org). I also recommend the Mercury Policy Project (www.mercurypolicy.org), an organization that promotes policies to eliminate mercury use and reduce mercury exposure.

Other Useful Websites

- www.cent4dent.com/html/mercury_issues/links.html
- www.icnr.com/uam/hgcourse/Contents.html
- www.mercuryexposure.org
- www.mercurylife.com
- www.mercurypoisoned.com
- www.tuberose.com

Index

About the Authors

Linda Freud is recognized by leading integrative physicians as perhaps the premier medical intuitive in the world. Her international reputation stems from her extraordinary ability to dramatically improve difficult medical conditions that often elude conventional practitioners and approaches. Linda's gift originates from her ability to channel angels and spirit guides with a pendulum using sophisticated physical, emotional, and metaphysical databases of information. Through this process, she receives incredibly accurate and detailed information on health issues that allow her to craft precise healing regimens derived from a broad array of natural remedies and supplements, as well as customized diets. As the testimonials in this book show, Linda is able to achieve consistently amazing results. She also provides channeled psychological counseling and past-life research that reveal soul-satisfying explanations for life's intangible emotional and spiritual quandaries. Linda sees clients at the Beneveda Medical Group in Beverly Hills, California (www.beneveda.com). Working with and under the medical license of Dr. Thom E. Lobe, M.D., she also assists other selected physicians, healers, and institutions on their challenging cases. This includes seeing clients at the Malibu Beach Recovery Center, a facility recognized for its unique holistic approach to drug and alcohol rehabilitation (www.malibubeach recovery.com). She has also worked with clients in Switzerland at the Kientaler-hof Center for Wellbeing and the Paracelsus Klinik. In addition, Linda has used her gift to design orthomolecular and homeopathic supplements for prominent companies. Linda can be reached at the Beneveda Medical Group at lfreud@ beneveda.com. Her website is www.thehealinggift.com.

David Freud is Linda's husband and partner in this extraordinary endeavor. Well regarded as a top medical researcher among integrative physicians and healers, he possesses a vast knowledge of natural healing modalities, including cutting-edge detoxification protocols for a range of environmental toxins. In the early 1990s, David began to amass alternative medical information that, in conjunction with Linda's gift, cured Linda and himself of complicated medical conditions, that could not be healed through conventional allopathic means. David created a series of massive databases that enable Linda to channel and treat the whole person, pinpointing unique and highly detailed levels of physical, emotional, and metaphysical information for each client. David continually updates the databases so that Linda and her clients have the benefit of the latest medical research. In addition, he lectures at medical conferences on health issues related to environmental toxicity and chronic degenerative disease.